WERNER'S OFFICE DIAGNOSIS

Werner's Office Diagnosis

Harold V. Werner, M.D.

Jackhal Books
Vega, Texas

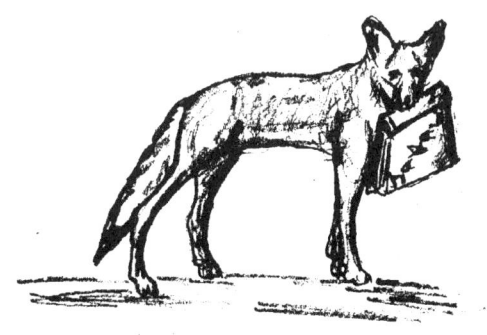

JACKHAL BOOKS
PO Box 357
Vega, Texas 79092

This publication is designed to provide accurate and authoritative information in regard to the subject matter covered. However, there is no warrant express or implied that the information is in every respect accurate or complete. In publishing this book the author and publisher disclaim any liability, loss or damage as a result, directly or indirectly, from using or applying any of the contents herein.

Harold V. Werner, MD
Professor of Medicine
Department of Medicine
Texas Tech University HSC
Amarillo, Texas

WERNER'S OFFICE DIAGNOSIS

ISBN 1-888856-01-7
Library of Congress Control Number: 2004106477

Copyright © 2004, by Harold V. Werner.

All rights reserved. No part of this publication may be reproduced or transmitted in any form or by any means, electronic or mechanical, including photocopy, recording, computer, or any information storage and retrieval system, without permission from the publisher.

Printed in the United States of America
Last digit is the print number: 9 8 7 6 5 4 3 2 1

DEDICATION To Jacky–my *SINE QUA NON*

Front cover:
Dr. Werner with model Corrina Dawn
Depicted is the total patient and especially her mouth and face, to express her symptoms–what she feels inside.
Depicted are the clinician's tools of diagnosis–eyes, ears, mouth, hands.

Back cover:
Sitting, left to right: Texas Tech internal medicine residents
Drs. Bradford, Smirnova, (Dr. Werner), Glover, Hough
Standing, left to right: Texas Tech third year medical students
Rush, Manjoros, Hulme, Chen, Thompson, Richardson

ACKNOWLEDGMENT

I thank fellow faculty members at Texas Tech for reading parts of earlier drafts and providing helpful suggestions:
 Drs. Misty Evans, Rush Pierce, Andrew Stenhouse and Steve Urban.

Thanks especially to Dr. Steven Kelleher for his helpful suggestions and many stimulating and provocative conversations.

Thanks to MIII Scott Frankfather for the suggestion to "ACE" the diagnosis.

Most of all I thank the students and residents at schools where I have trained and taught–Northwestern University (Chicago), Washington University (St. Louis), University of Missouri (Columbia) and Texas Tech University (Amarillo).

We learn the most from those we teach.

Table of Contents

Preface	1
Introduction	3
Abbreviations	6
Chapter 1 Principles of Office Diagnosis	9
Chapter 2 Abdominal Pain	17
Chapter 3 Chest Pain	33
Chapter 4 Constipation	48
Chapter 5 Cough	59
Chapter 6 Diarrhea	70
Chapter 7 Edema	85
Chapter 8 Fatigue	96
Chapter 9 Headache	107
Chapter 10 Joint Pain	120
Chapter 11 Low Back Pain (LBP)	136
Chapter 12 Presyncope	149
Chapter 13 Rash	161
Chapter 14 Shortness of Breath (SOB)	176
Chapter 15 Sore Throat (ST)	188
Chapter 16 Spells	199
Chapter 17 Sublibido	211
Chapter 18 Tremor	221
Chapter 19 Vertigo	232
Chapter 20 Weakness	244
Index	257

PREFACE

Clinicians have been taught to diagnose inefficiently for office practice. There are two reasons. You learn about diagnosis almost exclusively in hospitalized patients, and you learn how to diagnose by observing specialists (hospitalists, intensivists, cardiologists) and hospitalists diagnose diseases in these patients. So what is wrong with that?

First, patients in the hospital are different from those in the office. Patients are in the hospital because they have organic diseases, which you studied extensively in pathology. Organic disease means there has been damage to an organ (brain, heart, stomach, muscle, nerve), and the damage results in structural, chemical, immunological or microbiological changes. These changes potentially are detectable by some technology. Researchers originally "isolate" an organic disease from similar illnesses by using a new technology that detects one of these changes e.g. structural or chemical. As you would expect, clinicians today diagnose that organic disease accurately by using that same technology.

Second, you learn how to diagnose by observing a very specialized kind of diagnosis. When a patient is admitted to the hospital with a possible organic disease, specialists order many expensive technologies (tests). You watch the specialists use the history and physical exam only as a tool to find the most appropriate areas of the body to apply the technologies. The concept underlying diagnosis in the hospital is to find some technology that will diagnose the patient's organic disease. The best diagnostician in the hospital is the one consistently ordering the right technology first.

As a student you witness the amazing successes of this approach to positive diagnosis by technology, which is inherently necessary to diagnose organic diseases. Of the many tests ordered in a hospitalized patient, almost always some are positive, and a correct diagnosis is made. This technology is successful, however, only because almost all hospitalized patients have organic diseases. But fewer than 3% of all office patients with a new symptom are hospitalized. Thus from the perspective of office practice, you have learned only the method of diagnosis by technology. This specialized approach is useful to make a positive diagnosis in only a select group of patients (<3% of office patients) having difficult-to-diagnose organic diseases.

Given this background, it is not surprising that you enthusiastically apply this same technology to try to diagnose all illnesses in the office, not just the 3% hospitalized with organic diseases. Different from in the hospital, your test results are almost always negative, because few of the remaining 97% of office patients have organic diseases requiring testing. You often conclude wrongly that many of these office patients are not really ill, and they are wasting your time. Use of technology for office diagnosis is inefficient for you, costly for the insurance company or taxpayer, and unfair, or even dangerous for your patients.

In this book we show you how to use a second method to diagnose efficiently the causes of new symptoms in the other 97% of sick patients. The diagnostic process in the office is different from that in the hospital, simply because only 3% of office patients with a new symptom have a difficult-to-diagnose organic disease causing it. Even though 20% of new symptoms are caused by an organic disease, most are diagnosed easily in the office by physical exam–for example, infections such as otitis media, pharyngitis, URI, gastroenteritis, bronchitis, UTI. Most of the rest of the diagnoses are "non-organic illnesses" or syndromes such as tension-type headache, fibromyalgia, nonulcer dyspepsia, depression, somatization disorder, costochondritis, myofascial pain, migraine, panic attack, chronic fatigue, interstitial cystitis, frequency-dysuria syndrome, irritable bowel syndrome, prostatodynia.

Note that these common syndromes are not included in pathology courses. Different from organic diseases, a syndrome rarely has even one physical sign and <u>never</u> has an abnormal test. Any test that you order in a patient with one of these syndromes predictably will be negative. Thus it is <u>necessary</u> that a positive diagnosis of a syndrome (rather than a diagnosis of exclusion) can be only by the <u>method of history and physical exam</u>. The best diagnostician in office practice is the one most skilled in making clinical diagnoses using only the history and physical exam.

Understand what we are saying: In the hospital the nature of organic diseases <u>requires</u> that you use technology for positive diagnosis. In contrast, in the office the nature of syndromes <u>prohibits</u> use of technology to make a positive diagnosis. Because these syndromes do not have abnormal changes detectable by technology, their positive diagnoses can be <u>only</u> by history and exam.

To all clinicians, present and future: As in all of history, the sick and suffering person comes to you with a new symptom. The symptom arises from the sickness inside; thus the symptom is the only link from the internal illness to the clinician's ear. The patient wants you to interpret the symptom, to explain what caused the symptom, then to treat the cause, stop the illness, prevent its recurrence. In the last 2500 years this approach to office diagnosis by history and exam has not changed. Just as this method of office diagnosis has not changed, <u>the illnesses you see today in the office are the same ones that confronted Hippocrates.</u> The illnesses just have different names. Most of his diagnoses were easily diagnosed infections and syndromes, and most of yours will be also. Be proud of your role in continuing this 2500 year Hippocratic tradition. Use your clinical skills to their fullest to diagnose efficiently, and thereby to treat appropriately, almost all of your patients' illnesses.

INTRODUCTION

Imagine how easy diagnosis could be if there were only one disease, or even three diseases. Differential diagnosis would be easy. Most symptoms, however, have dozens of potential causes, and some have more than one hundred e.g. headache, dizziness, joint pain, diarrhea. Such a multitude of possible diagnoses is confusing when your patient has a new symptom. How can you quickly form a differential diagnosis when there are more than 100 causes? If only you could limit the differential diagnosis to a few diseases, then diagnosis in your individual patient would be easy. A simplified approach to diagnosis is suggested by the distribution of causes of new symptoms commonly presenting in our residents' internal medicine clinic in the years 1992-97.

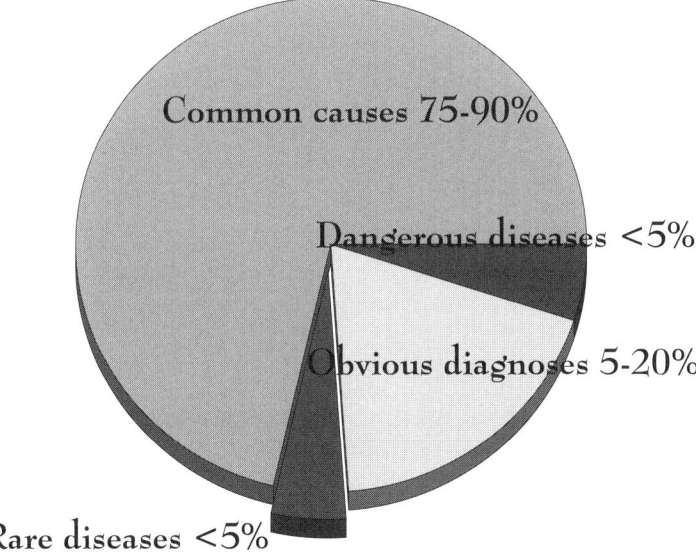

Note from the figure above that dangerous diseases and obvious diagnoses <u>combined</u> account for only 10-25% of diagnoses when the patient has a new symptom. According to these data, if you could be confident by your history and exam that your patient had neither 1) a dangerous disease nor 2) an obvious diagnosis, then almost always the diagnosis <u>must</u> be one of the 2-4 common causes (see the figure on the next page).

The key to diagnosis of any new symptom then depends on your knowing the 2-4 common causes of that symptom that regularly occur in most office patients. From our experience in the clinic, we tell you the common causes. Your approach to diagnosis is clear–first, be confident that your patient has neither a dangerous disease nor an obvious diagnosis. Then search for <u>only</u> the few characteristics of the symptom that differentiate among the common causes.

Note about concepts of diagnosis: The approach to diagnosis in the hospital is inductive. First, you collect <u>all the facts</u> (H&P, many labs), then form a <u>differential diagnosis</u>, order more tests, make a working diagnosis.

For office diagnosis we have inverted the process: First, at the start of each chapter we give you the <u>differential diagnosis</u> (the common causes) and the <u>facts</u> (the 1-2 symptoms or signs that differentiate among these common causes). Then you look for those specific "facts" in your patient to make a working diagnosis.

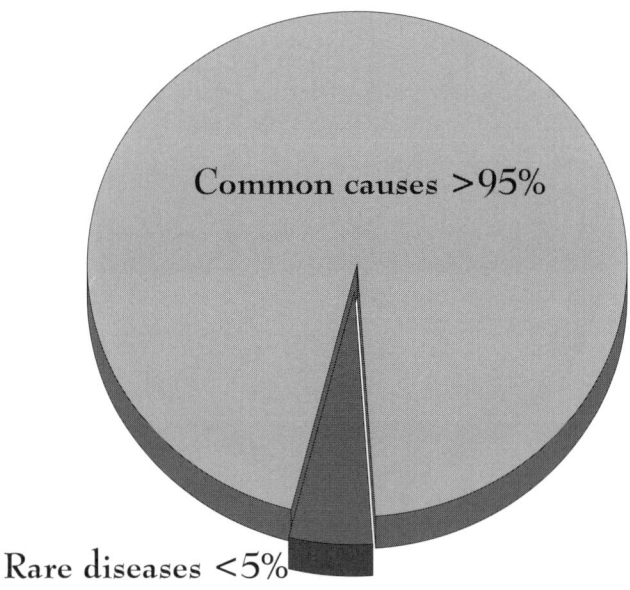

In this book, for each of 19 common symptoms seen in office patients, from our experience we tell you specifically what to look for in your patient:
1. Symptoms and signs of the <u>dangerous diseases</u> (Section B);
2. The <u>obvious diagnoses</u> (Section C);
3. The 2-4 <u>common causes</u> and their distinguishing characteristics (Section E); and
4. The <u>uncommon or rare diseases</u> (Section G).

Diagnosis by your history and physical exam is a lifetime skill. Because that is all you need for almost all office diagnoses, there is little in the book on laboratory tests. Also, you will find little on treatment because new and better therapies arrive almost monthly, quickly outdating any treatment suggestions we could make today.

This is not an ambulatory care textbook, but it is a <u>proven</u> common sense approach to diagnosis in the office that is easy and efficient for you, and safe and inexpensive for your patient. You will find nothing on preventive care, nor do we list the latest practice guidelines for diagnoses. When a patient comes with a new symptom, the patient and the HMO expect diagnosis and therapy soon. Only an academic purpose is served by postponing diagnosis and treatment for months or years, for example, until all DSM IV criteria for major depression, IHS criteria for migraine headache, or ARA criteria for rheumatoid arthritis are met.

Abbreviations Used in the Book:

- ≥ equal or greater than
- ≤ equal or less than
- < less than
- \> greater than
- ac before meals
- am before noon
- ACEI angiotensin-converting enzyme inhibitor
- AD aortic dissection
- AIDS acquired immune deficiency syndrome
- AIP acute intermittent porphyria
- ALS amyotrophic lateral sclerosis
- ANA antinuclear antibody
- ARDS acute respiratory distress syndrome
- ARF acute renal failure
- ASD atrial septal defect
- AV arteriovenous
- bid twice daily
- BM bowel movement
- BMI body mass index
- BP blood pressure
- BPH benign prostatic hypertrophy
- bpm beats per minute
- BPPV benign paroxysmal positional vertigo
- Ca calcium
- CAD coronary artery disease
- CABG coronary artery bypass graft
- CBC complete blood count
- CCB calcium channel blocker
- CCU cardiac care unit
- CFS chronic fatigue syndrome
- CHF congestive heart failure
- CMC carpometacarpal (joint)
- CMV cytomegalovirus
- CNS central nervous system
- COPD chronic obstructive pulmonary disease
- CPK creatine phosphokinase
- CRF chronic renal failure
- CSF cerebrospinal fluid
- CT computed tomography
- CTS carpal tunnel syndrome
- CVA costovertebral angle
- CVP central venous pressure
- CXR chest x-ray
- d day
- DBP diastolic blood pressure
- DDx differential diagnosis
- DIP distal interphalangeal
- DKA diabetic ketoacidosis
- DM diabetes mellitus
- DOE dyspnea on exertion
- DRE digital rectal exam
- DTR deep tendon reflexes
- DVT deep venous thrombosis
- EBV Epstein-Barre virus
- ED emergency department
- EEG electroencephalogram
- e.g. (Latin *exempli gratia*) for example
- EGD esophagogastroduodenoscopy
- EHEC enterohemorrhagic E. coli
- ENT ear, nose, throat
- EKG, ECG electrocardiogram
- ESR erythrocyte sedimentation rate
- FSH follicle stimulating hormone
- FTA-ABS fluorescent treponemal antibody absorption (test)
- FUO fever of undetermined origin
- GABHS Group A β-hemolytic streptococcus
- GAD generalized anxiety disorder
- GBS Guillain-Barré syndrome
- GE gastroenteritis
- GERD gastroesophageal reflux disease
- GI gastrointestinal
- GU genitourinary
- GYN gynecological
- H&P history and physical exam
- HBV hepatitis B virus
- HCM hypertrophic cardiomyopathy
- HCT hematocrit
- HCV hepatitis C virus
- HIV human immunodeficiency virus
- HPS hantavirus pulmonary syndrome
- HSV herpes simplex virus
- HTN hypertension
- HUS hemolytic uremic syndrome
- i.e. (Latin *id est*) that is
- IBD inflammatory bowel disease
- IBS irritable bowel syndrome
- IM infectious mononucleosis
- IPD idiopathic Parkinson's disease
- ICU intensive care unit
- JVD jugular venous distention
- JVP jugular venous pressure

K potassium
kg kilogram
KOH potassium hydroxide
lb pounds
LBP low back pain
LFTs liver function tests (ALT, AST)
LH luteinizing hormone
LMP last menstrual period
LP lumbar puncture
LLQ left lower quadrant
LMN lower motor neuron
LS lumbosacral
MAP mean arterial pressure
MCP metacarpophalngeal
MD major depression
MDI metered dose inhaler
Mg magnesium
MG myasthenia gravis
MI myocardial infarction
min minute
MM multiple myeloma
MOI mild orthostatic intolerance
MRI magnetic resonance imaging
MS multiple sclerosis
MT metatarsal
MTC medullary thyroid carcinoma
MTP metatarsophalangeal (joint)
MVP mitral valve prolapse
ng nanogram
Na Sodium
NSAID nonsteroidal anti-inflammatory drug
NUD nonulcer dyspepsia
OA osteoarthritis
OSA obstructive sleep apnea
OTC over the counter
p pulse
P phosphate
PAN polyarteritis nodosa
pc after meals
PCOS polycystic ovary syndrome
PDR Physician's Drug Reference
PE pulmonary embolus
PFD pelvic floor dysfunction
PID pelvic inflammatory disease
PIP proximal interphalangeal
PMH past medical history
PMI point of maximal impulse (heartbeat against the chest wall)
PMN polymorphonucleocytes (WBC)
PMR polymyalgia rheumatica
PMS premenstrual syndrome
PNDS postnasal drip syndrome
POTS postural tachycardia syndrome
PPI proton pump inhibitor
prn when necessary
PSA prostate specific antigen
PTH parathyroid hormone
PUD peptic ulcer disease
PVC premature ventricular contractions
PVD peripheral vascular disease
qid four times daily
RA rheumatoid arthritis
RAS renal artery stenosis
RBC red blood cells
RF rheumatoid factor
RLQ right lower quadrant
RLS restless leg syndrome
RMSF Rocky Mountain spotted fever
ROM range of motion
ROS review of symptoms
RPR rapid plasma reagin
RR respiratory rate
RSD reflex sympathetic dystrophy
RUQ right upper quadrant
Rx prescription
SAH subarachnoid hemorrhage
SARS severe acute respiratory syndrome
SBE subacute bacterial endocarditis
SBO small bowel obstruction
SBP systolic blood pressure, spontaneous bacterial peritonitis
SIADH syndrome of inappropriate antidiuretic hormone
SHBG sex hormone binding globulin
SLE systemic lupus erythematosis
SLR straight leg raise (test)
SOB shortness of breath
SSRI selective serotonin reuptake inhibitor
ST sore throat
stat immediately
STC slow transit colon
STD sexually transmitted disease
SVC superior vena cava
SVT supraventricular tachycardia
T temperature
TA temporal arteritis
TB tuberculosis

TC total cholesterol
TCA tricyclic antidepressant
TG triglycerides
TIA transient ischemic attack
tid three times daily
T1DM Type 1 diabetes mellitus
T2DM Type 2 diabetes mellitus
TMJ temporomandibular joint
TMT tarsometatarsal (joint)
TrP trigger point
TSH thyroid-stimulating hormone
TTP thrombotic thrombocytopenic purpura
US ultrasound
UA urinalysis
UMN upper motor neuron
URI upper respiratory infection
UTI urinary tract infection
VDRL Venereal Disease Research Laboratory (test for syphilis)
VIP vasoactive intestinal polypeptide
VS vital signs
viz (Latin *videlicet*) namely
WBC white blood cell
WNV West Nile virus
XR x-ray
y/o years old

CHAPTER 1
PRINCIPLES OF OFFICE DIAGNOSIS

If you are not capable of getting the right information out of the patient, you are a clinical menace at the bedside. No amount of double-think about "the scientific basis of medicine" or "the art of patient management" will gloss over this fact. FT de Dombal, 1972

> Important: Rapid, accurate diagnosis is supposed to take minutes, yet the amount of material in some chapters of the book may seem daunting at first glance. Don't be overwhelmed. Most of the content is in sections you will use only occasionally for reference–Sections B, D, G, H. For most new problems all you need is contained in Sections A, C, E (you can ACE the diagnosis). Accordingly the print type is larger in these frequently used ACE sections. Moreover, once you have used this diagnostic approach in some typical patients with that symptom, you no longer will need to use most of the material in each section. In almost all patients with that new symptom, all you will need for correct diagnosis is contained in the boxes in Sections A, C, E and F.

The format of the book is the same for each of the 19 common symptoms. Preceding each chapter are questions and answers. The questions are not meant to test your present knowledge. They are meant to "prime" your mind, to direct your thinking to the important few characteristics of the symptom for differentiating among the 2-4 common causes likely in your patient.

In the text we immediately give you the differential diagnosis (DDx) of the common causes, that is, the characteristics of the symptom that separate one common cause from another. From the moment you start talking with your patient, have this DDx in mind. The text for each symptom follows sequentially the actual process you use toward diagnosis.

Section A. Be certain of the symptom and its distinguishing characteristics.

You must understand precisely what your patient's symptom is. The words that most patients use to describe their symptoms do not have the same meanings to clinicians. For example, your patient may complain of "dizziness." In fact, it may be either vertigo, presyncope, or disequilibrium. Each of these has different causes. Section A of each chapter provides a few key questions. Accurate answers to these questions serve two purposes: first, to clarify what your patient's symptom is, and, second, to help you get from your patient the important characteristics of that symptom (listed above in the DDx, and in more detail in Section E) that separate one common cause from another. To achieve these two goals, you may need to ask 2-3 questions, or even none, if your patient volunteers the necessary information.

The suggested physical exam in each chapter is brief, and it is designed to help you elicit any one important sign alerting you to the presence of a dangerous disease (Section B) or of an easily diagnosed cause (Section C).

Section B. Be confident it's not a dangerous disease.

This list of symptoms and signs of dangerous diseases is not intended to be scrutinized each time you have a patient with a new symptom. It is a comprehensive list of dangerous causes that more often present in the ED than in the office, so use it only when your patient's clinical presentation is unusual and possibly dangerous. Fewer than 5% of your office patients will have a dangerous etiology causing the symptom, but you first and always must be confident by your H&P (and rarely, a test) that your patient is not in that 5% category.

Section C. Make a quick diagnosis if it's obvious.

After you have obtained the information in Section A by your H&P, you should be fairly confident if the diagnosis likely is one of the 2-4 common causes. Nevertheless, there are a few less common organic diseases for each symptom that are easily diagnosed (by a physical sign or a lab test). Depending on which symptom, these entities account for 5-20% of diagnoses. Some are even spot diagnoses with pathognomonic signs, and you want to recognize them early on in talking with your patient. Also, medication side effects always must be thought of first, as another easily treatable cause of your patient's symptom. You should have these less common, easily diagnosed causes in mind when you first begin talking with your patient, and if one of these is present, diagnose and treat immediately.

Section D. Identify your patient's worries and wants.

Each patient coming to you for help is suffering, frightened, and worried. Think of the symptoms as information originating from inside your patient for you to interpret, so you can help him. The symptom is a major part of the message helping you in diagnosis, but also you need to be sensitive to and interpret other aspects, other information, from his illness and from him–what's going on in his daily life. Your patient already has interpreted his symptoms, often incorrectly, and for the worst. If he had your knowledge and experience, he probably would know how benign his symptom or problem really is. But he doesn't have your knowledge and he is coming to you because he is worried and needs your help. He may not even know specifically what he is worried about, or he may not be able to express his worry.

In Section D of each chapter are listed worries and wants we have seen commonly in patients having that particular symptom. Your patient may have either a different worry or a different want, so try to discover, or intuit, during your history and physical exam, just what his concerns and needs might be. Then be sure to provide him your best answers to his worries and wants at his first visit, or as soon as you can. This is the best way to help your patient–to help him in ways that you would like to be

Chapter 1 Principles of Office Diagnosis 11

helped if you were <u>his</u> patient. Furthermore, by understanding as much as you can about his daily life, you can counsel him better about all his problems, present and future, especially lifestyle changes to prevent future diseases.

Section E. Know the characteristics of the symptom that differentiate among the common causes.

In this section we identify the commonest cause, as well as the other 1-3 common causes of that symptom we have found in office patients. Together these common causes account for 75-90% of diagnoses. First, we provide the few important characteristics of the commonest cause, especially related to the rate of onset to peak intensity of the symptom (abrupt, rapid, gradual, slow or insidious), whether it is either a new, or an episodic, or a chronic, persistent symptom, whether there are important concomitant symptoms, and the patient's age and sex.

Second, we list the few ways the symptom characteristics of the other 1-3 common causes differ from the commonest cause, but <u>not</u> the ways each is similar to the commonest cause. That is what diagnosis is all about, the <u>differences</u>; so don't clutter your mind with the similarities among causes. Search in your patient for the important characteristics of the symptom that separate one common cause from the other.

Section F. Use this summary for efficient diagnosis of a common cause.

Here is our rapid approach to diagnosis of that particular symptom, by summarizing the most important information you already have obtained in Sections A-E. This approach allows you, quickly and accurately, to make a working diagnosis, which in most instances will be one of the 2-4 common causes of that symptom listed in Section E.

Section G. Look for an uncommon cause only if the diagnosis is not a common cause.

In followup over the next days, weeks, months and even years, if your patient's clinical response to treatment or no treatment is what you expect from your working diagnosis, then your diagnosis likely is confirmed. It becomes your final diagnosis. If the clinical response does not conform to what you expect from your working diagnosis, and if you do not think it is one of the other few common causes listed in Section E, now and <u>only</u> now should you consult Section G. This is a comprehensive list of uncommon or rare diseases that occasionally may cause that symptom in your patient. Some of them you may never see in a lifetime of office practice, but if your patient has one of these "zebras," it is listed for you to consider it. You may want to order specific tests, or alternatively, refer your patient for an appropriate specialist consult.

Summary of Sections A-G:

Diagnosis of the cause of the usual new symptom in the office should take minutes.
1. Have in mind the differential diagnosis of the 2-4 common causes listed above Section A.
2. In Section A, be certain of the symptom. Unless there is something unusual about the presentation, <u>assume</u> the cause of the new symptom

is one of the 2-4 common causes. Then search in your patient for the few characteristics that differentiate these common causes.
3. While talking with your patient and doing the physical exam:
   a. Be alert for any <u>one</u> symptom or sign suggesting a dangerous cause (Section B); and
   b. Look for evidence (physical <u>sign</u>, <u>rarely</u> a test) that either an easily diagnosed condition or a medication might be causing your patient's symptom (Section C).
4. In Section E, more characteristics of the symptom are listed to help you differentiate among each of the 2-4 common causes.
5. Make a positive diagnosis–usually by the pattern of symptoms and absence of a physical sign–of one of the common causes, and treat it (Section F).
6. Expected response to your management in followup for days, months, or even years, helps to confirm your working diagnosis, but:
   a. If the clinical response is different from what you expect, <u>or</u>
   b. If you find any <u>one</u> new symptom or sign of a dangerous disease, <u>or</u>
   c. If any new pertinent laboratory abnormality occurs, then reassess your diagnosis and consider an uncommon or rare cause (Section G).

Example of Diagnosis in a Typical Everyday Patient
1. Use Section A to be certain of the symptom, e.g. headache. In the first seconds of talking with your patient, you should have a good idea whether this is your typical patient with headache. Use the first few pieces of information (age, sex, symptom) for example, "20 y/o woman with an episodic headache." <u>Assume</u> it is due to one of the 3 common causes, e.g. the commonest cause, tension-type headache. But you quickly learn she can't eat while having the headache (nausea) and she has to leave work and go to bed during the headache (disabled). Case closed–she almost certainly has migraine headaches.
2. Nevertheless, while talking with and examining your patient:
   a. Continually look for any one <u>sign</u> of an organic disease, and
   b. Be sure there is no obvious disease or a medication causing the headaches.
3. In followup of months to years be certain she responds appropriately to your management and that no sign of a dangerous disease arises.

Clues suggesting the presence of an organic disease or a potentially dangerous disease.
   Even though syndromes commonly are responsible for most new symptoms in the office patient, you first must be as confident as possible that an organic disease is not present in your patient. If you find any <u>one</u> of the following clues present, then your patient is <u>not a typical everyday patient</u>. Proceed as if an organic disease, or even a dangerous disease, is present–that is, use your technological approach to diagnosis or send your patient to the hospital.
   1. Onset of a new or different symptom in a patient >40-50 y/o (the older he is, the more likely it may be an organic, or dangerous, disease).
   2. Any <u>one</u> objective finding or sign on physical exam that can be related anatomically or physiologically to the symptom, e.g., jaundice in a patient with abdominal pain.
   3. A symptom, such as headache, that progressively worsens, either

Chapter 1 Principles of Office Diagnosis   13

in frequency or severity over days, weeks, or months.
4. Abrupt onset of the symptom, such as abdominal pain, and it continues at the same or greater severity.
5. Any unexplained bloody discharge (hemoptysis, hematemesis, hematochezia, occult stool blood).
6. A symptom that persistently worsens at night, such as low back pain or diarrhea, and awakens the patient.
7. A nonspecific symptom, such as a rash or arthralgias, that occurs concurrently with fever (never miss fever; get rectal temperatures q6h at home if there is any question there might be a fever).
8. Your patient "looks" ill or toxic.
9. Your patient volunteers malaise–"I feel sick" or "I feel ill" i.e. it's not just lack of energy or interest that keeps him from doing his usual activities.
10. Associated with the complained-of nonspecific symptom, you find any one potentially dangerous symptom–syncope, unexplained weight loss, anemia, night sweats, high ESR.
11. Your patient previously always was "healthy," that is, no history of many ED or office visits, and now he comes to you for help with a new symptom.
12. The nonspecific symptom is expressed in a straightforward, concerned, or frightened manner, i.e. not in bizarre terms, not with indifference, not in dramatic exaggerated terms.
13. The chronic symptom fluctuates, that is, it is not "constant" or "there all the time."
14. The symptom interferes with activities of daily living, including weekend or vacation activities.
15. Your patient is "refreshed" on awakening in the morning, but he's "all tired out" by mid-afternoon.
16. Symptoms are consistent anatomically and physiologically with abnormalities in the physical exam.
17. New onset of a mental disorder, e.g. MD, in a patient >50 y/o, always think of malignancy.
18. Onset of a new symptom associated with the same organ that caused the original symptom, e.g. previously only occasional cough, now he is also "short of breath."

Characteristics of the symptom to differentiate among its common causes.

Some words that we use casually in medicine can confuse diagnosis, and "acute" is one of those words. We use two words to describe the length of time that a symptom of a disease is present–chronic and acute. In diagnosis "chronic" can be a useful term, but "acute" meaning short-lived is not. Only in retrospect, after a short illness is over, can we say it was acute–for example, "He had acute abdominal pain," because it lasted 6 days. But when you saw the patient in your office on day 3 of his symptoms, saying the symptom is "acute" adds nothing to help you diagnose the cause of the abdominal pain, because at that moment you don't know if it will last only 3 more days, or it will become chronic, persistent daily pain and last years. Possible diagnoses of diseases that last days are very different from those lasting months or years. Rarely will you see the word "acute" used in this book.

What you really want to know for accurate diagnosis is precisely how

the symptom began and the time it took to reach its peak severity. Other words are more accurate and descriptive than "acute" to describe the mode or rate of onset of a symptom to its peak intensity:
a. Abrupt–peak severity at the same time the symptom began e.g. vascular causes (SAH)
b. Rapid–peak severity only after a few minutes or <1-2 hr from onset e.g. angina pectoris, panic attack
c. Gradual–peak severity only after hours or <1-2 days from onset
d. Slow–peak severity only after a number of days from onset
e. Insidious–the symptom has been present for months or even years, so the patient has no distinct memory of when the symptom began or the circumstances surrounding its onset

In the patient described above with 3 days of abdominal pain, you want to know whether the onset to peak intensity was either abrupt, rapid, or gradual. With such a recent onset the patient always should be able to specify when and how the pain began and important circumstances that occurred in the hours preceding the pain. As important as knowing the precise mode of onset of a symptom is whether the symptom is:
i. New onset (first or second time the patient has had the symptom)
ii. Episodic (asymptomatic periods of days, weeks or months between attacks)
iii. Chronic (persistent, and present almost daily)

In addition to the rate of onset of the symptom and its course, contrasting one or more of the following patient characteristics can help you differentiate the common causes of that symptom.
  a. Age <40-50 y/o or >50 y/o
  b. Man or woman
  c. Associated symptoms or none (that is, is it an isolated symptom or does it occur with other related symptoms)
  d. Local (focal) or regional or generalized (pain or weakness)
  e. Unilateral or bilateral symptoms
  f. Fluctuating or constant symptom
  g. Symmetrical or asymmetrical symptom

Certainties ("Always" and "Nevers") in talking with your patient

a. Always envision your patient as your sister or mother or grandfather, and treat your patient in all respects as you would treat that close relative.
b. Always treat your patient as you would want to be treated i.e. gently, empathetically.
c. Always introduce yourself and use the patient's last name: Mrs. Smith, Mr. Jones (unless the patient requests otherwise).
d. Always use the 8 magic words: "When you say _____, what exactly do you mean?" to determine precisely the patient's meaning of some word or phrase he uses to describe his symptom, associated symptoms, or important events preceding his sickness. We may use this question 4-5 times with a difficult problem e.g. dizziness.
e. Always, after you have first introduced yourself and taken a brief history at the initial visit, have all of your patient's clothes removed (except panties or undershorts) and your patient gowned for the physical exam.
f. Always see that your patient is comfortable, make the room as quiet

Chapter 1 Principles of Office Diagnosis   15

as possible, have adequate light, and adjust the table to the correct level for you to examine accurately.

g. Always explain what it is you are going to do, and why, especially if there is any question or hesitation from your patient.
h. Always examine the supine patient from the patient's right side.
i. Always push the left breast aside (gently, appropriately) to palpate, percuss or auscultate at the apex for maximal impulse, heart sounds, murmurs.
j. Never palpate, percuss or auscultate through the gown, sheet or clothes.
k. Never, never argue with a patient (or family member): Reason, yes; argue, no.
l. Never forget that your elderly or sick patients were once your age and had your present excellent health; try to see in your "mind's eye" that formerly young and healthy person and know that someday "There go I."
m. Never can you over-use the six-letter word, please, during your exam. "Please sit up." "Please close your left eye." "Hold your breath now, please." It's polite and converts a command into a request. Please don't order–please ask.
n. Never forget your human limitations–both in diagnosis and in life. Be humble, but appropriately confident in your clinical skills.

I never met a person who wasn't smarter than me about some things.
Will Rogers (paraphrased)

Section H. Glossary

At the end of each chapter, we provide a glossary of terms commonly used either in the literature or in this book. Many of these terms have been used by clinicians for hundreds or even thousands of years, sometimes for exactly the same things we now use them–and sometimes not. Use each term precisely and correctly. Knowing its origin sometimes can be helpful in remembering its meaning and in using the term correctly. Sloppy use of language can lead to imprecise thinking and inaccurate diagnosis.

1. **Clinician** (Greek *kline* meaning "a couch or bed," referring to one caring for the sick person in bed.) Now it refers to any medically trained person who diagnoses and treats patients–distinguished from the academician and laboratory researcher.
2. **Diagnosis** (Greek *diagnosiskein*, meaning "to distinguish.") To the Greeks, it was a process of discriminating between two or more possibilities, and we still use it that way. The general process is the same whether we are trying to identify the cause of chest pain (either an organic disease or a syndrome) or the cause of your car not starting (no fuel or a dead battery).
3. **Disease** (French *des* meaning "away from" and *aise*, "ease.") Early use was for anything affecting one's ease or normal state. Now the more restricted meaning in medicine refers to measurable or observed changes in structure or function of some organ, hence the designation "organic disease."
4. **Disorder**– derangement or abnormality of function
5. **Doctor** (Latin *docere* meaning "to teach.") In keeping with the meaning of the word, teach your patients to help themselves.

6. **Entity** (Latin *ens* meaning "a being.") It implies an independently existing thing, not exactly what organic diseases are, though we act as if they are.
7. **Etiology** (Greek *aitia* meaning "a cause" and *logos*, "a discourse.") It is a study of causes, thus etiology is not a synonym for "cause," but commonly we use it that way today.
8. **Organic** (Greek *organikos*, meaning "pertaining to an organ or organs.") An organic disease is an illness with abnormal structure or function (demonstrable by technology) of an organ.
9. **Patient** (Greek *patior* meaning "to suffer.") A patient is one who is suffering physically or mentally, and comes to you for help in diagnosing and treating her illness. Some paramedical professionals e.g. psychologists, use the term, "**client**" (Latin *cliens*, meaning "dependent or under another's protection.") It is a term best used to describe persons purchasing goods or services, e.g. used cars, stocks and bonds, clothes, legal advice.
10. **Symptom** (Greek *symptoma* meaning "anything that has befallen one, by chance or mischance.") Note the implication of something coming from outside to afflict the person. Today a symptom is some feeling or sensation (pain, anxiety, dyspnea) arising from inside the patient and providing clues to the cause (explanation) of the symptom or distress.
11. **Syndrome** (Greek *syn* meaning "together" and *dromos* "a running.") It is a group of symptoms observed to occur together in a large number of people who are ill. Implied is that these people do not have an organic disease i.e. no abnormal test of a damaged organ to explain the illness. Some call them "nonorganic illnesses." We call them syndromes because they are heterogeneous in causation and frequently include some "undiscovered" organic diseases. For example, 30 years ago IBS included patients that we now know had the organic diseases, lactase deficiency and giardiasis.
12. **Therapy** (Greek *therapeno* meaning "I wait upon.") It suggested service or attendance to the sick and suffering person, and it still does.

For more on medical word meanings and origins see references used:

Dorland, W.A.N. Dorland's Illustrated Medical Dictionary, 30th Ed. Philadelphia: WB Saunders, 2003.

Haubrich, W.S. Medical Meanings: A Glossary of Word Origins, 2nd Ed. Philadelphia: American College of Physicians, 2003.

Chapter 2 Abdominal Pain

Questions on Abdominal Pain

A. When your patient complains of abdominal pain or "My stomach hurts," you should determine 3 things before going further in diagnosis of cause. They are:
   1.
   2.
   3.
B. Specifically, the 2 questions you ask your patient to determine whether it is episodic abdominal pain as opposed to "new onset" abdominal pain are:
   1.
   2.
C. Before diagnosing one of the 4 common causes of intra-abdominal pain, you must be confident that it is not organic disease of one of 3 extra-abdominal organ systems causing referred pain:
   1.
   2.
   3.
D. You can use 2 findings (1 on history, 1 on physical exam) to distinguish the 2 common causes of <u>new</u> abdominal pain. The 2 causes and the 2 findings for each cause are:
   1.
      a.
      b.
   2.
      a.
      b.
E. Three historical findings differentiate the 2 common causes of <u>episodic</u> abdominal pain. The 2 causes and the 3 findings for each cause are:
   1.
      a.
      b.
      c.
   2.
      a.
      b.
      c.
F. Your patient has continuous or nearly continuous abdominal pain for months. The pain is unaffected by eating, defecation, or menses, and you find no objective signs. Its prevalence is about 2%, and it is named:

G. Abdominal pain is the commonest cause (16%) of <u>new or episodic</u> pain visits to the office. The percent of these patients who have a dangerous or a surgical cause of the pain is:

Answers on Abdominal Pain

A. Determine that the pain is originating intra-abdominally; next, that the pain is from the bowel versus solid abdominal organs e.g. liver, kidney
   1. "Show me where the pain is" and he points to the abdominal area and not the flank or back or pelvic area
   2. Be sure it's not referred pain to the abdomen. Think it might be referred pain:
      a. If it is "sharp" or burning or lancinating pain that changes with movement of the body or a Valsalva maneuver e.g. cough (rather than deep dull diffuse visceral pain associated with intra-abdominal disease); and
      b. If on deep palpation the degree of tenderness is much less than you would expect from the intensity of the patient's pain complaint
   3. Try to be confident the pain is originating from the GI tract or bowel rather than from a solid abdominal organ. Bowel pain characteristics are:
      a. Earliest pain is a mild discomfort and located midline; later it becomes crampy or colicky pain (rather than more constant pain) and usually is lateralized, rather than midline
      b. Accompanying bowel symptoms are common *viz* flatus, fluctuating distention, change in BMs to diarrhea or constipation

B. Distinguishing new onset pain from episodic pain
   1. Ask "When is the last time you had a similar abdominal pain, even though it might have been a lot less severe?" and "When before that time?" Positive answers to both questions suggest episodic pain
   2. "How many times do you think you have had such a similar pain in the past month (or year, or 5 years, or 10 years)?" Once or twice every few months–now you know it is episodic pain

C. Look for signs and symptoms of organic disease that can cause referred pain to the abdomen
   1. Cardiopulmonary pain occurs with activities causing increased cardiac output (myocardial ischemia) or with deep inspiration (pleuritic); there are associated symptoms of cardiac or pulmonary disease, such as dyspnea, tachypnea, orthopnea, edema
   2. Genitourinary–there may be flank pain or CVA tenderness on percussion; or severe colicky pain in the abdomen but no change in bowel sounds, distention, flatus. (Note that when we say pain is "radiating" to a certain site, it means the pain seems to be originating at this distant site–it doesn't necessarily mean there is a linear band of pain from one site to another). Symptoms suggesting UTI may be present *viz* dysuria and frequency, and abnormal urinalysis confirms the UTI
   3. Gynecological disease–anytime there is new onset "abdominal pain" in a woman of reproductive age, especially if the pain is in the mid-lower abdominal region; patient <50 y/o, get a pregnancy test, first and always

D. Common causes of new abdominal pain and their distinguishing characteristics
   1. Nonspecific abdominal pain
      a. May have nausea and occasionally minimal vomiting
      b. No sign on exam

Chapter 2 Abdominal Pain 19

 2. Acute gastroenteritis (GE)
    a. Nausea, prominent vomiting and diarrhea commonly; other symptoms of infection e.g. mild fever, myalgias, headache
    b. Hyperactive bowel sounds
E. Common causes of <u>episodic</u> abdominal pain and their distinguishing characteristics
 1. Nonulcer dyspepsia
    a. Discomfort or pain starts midline, epigastric and it stays midline (no lateralization)
    b. No change in bowel habits or stool appearance (no diarrhea or constipation) with onset of pain
    c. No relief of pain with BMs
 2. Irritable bowel syndrome (IBS)
    a. Abdominal pain at <u>any</u> abdominal site
    b. With onset of pain there is concomitant change in BMs, either diarrhea or constipation
    c. Partial or total relief of pain with BMs
F. Functional abdominal pain syndrome (FAPS)–Think of FAPS if abdominal pain almost daily for months and is an <u>isolated</u> symptom with minimal relationship to other GI functions
G. Recognize the rarity of dangerous causes of abdominal pain in the office
   It is 3-5%–thus, most patients with new or episodic abdominal pain seen in the office will have one of the 4 common causes listed above, or an obvious cause such as abdominal wall pain

Abdominal Pain

Differential diagnosis: the 4 common causes of abdominal pain
1. Nonspecific abdominal pain (NSAP)–<u>new</u> onset; minimal other symptoms
2. GE–<u>new</u> onset; symptoms of infection e.g. fever, headache, vomiting, diarrhea; hyperactive bowel sounds
3. Nonulcer dyspepsia (NUD)– <u>episodic</u>, epigastric pain; no change in bowel habits; BMs do not affect the pain
4. IBS–<u>episodic</u> pain; associated with diarrhea or constipation; some pain relief with BMs

A. **Be certain of the symptom and its distinguishing characteristics.** Your patient's problem or chief complaint is "My stomach hurts."
1. First, try to be sure it is pain originating intra-abdominally (degree of tenderness on palpation correlates with the intensity of the pain complaint), that is, it's not referred pain (sharp or burning pain related to body movements or cough). Once you are sure it is intra-abdominal pain, determine whether it is pain likely caused either by bowel disease (colicky or cramping pain; the earliest discomfort or pain begins midline; there are associated changes in bowel functions–distention, flatus, increased BM) or by other solid abdominal organs (more constant pain; not midline; less associated with changed bowel functions)
2. Have your patient show you where he feels the pain coming from now. <u>Don't</u> ask him to point with one finger, but if he voluntarily points to a focal area of the abdomen, think it might be benign abdominal wall pain if other bowel symptoms are minimal or absent. If he is significantly ill with other bowel symptoms, however, his pointing with one finger suggests somatic pain and a possible surgical cause. Also, be sure it is not pain referred to the abdomen from disease of the spinal column, thorax (lung, heart, esophagus), GU tract or pelvis (GYN). If it is pain referred from one of these sites, other signs and symptoms emanating from these extra-abdominal organs should be important parts of the clinical picture, with abdominal pain just one of the symptoms. At this point you should be confident the pain is originating intra-abdominally, and that the pain is due to bowel disease.
3. Determine if it is either new onset pain or episodic pain or chronic, almost daily pain. Ask him "Precisely when did this pain start?" or "Exactly when was the last time you did not have any stomach pain?" New pain means it began in the last 7 days, but most often it will have started within the past 48 hours. To determine if it is episodic pain, ask: "When is the last time you had abdominal pain anything like this one, even though it might have been a lot milder in the past?" and "When did you have similar stomach pains before that previous time?" If both answers are positive, he likely has

Chapter 2 Abdominal Pain 21

episodic abdominal pain. If he has pain lasting much longer than a few weeks, he probably has chronic abdominal pain, which has different causes and a different approach to diagnosis (See Section G.3)

Be certain:
1. The symptom is pain originating in the abdomen (not referred pain)
2. Whether it is either new pain or episodic pain
3. Whether its onset to peak severity was abrupt, rapid (<1-2 hours) or gradual (hours-days)
4. If other bowel symptoms (diarrhea, constipation, vomiting) are present
5. If there is any relationship between the pain and BMs.

(If it is chronic, persistent almost daily abdominal pain, see Section G.3 in the text.)

---

4. Next, understand this particular bout of abdominal pain. "How were you feeling the hours before the pain started?" and "Precisely where was the earliest pain or discomfort?" Usually bowel pain begins as a deep, dull discomfort in the midline, and only hours later does the pain become severe and lateralized. Determine where the earliest discomfort was located because it can help identify the part of bowel that is diseased–epigastric location (disease of esophagus, stomach or duodenum), periumbilical (disease of the small intestine), lower abdomen (disease of colon)

   "Tell me everything you can think of about this pain"–you must understand how the pain began and rate of progression until it got its worst; other symptoms that preceded or followed the beginning of the pain, and exactly when the other symptoms began, especially <u>when vomiting began in relation to pain onset</u>; food intake before and during the pain and food effect on the pain; bowel movement effect on the abdominal pain i.e. if BM makes the pain better or worse–"What usually happens to the pain when you have a bowel movement?"

5. Physical examination
   a. Watch attentively: does he get up on the exam table with normal movements; does he lie comfortably, or is there restless writhing (suggesting obstruction), or does he refuse to move (suggesting peritonitis)? Is there <u>objective</u> abdominal distention? To examine for pyelonephritis: with him supine place one of your hands under each flank, then alternately percuss (dorsum of the hand flat on the examining table, firmly flex your fingers at the MCP joints to percuss) his lower posterior ribs as the control site for tenderness to compare the tenderness you elicit when percussing each ipsilateral CVA area
   b. Auscultate for either absent bowel sounds or hyperactive bowel sounds. For the latter, you are not listening for borborygmi, but an

almost constant, often distant rumbling sound indicating hyperactivity. Press deeply, but slowly with your stethoscope to hear better, and also to determine the degree of tenderness

c. Palpate for guarding, rigidity, as well as tenderness at the site of pain. If tenderness is much less than suggested by the severity of the pain complaint, think of referred pain. If your patient appears minimally ill and the pain is focal, i.e. he voluntarily points with 1-2 fingers, think of abdominal wall pain and test for it: with his arms folded across his chest, and while he is supine, hold his knees with your right hand, and press gently on the site of pain with your left hand. Then, have him tense the abdominal wall by doing a "sit up" slowly. Aggravation of the pain localized to that site is a positive Carnett's sign and strongly suggests an abdominal wall source of the pain. Treat with an anti-inflammatory drug or inject the site with an analgesic

d. Pain on internal rotation of the hip with him supine (obturator sign) suggests an inflamed pelvic appendix or abscess; and pain on forced extension of the right hip while he is recumbent on his left side (Cope's iliopsoas sign) suggests an inflamed retrocecal appendix or abscess

e. Always perform a rectal and pelvic exam if you are uncertain of the diagnosis, or if you want a rectal temperature or feces sample to test for occult blood

By now you should be confident it is intra-abdominal pain, it is either new or episodic or chronic pain, and it is due to bowel disease or dysfunction. In almost all instances you now have the information you need for diagnosis of the obvious causes (Section C) and the common causes (Section E). In the rare instance that your patient appears different clinically from the usual office patient with abdominal pain, be certain (Section B) that he does not have a symptom or sign of a dangerous disease.

B. **Be confident it's not a dangerous disease.**

1. Send immediately to the ED by ambulance if there is:
   a. Evidence of a catastrophic event e.g. signs of shock, hypotension, tachycardia, cold and clammy extremities, pallor, syncope, think of MI, PE, Addisonian crisis, acute arsenic poisoning ("garlicky" breath)
   b. Abrupt onset of severe abdominal pain (these patients almost never come to the office, but the spouse may frantically telephone you, just get him to the ED by ambulance), think of ruptured aortic aneurysm, perforated PUD, mesenteric infarction, ruptured ectopic pregnancy, esophageal rupture, gastric volvulus
   c. Patient > 50 y/o with severe pain radiating to a flank or genitalia (suggesting in a young person, pyelonephritis, ureteral stone, testicular torsion), think of rupturing abdominal aneurysm
   d. Cyanosis in a patient > 50 y/o, think of vascular causes e.g. MI, leaking aortic aneurysm, mesenteric infarct
   e. Patient >50 y/o with severe pain but minimal abdominal tenderness, think of mesenteric ischemia, MI
   f. Abdominal pain and prominent dyspnea, think of MI, pneumonia, PE
   g. New onset abdominal pain, high serum ketones and serum bicarbonate <6-8, think of DKA as the cause of the abdominal pain; bicarbonate >8, think of abdominal disease causing the DKA
2. Admit at once to the ED or hospital if there is:
   a. Severe pain, vomiting, progressively worsening distention, that is, anytime your patient is obviously very ill
   b. Constant (not colicky) mid-epigastric or RUQ pain with onset in the evening or night, think of biliary colic or perforated PUD; if it persists more than 3-4 hours, especially if there is severe vomiting, think of acute cholecystitis or acute pancreatitis

Chapter 2 Abdominal Pain 23

    c. New onset abdominal pain that has been constant for more than 5-6 hours, especially if onset of vomiting followed pain onset more than 1-2 hours, think of surgical causes e.g. appendicitis
    d. Gradual onset of discomfort in the midline, then it becomes more severe and localizes laterally, think of acute appendicitis (RLQ) or acute cholecystitis (RUQ)

Be certain in the first few minutes of the exam that there is no evidence of any <u>one</u> dangerous symptom or sign associated with the abdominal pain:

1. Unstable vital signs e.g. hypotension, unexplained tachycardia or tachypnea
2. Any very ill-appearing patient
3. Either abrupt or rapid (minutes) onset of severe pain
4. New abdominal pain in a patient >50 y/o
5. Significant abdominal distention and vomiting
6. New, progressively worsening severe abdominal pain persisting more than 5-6 hours
7. Constant, new abdominal pain intensified by cough or body movement
8. Absent bowel sounds or rigid abdomen in an ill patient
9. Rushes of high-pitched tinkling bowel sounds simultaneous with severe colicky pain

Any suggestion of a dangerous disease, send your patient to the ED.

---

    e. Pain at onset is fairly localized, then it becomes diffuse, think of perforated PUD (upper abdomen) or ectopic pregnancy (lower abdomen)
    f. Worsening severe pain, then it gradually lessens, think of a perforated viscus
    g. Abdominal pain and LMP more than 5-6 weeks ago, think of ectopic pregnancy
    h. Rushes of hyperactive or high pitched, tinkling bowel sounds occurring simultaneous with episodes of colicky (intermittent) pain, think of SBO
    i. Fecal vomitus, think of SBO
    j. Significantly distended abdomen with severe colicky pain, think of bowel obstruction
    k. A palpable mass, think of appendicitis or Crohn's disease (young person), or (in the elderly) cholecystitis, diverticulitis, bowel obstruction, malignancy
    l. Constant pain intensified by movement or cough, think of appendicitis, peritonitis
    m. A previous episode of upper abdominal pain, but this one lasts hours and the pain intensifies on deep inspiration, think of acute cholecystitis
    n. Severe colicky pain either located centrally (periumbilical) or bilaterally symmetrical (but rarely unilaterally), think SBO
    o. Severe pain awakening the patient from sleep, think of biliary colic, perforated PUD, appendicitis
    p. Severe abdominal pain without vomiting, but there is blood and mucus in the rectum, think of intussusception
    q. Sudden distaste for food and new onset abdominal pain, think of appendicitis
    r. Abdominal pain and a pulsating mass in an elderly patient, think of aortic aneurysm
    s. Abdominal pain without vomiting may still be life threatening e.g. large bowel obstruction, ruptured ectopic pregnancy, intra-abdominal hemorrhage, vascular catastrophe
    t. Abdominal pain and hematochezia, think of vasculitis, neoplasm, IBD, ischemic colitis, solitary rectal ulcer syndrome
    u. Elderly patient with vague abdominal symptoms but altered mental status, always think of surgical abdomen, pneumonia, urosepsis

24 WERNER'S OFFICE DIAGNOSIS

    v. Chronic ascites and new abdominal pain, think of bacterial peritonitis
    w. "Gastroenteritis" in the spring or summer but also high fever and severe headache, think of RMSF (rash may occur only days later)
    x. Ecchymosis of the flank (Turner's sign) or umbilicus (Cullen's sign), think of retroperitoneal hemorrhage, ectopic pregnancy
    y. SOB and abdominal pain exacerbated by deep inspiration, think of pleuritic pain referred to the abdomen (pneumonia, PE, pneumothorax, diaphragmatic pleurisy)
    z. RUQ pain, fever, increased alkaline phosphotase, think of acute cholangitis

3. Admit to the hospital or have a specialist consult as soon as appropriate if there is:
   a. Any patient > 50 y/o (and the older the more urgent) with new abdominal pain of uncertain etiology
   b. Abdominal pain and unexplained tachypnea, think of DKA or a pulmonary cause (PE, pneumonia)
   c. Abdominal pain of recent onset but it has occurred before, think of causes of episodic abdominal pain that might become dangerous or surgical-- biliary colic, cholecystitis, intermittent SBO, PUD, diverticulitis, pancreatitis, mesenteric ischemia, angina pectoris
   d. Episodic abdominal pain with occult blood or hematochezia, think of IBD
   e. Episodic severe "gastroenteritis" with hyperactive bowel sounds, think of partial intestinal obstruction, IBD
   f. Patient >40-50 y/o with abdominal pain that occurs only with increased cardiac output (exercise, large meal), think of angina pectoris, ischemic bowel
   g. HIV-positive patient with CD4 cell counts <100/mm^3 and unexplained abdominal pain, think of unusual infections, lymphoma
   h. Patient taking glucocorticoids now has new onset mild abdominal pain, be cautious that steroids may mask symptoms of a dangerous or surgical abdominal disease
   i. Patient with bone marrow transplant and new abdominal pain, think of graft-versus-host disease (earliest symptom is severe, watery secretory diarrhea)
   j. Abrupt onset severe <u>continuous</u> RUQ pain that lasts 2-4 hours, think of biliary colic
   k. Persistent fever and abdominal pain for days, think of PAN, FMF, relapsing fever

C. **Make a quick diagnosis if it's obvious.** Is it an easily diagnosed non-GI cause or a medication that is responsible for the abdominal pain? In most patients you will be <u>highly</u> confident of a common cause of the symptom by now. If not, one or more of the following tests may exclude an organic disease and increase your confidence in your working diagnosis: CBC, Chem 7, UA, urine hCG, vaginal culture for chlamydia and gonorrhea, lipase, LFTs, abdominal US.

Recognize any easily diagnosed <u>new</u>, <u>non-GI</u> abdominal pain:

1. GU– pyelonephritis, prostatitis, nephroureterolithiasis, UTI
2. GYN–ectopic pregnancy, salpingitis, endometriosis
3. Spot diagnosis–abdominal wall pain, referred dermatomal pain
4. Medication side effect–any recently begun new medication

---

1. GU disease is suggested by concomitant symptoms of kidney, ureter, or bladder disease, and by relative absence of bowel symptoms
   a. Acute pyelonephritis is suggested by flank pain and confirmed by CVA tenderness, which is much greater intensity than tenderness to percussion over his ipsilateral adjacent ribs
   b. Ureteral stone is suggested by extremely severe colicky pain; this referred pain may occur only in the suprapubic area or in the testes
   c. UTI is suggested by dysuria and frequency, and confirmed by an

Chapter 2 Abdominal Pain 25

      appropriately abnormal UA
- d. Prostatitis causes lower abdominal pain and symptoms suggesting UTI; also there is fever and a very tender prostate on DRE
- e. Epididymitis causes gradual onset (6-24 hours) of lower abdominal pain; there is swollen, tender epididymis, and elevating the hemiscrotum reduces the pain
- f. Incarcerated inguinal hernia causes anorexia and vomiting; the upper spermatic cord and external inguinal ring are not swollen or tender

2. GYN diseases are commonly misdiagnosed. Anytime your patient is a woman of reproductive age, think GYN disease. If there is new onset mid- lower abdominal pain, more than 30% of the time it will be one of the following: salpingitis i.e. PID, UTI, dysmenorrhea (cyclical pain), ovarian cyst (bleeding or torsion), ectopic pregnancy or incomplete abortion, endometriosis (cyclical pain), mittelschmerz (cyclical pain), interstitial cystitis (cyclical with menses)
Key to diagnosis of GYN causes is the following:
   - a. A thorough GYN history including periods, especially the last one and when due; possibility of pregnancy; vaginal discharge; symptoms of pregnancy e.g. fainting or presyncope; <u>always</u> obtain a lab test for pregnancy in a woman <50 y/o with new unexplained abdominal pain
   - b. Limitations to the GYN physical exam:
     - (1) Rectal exam shows right-sided tenderness less commonly with appendicitis than with PID, ovarian lesions or an ectopic pregnancy; so right sided tenderness is <u>not</u> diagnostic of appendicitis
     - (2) Bimanual exam showing tenderness on moving the cervix indicates PID or ectopic pregnancy, but the sign is positive in only 50% of each

3. Abdominal wall pain–focal abdominal pain and positive Carnett's sign in a mildly ill patient
   - a. Dermatomal pain
     - (1) Varicella-zoster infection–pain and hyperesthesia may precede the vesicular rash by 5-7 days
     - (2) Compressive radiculopathy (sensory) due to OA, herniated disk, spinal tumor (pain is provoked by or intensified by palpation of, or movements of, the spine)
   - b. Focal wall pain
     - (1) Rectus sheath hematoma–follows coughing, vomiting, weight lifting; common site is midline and midway between the umbilicus and symphysis pubis
     - (2) Hernia sites of the abdomen–umbilical, epigastric (midline above umbilicus), spigelian (midabdomen, at the lateral edge of the rectus sheath); with the patient supine, hernia size should decrease markedly unless it is incarcerated; with him standing and performing a Valsalva maneuver, hernia protrudes
     - (3) Cutaneous nerve entrapment–positive Carnett's sign; tender trigger points along the lateral margins of the rectus abdominis muscle
     - (4) Myofascial pain syndrome–positive Carnett's sign; 1-2 cm diameter tender TrP
     - (5) Idiopathic–too tight belt or too constrictive clothing

4. Medications–<u>any new</u> medication should be suspect; all -mycins (including azithromycin), triple therapy for *H. pylori*, abacavir or valaciclovir, cisapride, colchicine, NSAIDs, ethambutol, fenfluramine, fluconazole, methotrexate, nifedipine (mesenteric ischemia), omeprazole, oral contraceptives, erythropoietin, terbenifine, tocopherol (vitamin E), digoxin, warfarin, theophylline, dilantin; 12-36 hours after stopping narcotics

D. **Identify your patient's worries and wants.** About 30% of the adult population has at least one bout of abdominal pain yearly, and fewer than one-third of these consult about it. During your interview and exam, try to intuit or discover why your patient is here today, and not previously, for this problem. Don't necessarily ask directly, but try to get some ideas from your patient's responses to questions about his perception of the abdominal pain itself. You can't completely help your patient unless you know what he really worries about and wants from you. That's why he is here to see you--to satisfy his worries and wants! Here are only some of the possible worries and wants of your patient with abdominal pain. You must discover his specific, unique ones

1. Common worries are:
   a. That the cause of the abdominal pain is a dangerous etiology e.g. appendicitis, cancer, ectopic pregnancy
   b. That the cause is some rare disease e.g. toxic chemicals, parasites from drinking water
   c. What other unique fears or anxieties might be troubling your patient? For example, he may have had IBS for years, and only now does he come for help. What has changed? Perhaps a friend or relative, who had similar episodic abdominal pain, recently has been diagnosed with colon cancer. There are many other possibilities–think of them

---

During your exam, discover your patient's worries (e.g. appendicitis, cancer, ectopic pregnancy) and wants (tests, reassurance it is not dangerous, pain relief) so that you can respond to his specific needs as soon as possible.

---

2. Your patient wants:
   a. You to perform a thorough physical exam focused on possible causes of the abdominal pain and he wants appropriate tests and imaging studies
   b. A plausible explanation of the cause of the abdominal pain
   c. Confident reassurance from you that it is not a dangerous or rare etiology. Tell him--"The good news, it's not appendicitis" (or whatever you believe his real worry is)
   d. To know the prognosis, short term (effects on job, home life, marriage; how soon he will be back to normal) and long term (if recurrences are possible; how to prevent recurrences; if it will cause any disability)
   e. Treatment to stop the pain now and to prevent recurrences e.g. TCA for IBS
   f. A referral (gastroenterologist, surgeon) if he believes you are not confident of the diagnosis

E. **Know the symptoms that differentiate the 4 common causes of episodic or new abdominal pain.**
   1. The commonest etiology is called nonspecific abdominal pain (NSAP), which accounts for more than 50% of all new abdominal pain seen in the office
      a. Characteristics of NSAP
         (1) It is a <u>new</u>, mild-moderately severe abdominal pain, and its onset was gradual over a few hours
         (2) Other GI symptoms do not fit a pattern suggesting any organic disease, e.g. appendicitis or cholecystitis, and the symptoms are

Chapter 2 Abdominal Pain 27

not progressively worsening. Occasionally there are individual symptoms of concern: 50% may vomit; there even may be RLQ pain but it definitely began there and stayed there; rarely, there may even be mild guarding or rebound, but not both together
   (3) Make the working diagnosis of NSAP only after you are confident organic disease is not responsible for your patient's abdominal pain
  b. What suggests it might not be NSAP

The causes of most new or episodic abdominal pain in the office patient <50 y/o are:
1. Nonspecific abdominal pain (NSAP)–new onset; minimal other symptoms
2. GE–new onset; symptoms of infection e.g. fever, headache, vomiting, diarrhea; hyperactive bowel sounds
3. Nonulcer dyspepsia (NUD)– episodic, epigastric pain; no change in bowel habits; BMs do not affect the pain
4. IBS–episodic pain; associated with diarrhea or constipation; some pain relief with BMs

---

   (1) Any time any symptom or sign suggests a dangerous cause (see above, Section B), or
   (2) If any one of the following findings suggesting appendicitis is present:
      (a) Pain migrates, i.e. the mild discomfort started in the midline (periumbilical) and then, over a few hours the pain became much more severe and moved to the RLQ
      (b) Vomiting did not start until 1-2 hours after the original midline discomfort began
      (c) Nausea, vomiting, anorexia are all present
      (d) Body movement or coughing intensify the pain, especially RLQ pain
      (e) Focal tenderness in the RLQ (McBurney's point)
      (f) Both guarding and rebound tenderness
      (g) Rectal exam shows tenderness only on the right side
   (3) If your patient is > 50 y/o, never attribute abdominal pain to NSAP without caution, some workup and careful followup. Even though 16% of those >50 y/o with new abdominal pain have NSAP, in those >70 y/o with new or episodic abdominal pain, 24% have occult malignancy and 10% have a vascular cause (MI, leaking aneurysm, mesenteric ischemia). The elderly patient may have a higher pain threshold or be on steroids or analgesics for another condition and mask the pain. They get different diseases causing abdominal pain and present differently from younger adults. Be very cautious with a patient >50 y/o with new onset abdominal pain
   (4) If your patient is a woman of reproductive age with lower abdominal pain (though 40% will have NSAP) search for signs and symptoms of GYN disease and always get a pregnancy test

2. Common look-alikes and how each differs from NSAP
   a. Gastroenteritis (GE)
      (1) It also is <u>new</u> abdominal pain
      (2) The pain is a cramping, moderately severe pain and it is of gradual onset over hours until peak severity. One or more associated GI symptoms (vomiting, diarrhea, mild anorexia) are common; vomiting <u>precedes or starts at about the same time</u> as the abdominal pain; diarrhea often is prominent
      (3) Hyperactive bowel sounds are present during the early stage. If the bowel sounds are not constant and hyperactive, be concerned that it might not be GE. Recognize, however, the hyperactive sounds are a constant "rumbling" and may be distant, soft, and difficult to hear. Slowly, press deeply with your stethoscope. These hyperactive bowel sounds are not like those due to SBO, which are loud or tinkling and come in rushes at the same time the colicky (intermittent) pain comes
   b. Nonulcer dyspepsia
      (1) It is <u>episodic</u> pain or discomfort "centered" in and around the midline of the upper abdomen, and the discomfort remains midline; it neither lateralizes nor becomes more severe
      (2) This "discomfort" he complains of may really be:
         (a) Early satiety–stomach is full out of proportion to the amount of food eaten; or
         (b) Fullness–unpleasant feeling that there is slow digestion, i.e. persistence of food in the stomach; or
         (c) Bloating–upper abdominal tightness, but not visible abdominal distention; or
         (d) Nausea–queasy feeling that he might vomit
      (3) Prompt referral for endoscopy should be done to exclude PUD, reflux esophagitis, or gastric cancer in the following patients with new onset dyspepsia:
         (a) All patients >45 y/o
         (b) Those <45 y/o, but who also have an unexplained dangerous symptom: melena, fecal occult blood, dysphagia, unexplained weight loss, pain that is constant or severe or radiates to the back, recurrent vomiting or hematemesis or unexplained anemia
      (4) For the rest of the patients <45 y/o, initial treatment could be either with an H_2-receptor antagonist or PPI. If typical reflux symptoms (heartburn or acid regurgitation) occur alone, or as a dominant symptom of dyspepsia, a short trial of high dose PPI is best
   c. IBS
      (1) IBS is <u>episodic</u> pain and the first episode of abdominal pain is almost always at age < 45 y/o. The pain is gradual onset with peak severity of pain hours or days after its onset
      (2) Almost always the abdominal pain has associated with it diarrhea or constipation, that is, some change in frequency of BMs or change in stool consistency; and BMs provide some or total relief from the pain
      (3) Never attribute fecal occult blood or hematochezia to IBS

F. Use this summary for efficient diagnosis of a common

Chapter 2 Abdominal Pain 29

cause. With the information from Sections A-E in mind, here is the rapid approach to diagnosis of new or episodic abdominal pain.
1. You already have determined:
   a. In Section A, by H&P, that it is intra-abdominal pain and not focal abdominal wall pain or pain referred to the abdomen.
   b. In Section B, that there is no evidence in the H&P of any one dangerous cause of the abdominal pain.
   c. In Section C, that there is no evidence either of GU or GYN disease, or a medication causing the abdominal pain.
2. From the focused H&P almost always you should quickly be confident of a working diagnosis. Confident final diagnosis is made only in followup the next few days, weeks or months when the response to treatment or nontreatment is appropriate to your working diagnosis.
   a. If the new pain is mild to moderate, the pain began at about the same time as nausea and vomiting or the pain only began after the nausea and vomiting, and there are hyperactive bowel sounds and diarrhea, diagnose gastroenteritis.
   b. If the pain is new and the intensity is similar to gastroenteritis, but there is no diarrhea or hyperactive bowel sounds, diagnose NSAP.
   c. If it is episodic and upper abdominal pain suggesting dyspepsia, and your patient is <45 y/o without dangerous signs, then treat with an H_2-blocker or PPI; refer for endoscopy older patients and those with a dangerous sign.
   d. If the episodic abdominal pain has its onset associated with either diarrhea or constipation, and BMs provide some or total pain relief, diagnose and treat IBS.
3. Answer your patient's worries and wants that you determined early on during the exam (Section D). Have you done everything you can to help him?
4. You now have a working diagnosis, but only with followup can you be more confident it is correct. In return visits you are always testing by H&P that your working diagnosis is correct.

G. Abandon your working diagnosis and look for an uncommon cause only if:
1. Any one dangerous symptom or sign (see above, Section B) occurs in followup of days, weeks, months, or years. Quickly obtain a consult or send the patient to the hospital as appropriate
2. The abdominal pain does not respond to treatment as you expect or the natural history of your working diagnosis does not occur. Either NSAP or GE should be getting better in 2-3 days from the onset of the pain, but definitely not progressively worsening. If the pain began 12-36 hours ago, have him notify you in 12-24 hours with a progress report. Each entity should be completely well in 1-2 weeks. If this degree of improvement is not occurring, then re-examine him

Don't spend time and money looking for one of the following etiologies until you are sure your patient doesn't have one of the 4 common causes of episodic or new abdominal pain above. If he doesn't have one of those causes, it may be that the correct cause was one of the less common etiologies listed below. These are important to recognize, because each has different treatment or prophylaxis. Most are causes of episodic pain and the patient is well between bouts of pain
   a. Extra-abdominal causes
      (1) Conditions that may mimic GE:
         (a) Narcotic withdrawal–then 12-36 hours later, a clinical picture like GE
         (b) Hypercalcemia of any cause
         (c) Ingestion of any amount of alcohol may cause early chemical gastritis, possibly hematemesis

- (d) Iron overdose causes corrosive chemical GE 1-2 hours after ingestion
- (e) Addison's crisis–pain, hypotension, weight loss
- (f) Mushroom poisoning causes severe chemical GE soon after ingestion
- (g) Ingestion of acid or alkali causes esophagogastritis
- (h) Diabetic ketoacidosis itself causes abdominal pain but only when bicarbonate is very low e.g. <8; usually the pain is due to abdominal disease that causes the DKA
- (i) Drug-induced colitis (oral contraceptives, NSAIDs)
- (j) HUS and TTP–likely the same disease; GE may precede symptoms of hemolysis, ARF, purpura, CNS sequelae

---

If your patient's symptoms do not respond as expected to your management, he may have an uncommon or rare cause listed in Section G.2 that you can diagnose and treat. Or you may want to refer your patient to a specialist.

---

(2) Diseases that may mimic IBS
  - (a) Lead poisoning–crampy episodic pain with constipation, paresthesias, anemia
  - (b) AIP–gradual onset (days) of abdominal pain, often with constipation worsening with pain onset; think of AIP if episodic pain occurs after negative laparoscopy
  - (c) Tertiary syphilis (tabes dorsalis)–nausea, vomiting, pain; Romberg test positive
  - (d) FMF– episodic severe abdominal pain and fever in a young patient of Mediterranean ancestry
  - (e) Hereditary angioneurotic edema–episodic colic, bloating, vomiting; nonpitting swelling and burning skin of the orofacial area or extremities; obtain C4 level
  - (f) Abdominal migraine–probably part of the cyclic vomiting syndrome; onset with abdominal pain, then prominent vomiting for hours, which decreases over 3-5 days; relate abdominal pain to concomitant migraine headaches (Am J Gastroenterol 94, 2855, 1999)
  - (g) Abdominal epilepsy–episodic abdominal pain, nausea, diarrhea, associated with confusion, dizziness, headache, visual changes; get a sleep EEG study
  - (h) Sickle cell anemia–diffuse bone pain with abdominal pain and ileus
  - (i) Collagenous colitis–woman >50 y/o with onset of episodic pain and watery diarrhea; in a man >50 y/o with the same picture, think of lymphocytic colitis
  - (j) Cryoglobulinemia–episodic crampy pain with enterocolitis
  - (k) Celiac axis compression syndrome–patient <40 y/o with postprandial epigastric pain, diarrhea, weight loss and epigastric bruit

(3) Other extra-abdominal causes of abdominal pain
  - (a) Thoracic
    - (i) Pneumonia, recurrent PE
    - (ii) Myocardial ischemia, angina pectoris
  - (b) Endocrine-metabolic
    - (i) Uremia–pain, constipation, pseudoobstruction, intussusception
    - (ii) Carcinoid syndrome–diarrhea, wheezing, flushing
    - (iii) Hypertriglyceridemia (chylomicronemia syndrome) >1000 mg/dL causing acute pancreatitis
    - (iv) DM– causes either episodic or chronic pain due to diabetic neuropathy or mesenteric ischemia
    - (v) Chronic Addison's disease–anorexia, weight loss, orthostatic hypotension
    - (vi) Hyperparathyroidism–anorexia, vomiting, constipation
    - (vii) Hypoparathyroidism–diarrhea or steatorrhea, intestinal tetany, pseudoobstruction
    - (viii) Hypothyroidism–constipation, distension and abdominal discomfort
  - (c) Hematologic
    - (i) Henoch-Schönlein purpura–pain, vomiting, diarrhea may precede the purpuric rash
    - (ii) Hemolytic anemia–anemia, high LDH, low haptoglobin
    - (iii) Acute leukemia–high WBC

Chapter 2 Abdominal Pain 31

            (iv) Behcet disease–oral ulcers and presentation suggesting Crohn's disease
            (v) Churg-Strauss syndrome–nausea, vomiting, GI hemorrhage
        (d) Connective tissue diseases
            (i) Polymyositis, dermatomyositis–dysphagia, early satiety, bloating, myalgias, high CPK
            (ii) Progressive systemic sclerosis (scleroderma)–small intestine dysfunction (malabsorption, steatorrhea, weight loss) and postprandial periumbilical pain
            (iii) Seronegative spondyloarthropathies–chronic mild diarrhea, cramping abdominal pain, LBP
            (iv) SLE–multiple causes of abdominal pain (lupus peritonitis, terminal ileitis, pancreatitis, enteritis, intussusception)
            (v) Neurofibromatosis–GI bleed, obstructive type pain
        (e) Miscellaneous
            (i) Tuberculosis–pain, fever, weight loss, night sweats
            (ii) Hypersensitivity reactions
            (iii) Snake bite, spider bites
            (iv) TA– anorexia, weight loss, patient >50 y/o
    b. Intra-abdominal, non-bowel causes–any disease of liver, gall bladder, diaphragm, spleen, kidney, ureters, retroperitoneal area, aorta, uterus, ovary, bladder
    c. Intra-abdominal, bowel causes–symptoms mimic IBS
        (1) Lactase deficiency–bloating and diarrhea following ingestion of lactose-containing foods
        (2) Giardiasis–diarrhea, severe flatulence, weight loss
        (3) Whipple's disease–malabsorption, fever, lymphadenectasis, arthralgias; >40 y/o Caucasian man
        (4) Trichinosis–diarrhea, myalgias, fever, eosinophilia
        (5) Amebiasis–diarrhea with positive occult bloody stools
        (6) Celiac sprue–chronic diarrhea, flatulence, weight loss, rash
        (7) Eosinophilic enteritis–weight loss, diarrhea, eosinophilia
        (8) Bile acid malabsorption–diarrhea; Rx cholesytramine
        (9) Bacterial overgrowth, intestine–malabsorption, diarrhea, weight loss, macrocytic anemia; Rx tetracycline
3. Chronic persistent, almost daily, abdominal pain for months–approach to diagnosis:
    a. If there is any one dangerous sign or symptom e.g. fever >101°F or 38.3°C (get rectal temps tid at home), increased WBC, ascites, abdominal mass, night sweats, lymphadenectasis, jaundice, unexplained weight loss, pathologic fracture, unexplained anemia, melena or cachexia; think of malignancy, chronic pancreatitis, IBD, autoimmune diseases, infiltrative diseases, degenerative neurological or muscular disorders, abscess
    b. If there is not one sign of organic disease, and there is little or no relationship to eating, defecation, menses, or to other physiological events; think of
        (1) Functional abdominal pain syndrome (FAPS) which occurs in 2% of the adult population, and there may be significant loss of daily functioning attributed to the chronic pain; abdominal pain is the dominant symptom with minimal other bowel symptoms
        (2) Somatization disorder–onset <40 y/o; pain in multiple other organ systems
        (3) MD–commonly has multiple somatic complaints, including abdominal pain with anhedonia and depressed mood

H. Use the glossary for precise thinking and accurate diagnosis.

1. **Acute**--"acute abdomen" is medical slang and it is not helpful for diagnosis; acute and chronic are the only terms that we use regarding the "time course" of any illness, but we don't know our individual patient has an acute disease, except in retrospect; "new" or "episodic" are words that provide important information regarding the pain, as does the time to peak pain from its onset–"abrupt" "rapid," "gradual," and "insidious."
2. **Allodynia** (Greek *allo* meaning "other or differing from the usual" and *odyne*, "pain.") Pain resulting from a stimulus that usually would not cause pain.
3. **Analgesia** (Greek *an* meaning "without" and *algesia*, "pain.") An agent that stops pain.
4. **Anesthesia** (Greek *an* meaning "without or lack of" and *aisthesis*, "feeling or sensation.") No feeling from a given stimulus.
5. **Anorexia** (Greek *an* meaning "without or lack of" and *orexis*, "appetite.")
6. **Appetite** (Greek *ap* meaning "toward" and *petitus,* "desire.") Desire or craving for

pleasurable things e.g. food, drink, sex, hobbies; culture is the important determinant of appetite. Animals don't have appetite, only hunger to maintain life. Hunger does not cause obesity, only culturally driven inappropriate appetite causes most obesity.

7. **Borborygmus, plural, borborygmi** (Latin for "rumbling or growling bowels." Its origin very likely is onomatopoeia (Greek *onomatos* meaning "a name" and *poiein*, "to make") that is, forming a word in imitation of natural sounds.
8. **Choledocholithiasis** (Greek *chole* meaning "bile," and *doche*, "a receptacle" and *lithiasis*, "stones.") Literally it means bile stones in the gallbladder, but *choledochus* is Latin for common bile duct, so choledocho- now means "pertaining to the common bile duct," thus, choledocholithiasis now means stone in the common bile duct.
9. **Colic** (Greek *kolikos* meaning "related to the colon.") Now it implies colicky pain, a wave-like buildup in intensity of pain, and then some relief before another buildup in pain occurs; colicky pain suggests GI tract or bowel disease.
10. **Dyspepsia** (Greek *dys* meaning "difficult or impaired" and *pepsis*, "digestion.") It refers to epigastric discomfort following meals.
11. **Focal** (Latin *focus* meaning "fireplace.") It implies is a very small area, as opposed to local, from Latin *localis*, generally signifying a larger region; both are opposed to general, from Latin *generalis* suggesting many or all parts of the organism.
12. **Hernia** (Greek *hernos* meaning "a sprout-like protruding bud of a plant.") Any unsightly bulge from the body.
13. **Hunger** (Anglo-Saxon *hungor*, a physiological overwhelming drive to eat in order to survive.) All species have hunger.
14. **Hyperalgesia** (Greek *hyper* meaning "above" and *algesis*, "pain.") It is heightened sensitivity to perception of pain from a given noxious stimulus.
15. **Hyperesthesia** (Greek *hyper* meaning "above" and *aisthesis*, "feeling or sensation." Increased sensitivity (to pain, light, or sound) to a given stimulus.
16. **Hypoesthesia** (Greek *hypo* meaning "below" and *aisthesis*, "feeling or sensation.") Abnormally decreased sensitivity to a given stimulation.
17. **Intussusception** (Latin *intus* meaning "within" and *suscipere*, "to receive.") Prolapse of a part of intestine into the lumen of an immediately adjoining part causing bowel obstruction.
18. **Lancinating (pain)** (Latin *lancinare* meaning "to stab.") It is pain characterized by a sensation of sharply cutting, piercing, or stabbing.
19. **Migration (of pain)** (Latin *migratio* meaning "movement.") It is pain that begins at one site, disappears or lessens as it moves to another site e.g. appendicitis, cholecystitis.
20. **Mittelschmerz** (German *mittel* meaning "middle or mid" and *schmerz*, "pain.") It is mild intermenstrual pain, at ovulation.
21. **Obstipation** (Latin *obstipatio* meaning intractable constipation).
22. **Parietal** (Latin *paries* meaning "an encircling wall" or *parietalis*, "the wall of a body cavity.")
23. **Radiation (of pain)** (Latin *radiare* meaning "to furnish with spokes.") it is pain originating at one site, remains at that site, but it also is felt at one or more other distant sites at the same time.
24. **Referred (pain)** is misperceived by the brain as a dull ache coming from the body surface i.e. skin or muscle; this cutaneous area has its somatic innervation in the same spinal roots that supply visceral afferents to the diseased organ.
25. **Salpingitis** (Greek *salpinx* meaning "trumpet.") It refers to a tubular anatomic structure with a flared bell-shaped end e.g. fallopian tube; pelvic inflammatory disease (PID) is a more general term.
26. **Satiety** (Latin *satis* meaning "sufficient" and *ety*, "condition of.") It is complete gratification of appetite, no further desire to ingest food or liquid.
27. **Sitophobia** (Greek *sitos* meaning "food" and *phobein*, "to fear.") It refers to eating very little with much weight loss, because when he eats he gets such severe pain from mesenteric ischemia.
28. **Umbilicus** (Latin word for "belly button," probably originated from *umbo*, "the boss of a shield" or the ornamental stud at the center of a soldier's shield).
29. **Visceral** (Latin *visceralis* or *viscus*). It refers to any large organ in the 3 major body cavities, but especially now to organs in the abdomen.

Chapter 3 Chest Pain

Questions on Chest Pain

A. To be confident the chest pain is due to intra-thoracic disease (heart, lung, mediastinum), first exclude localized or referred pain as causing the chest pain:
   1.
   2.
   3.
B. In your patient's description of the chest pain, you specifically try to identify a respirophasic component–that is, that deep inspiration brings on or intensifies the chest pain. Pleuritic chest pain is one kind of respirophasic pain
   1. Name another cause of respirophasic chest pain:
   2. Pleuritic chest pain has 3 characteristics:
      a.
      b.
      c.
   3. There are 5 common causes of pleuritic chest pain, each beginning with "P":
      a.
      b.
      c.
      d.
      e.
C. The commonest cause of chest pain in the office patient and its 3 major distinguishing characteristics are:
   1.
      a.
      b.
      c.
D. The other 3 common causes of chest pain and their distinguishing characteristics are:
   1.
      a.
      b.
   2.
      a.
      b.
   3.
      a.
      b.
E. In order not to miss diagnosing angina pectoris, you look for 4 characteristics of the chest pain:
   1.
   2.
   3.
   4.
F. Five characteristics of "nonangina" or atypical or nonspecific chest pain are:
   1.
   2.
   3.
   4.
   5.
G. You must be able to differentiate "shortness of breath" from dyspnea in a patient with new or episodic chest pain, because:

Answers on Chest Pain
A. Localized or referred pain is suggested by typical findings
  1. Chest wall pain is focal pain; it is brought on or intensified by deep inspiration (but it is not pleuritic pain), coughing or sneezing, and by provoking onset or increasing the intensity of the pain by you or the patient pressing firmly at the site of pain
  2. Referred pain from neck, shoulder, or spine disease–movements of the head, neck, arms, or torso, brings on or intensifies the chest pain
  3. Referred pain to the chest may be recognized by associated symptoms suggesting disease of liver, diaphragm, gallbladder, stomach or duodenum
B. Pleuritic pain is just one kind of respirophasic chest pain
  1. Either chest wall pain or referred pain from back or shoulders
  2. Three characteristics of pleuritic chest pain
     a. Pleuritic pain is unilateral and localized to a small area, that is, the patient voluntarily points with 1-2 fingers at the site of pain
     b. It is sharp or knife-like in character
     c. Because it is caused by irritation of the parietal pleura deep inside the chest wall, your pressing on the chest wall should not provoke or intensify the pain
  3. Common causes of pleuritic chest pain: The 5 "Ps" are pleurisy, pneumonia, pneumothorax, pulmonary embolism, pericarditis. Note that if you can be highly confident the chest pain is pleuritic, the likelihood of the chest pain being due to cardiac ischemia is very low. So try your best to find a respirophasic component early on in talking to and examining your patient with chest pain
C. The commonest cause of chest pain in the office
  1. Chest wall pain
     a. New onset pain at any age
     b. Respirophasic (but not pleuritic), i.e. pain occurs and intensifies during deep inspiration
     c. There is point tenderness on the chest wall, and pressing at that site exactly reproduces the pain
D. Each of the other 3 common causes have episodic chest pain, which is not respirophasic
   a. Angina pectoris
      (1) Onset >30-40 y/o
      (2) Pain occurs only during any action significantly increasing cardiac output
   b. Panic attack
      (1) Onset <30-40 y/o
      (2) Chest pain occurs only during a panic attack with typical associated symptoms e.g. dyspnea, fear of dying
   c. Nonspecific chest pain
      (1) Onset <30-40 y/o
      (2) Isolated chest pain can occur at any time. Characteristics of "nonangina" are present (see Answer F, below), and symptoms of ischemia or panic attack are absent
E. Four characteristics of angina pectoris
  1. It is episodic chest pain
  2. It is any pain located between the earlobes and the umbilicus, and
  3. The pain occurs during or immediately after some increased cardiac output (running, sex, hurrying up stairs, anger), and

Chapter 3 Chest Pain

    4. It rapidly peaks and plateaus in a few minutes; upon stopping the precipitating activity, the pain rapidly disappears over 5-10 minutes
- F. Characteristics of atypical or nonspecific chest pain, any one or more may occur in your patient
  1. Abrupt onset and abrupt disappearance of the pain
  2. Pain is unrelated to activities causing increased cardiac output
  3. Pain lasts seconds, or hours, or days, or "it's there all the time"
  4. It is precordial pain, that is, he <u>voluntarily</u> points with 1-2 fingers over the heart, and especially if he points to the heart apex
  5. Pain is relieved by <u>increased</u> activity or by bending or twisting his body or changing positions
- G. Dyspnea almost always signifies either heart or lung disease

    All patients with dyspnea will have shortness of breath (SOB). But some patients with SOB and chest pain do not have dyspnea. If the onset of SOB (<u>not</u> dyspnea) is in a patient <40-50 y/o, think especially of panic attack. With panic attack there is not the labored or hard work of breathing that is dyspnea. Instead, it is a "feeling" that he is "not getting enough air in." Your exam shows no adventitious sounds (crackles, wheezes), breath sounds are normal, cardiac exam is normal and there are no signs of CHF

Chest Pain

Differential diagnosis: the 4 common causes of chest pain
1. Chest wall pain–<u>new</u> onset; respirophasic but not pleuritic; focal chest wall tenderness
2. Angina pectoris–<u>episodic</u>; onset >30-40 y/o; pain is ischemic, not respirophasic
3. Panic attack–<u>episodic</u>; onset <30-40 y/o; typical symptoms of sympathetic hyperarousal
4. Nonspecific chest pain–onset <30-40 y/o; <u>episodic or chronic</u>; not respirophasic or ischemic or chest wall pain

A. **Be certain of the symptom and its distinguishing characteristics.** Your patient's problem or chief complaint is "I get this sharp pain in my chest." The following questions should take 1-2 minutes only, but if he is in significant distress from the pain, don't ask questions, get him to the hospital at once.
1. Be certain the problem is pain originating from his chest. "Show me where the pain is the worst," and "Where did it start?" Don't ask him to point with one finger, but if he does it suggests somatic pain and, therefore, likely a nonischemic cause of the chest pain. If he does point with 1 or 2 fingers, say "Press on your chest at that point." Commonly, this pressure provokes or aggravates the chest pain as shown by his facial expression. If his pressing does not provoke pain, then you should press in that area, as well as all other areas of the chest wall, trying to elicit tenderness or to replicate his pain <u>exactly</u>.
2. Assuming no localized tenderness to the chest wall–"Think back to before the pain started–how were you feeling?" You are looking for associated symptoms of either the cardiac, pulmonary, GI or musculoskeletal system, or autonomic symptoms of panic attack.
   a. "Tell me exactly what the pain felt like." There are many imprecise terms used by patients to describe the pain, for example, some say "sharp" pain when they mean it is "severe." You must understand precisely what he was feeling–you can never overuse the question –"What do you mean by . . .?"–until you are certain you understand exactly what the patient felt when he had the pain. "From the moment the pain began, how long did it take until it was its most severe?" and "What exactly were you doing just before the pain began?" You want to know if there was any activity causing increased cardiac output.
   b. Next, "Could you find any way to lessen the pain or even make it go away?" "Whenever I get a chest pain like that, I take some deep breaths to get more oxygen to my heart. What happened when you did that?" If he did not previously do that–"Take some deep breaths–does that make the pain better?" You are trying to identify respirophasic pain, that is, the pain occurs only with, or is intensified by, usual or deep inspirations. Pleuritic pain is

Chapter 3 Chest Pain 37

respirophasic and it is localized and sharp or knife-like in character; chest wall pain also is respirophasic but it is not pleuritic. Major causes of pleuritic chest pain (5Ps) are pleurisy, pneumonia, pneumothorax, pulmonary embolism, pericarditis. Thus, if you can determine it is respirophasic pain, the likelihood of ischemia causing the chest pain becomes very low. "Could you find any position or movement that made the pain better or worse?" Ischemic pain should be unaffected by position or movements. Pericarditis is suggested by improvement of the pain when he leans forward.

  c. Finally, determine if this is a new chest pain or a recurrence of a

---

Be certain:
1. The symptom is chest pain (not referred pain)
2. Whether it is either new pain or episodic pain
3. Whether its onset was abrupt, rapid or gradual
4. If the pain is respirophasic
5. If some activity preceded the pain
6. Whether there were associated symptoms

---

past identical or somewhat similar chest pain. "When is the last time you had a chest pain _anything_ like this?" and "When did you have it before then?" Positive answers to both questions suggest it is episodic chest pain.

3. Physical exam
  a. If pleuritic pain is present–auscultate for a localized area of absent breath sounds (pneumothorax), focal crackles (pneumonia), pleural friction rub that disappears on breath holding (PE), friction rub during breath holding (pericarditis).
  b. Respirophasic pain that is _not_ pleuritic pain suggests chest wall pain.
    (1) Palpate all chest wall areas where musculoskeletal pain can arise _viz_ sternum, costochondral junctions, sternoclavicular joints, xiphoid.
    (2) To provoke or intensify possible referred pain, evaluate various movements of the cervical spine, thoracic spine, shoulders, clavicle.
  c. Cardiac valve damage can cause chest pain, so auscultate especially for the systolic murmurs of aortic stenosis or HCM; diastolic murmur of aortic regurgitation, and loud S2 of pulmonary hypertension (S2>S1 at cardiac apex).

By now you should be confident it is chest pain, whether it is either a new pain or episodic pain, if it is respirophasic chest pain, and if any activity preceded the onset of pain. In almost all instances you now have the information you need for diagnosis of the obvious causes (Section C) and the common causes (Section E). In the rare instance that your patient appears different clinically from the usual office patient with chest pain, be certain (Section B) that he does not have a symptom or sign of a dangerous disease.

B. Be confident it's not a dangerous disease.

1. Send immediately to the ED by ambulance if there is:
   a. An overall appearance of severe distress, e.g. he is very ill with unbearable pain, chest heaviness with dyspnea
   b. Evidence of a catastrophic illness e.g. hypotension, marked diaphoresis, cold and clammy extremities, pallor, presyncope or syncope
   c. Abrupt onset of severe chest or back pain, think of AD, pneumothorax, PE, perforated GI viscus
   d. A distressed patient with abrupt onset of unexplained dyspnea or tachypnea or pleuritic chest pain, think of PE or pneumothorax
   e. A patient >50 y/o or one with long-standing DM who has new onset of syncope or confusion and minimal or no chest pain, think of MI
   f. Distressed patient with dyspnea, chest pain, pulsus paradoxus, think of cardiac tamponade, severe asthma attack.
   g. Severe pain that radiates or migrates up the chest or back and down the arm or leg, think of AD (palpate for asymmetric pulses)
   h. A patient <30-40 y/o with symptoms suggesting MI, think of drug-induced infarction e.g. cocaine
   i. Signs and symptoms of shock but BP >140/90, think of MI, AD

Be certain in the first minutes of your exam that there is no evidence of any one dangerous symptom or sign associated with the chest pain:

1. Patient is obviously ill and distressed
2. Unstable vital signs e.g. hypotension
3. New onset of very severe pain
4. Chest pain is unbearable
5. Unexplained pleuritic pain and abrupt onset of either dyspnea or tachypnea
6. Unstable angina pectoris

Any suggestion of a dangerous disease, send your patient to the ED.

---

2. Admit at once to the ED or hospital if there is:
   a. A distressed patient with abrupt onset, severe knife-like or stabbing constant localized (pleuritic) pain, with or without dyspnea, think of pneumothorax, PE
   b. A patient with retching or vomiting that precedes the chest pain, think of esophageal rupture (Boerhaave's syndrome)
   c. Pleuritic chest pain of gradual onset (may be no dyspnea) that may be worsened or first noticed when supine, and relieved by sitting up, think of pericarditis
   d. A patient >45-50 y/o with new unexplained chest pain (nonpleuritic) of any description, located retrosternal or left chest, think of MI or unstable angina pectoris
   e. A patient with new onset of angina pectoris, that is, it is unstable angina pectoris
   f. Previously diagnosed angina pectoris that is worsening, e.g. increased frequency, less exertion causing similar degree of pain, increased severity of pain with the same exertion or nocturnal angina or rest angina, by definition it is unstable angina
   g. Your patient is in mild distress with pleuritic chest pain and concomitant dyspnea, fever, focal late inspiratory crackles, cough, think of pneumonia
   h. Episodic chest pain always occurring with severe headache, but no obvious factor precipitating increased cardiac output, think of carbon monoxide poisoning
   i. Chest pain that sounds ischemic but there is absolutely no cause of increased cardiac output, think of variant (Prinzmetal's) angina, unstable angina pectoris
3. Admit to the hospital or have a specialist consult as soon as appropriate if there is:
   a. Respirophasic chest pain or focal wheezing in a patient with possible malignancy or a history of malignancy, think of metastases e.g. lung or pleura
   b. Insidious onset of pleuritic chest pain along with associated symptoms of cough,

Chapter 3 Chest Pain 39

   unexplained weight loss, night sweats, fever, think of TB
   c. Pleuritic chest pain 2-10 weeks following MI, think of Dressler's syndrome (concomitant fever and pericardial effusion)
   d. New chest pain after recent CABG, think of postcommissurotomy syndrome (pleuritic pain) or graft occlusion causing new anginal pain (nonpleuritic, ischemic pain)
   e. Chest pain that awakens the >40-50 y/o patient, think of nocturnal angina (angina decubitus) or OSA (Mayo Clin Proc 69, 244, 1994); if <30-40 y/o, think of panic attack or esophageal spasm
   f. Young person with nonpleuritic chest pain, think of HCM, MVP, cocaine, amphetamine, precordial-catch syndrome (benign); if pleuritic pain, think of pneumothorax, pneumonia, PE; still the commonest cause in the young patient in the office is either pleuritis (pleurisy) or nonspecific chest pain
   g. Elderly patient with angina pectoris and a systolic murmur radiating to the carotids, think of tight aortic stenosis
   h. Patient <50 y/o with a systolic murmur that diminishes on squatting and increases on standing up, and chest pain or presyncope during or only after exertion stops, think of HCM
   i. Chest pain onset at rest (usually relieved by nitroglycerin) associated with transient ST segment elevation, think of Prinzmetal's variant angina
   j. Causes of ischemic chest pain at rest, think of: severe HTN; hyperkinetic states e.g. thyrotoxicosis, pheochromocytoma, severe anemia, high altitude, Paget's disease; aortitis or vasculitis impeding coronary blood flow; paroxysmal rapid ventricular rates with shortened diastole; unstable angina or MI
   k. Worsening of chest pain after nitroglycerin, think of HCM
   l. Episodic pleuritic pain, abdominal pain and fever in a patient <25 y/o, think of FMF

C. **Make a quick diagnosis if it's obvious.** Next, is it an easily diagnosed condition or a medication that may be responsible for the chest pain? In most patients you will be highly confident of a common cause of the symptom by now. If not, one or more of the following tests may exclude an organic disease and increase your confidence in your working diagnosis: CBC, Chem 7, LFTs, EKG, CXR
   1. Pain resulting from a lung disease almost always is pleuritic chest

---

Recognize any easily diagnosed cause of chest pain:
1. Pleuritis–new, rapid onset of pleuritic pain and no evidence of pneumonia i.e. no crackles or dyspnea
2. Tracheobronchitis–new, gradual onset of nonpleuritic pain associated with productive cough, mild sore throat, fever, minimal chills; no crackles or dyspnea (different from pneumonia)
3. GERD–episodic, rapid onset nonpleuritic pain in a patient <45 y/o with typical GI symptoms relieved with a PPI
4. Spot diagnoses–Dressler's syndrome, *H. zoster* rash, pendulous breasts, brassiere syndrome
5. Medication side effect

---

pain and it alarms the patient because is new onset
   a. There are five major causes of pleuritic chest pain and each starts with a "P": PE, pneumothorax, pericarditis, pneumonia, pleurisy. The first three should already have been sent to the ED or ICU as dangerous causes (see Section B). Pleuritic pain is one form of respirophasic pain, and it usually is unilateral and described as a

sharp, stabbing, knife-like, or sticking pain causing splinting and brief, shallow respirations. Neither finger pressure at the pain site nor movements of the torso or arms should provoke or aggravate pleuritic pain.
   b. Pneumonia has additional symptoms of lung infection. Very distinctively there is dyspnea and late inspiratory crackles (they do not clear with deep cough), often focal and unilateral; also high fever, productive cough, myalgias, malaise, high WBCs.
   c. Pleuritis (pleurisy), commonly viral, may have myalgias, fever and cough also, but neither crackles nor dyspnea. Your patient may have difficulty breathing due to splinting caused by the pain, so he may complain of SOB, but it is not dyspnea.
2. Tracheobronchitis
   a. It is new onset of nonpleuritic chest pain
   b. There are associated symptoms of a lower respiratory tract viral infection (early dominant symptom is dry cough, then later a mucopurulent-producing cough) following a 24-hour prodrome of mild pharyngitis, rhinorrhea, mild fever, headache, myalgias; the trachea may be tender to palpation and movement
   c. Pneumonia is absent i.e. no dyspnea or focal inspiratory crackles.
3. GERD causing esophageal spasm or dysmotility
   a. Typical GERD symptom is heartburn (pyrosis) due to regurgitation of stomach contents into the esophagus. GERD may occur alone or as the dominant symptom of dyspepsia, i.e. recurrent episodes of discomfort centered in the midline above the umbilicus and felt as early satiety, fullness, bloating or nausea. Prompt response to high dose PPI usually is diagnostic for GERD
   b. GERD may cause esophageal spasm and nonpleuritic, episodic chest pain. In a patient >45 y/o with new onset of dyspepsia, perform EGD to exclude malignancy and other GI causes of chest pain. In a patient with similar symptoms but <45 y/o, response to aggressive PPI therapy would be appropriate, unless the H&P suggests ischemia is causing the chest pain. (See Section G.4 for characteristics suggesting an esophageal etiology for the chest pain)
4. Spot diagnoses
   a. Dressler's syndrome has new onset pleuritic pain within 6 weeks after an MI or cardiac surgery
   b. H. zoster rash has chest pain that may precede the rash by 5-7 days, and it is dermatomal type pain not crossing midline
   c. Pendulous breast and brassiere syndromes
5. Medications associated with chest pain–alpha blockers, beta blocker e.g. propranolol, beta-blocker withdrawal, bromocriptine, cocaine, ephedrine, ergotamine, fenfluramine, granulocyte colony stimulating factor, hydralazine, mesalazine, methysergide, mexiletine, minoxidil, nicotine patch, nicotinic acid, nifedipine, ondansetron, oxytocin, procainamide, pergolide, all triptans, thyroxine excess (during treatment of hypothyroidism); angina pectoris may be precipitated by amphetamines, cocaine, OTC cold remedies

D. **Identify your patient's worries and wants.** Chest pain is very common, and few patients consult about it. Try to intuit or discover why your patient is here today, and not previously, for this problem. Especially try to understand why your patient with stable angina pectoris is here today. What is he worried about? Has it become unstable angina? Don't ask directly, try to get some

Chapter 3 Chest Pain 41

ideas from your patient's responses to questions about the chest pain itself. You can't completely help your patient unless you know what he really worries about and wants from you. That's why he is here to see you--to satisfy his worries and wants! Here are only some of the possible worries and wants of your patient with chest pain. You must discover his specific, unique ones

1. Common worries are:
   a. That the cause of the pain is a dangerous etiology e.g. MI, PE, blood vessel "bursting"
   b. That the etiology is some rare disease e.g. Lyme myocarditis, Hantavirus, WNV
   c. What other fears or anxieties might be troubling your patient? For example, he may have had chest pain for many years, and only now does he come for help. What has changed? Perhaps a friend or relative, who had similar episodic chest pains, recently died suddenly with an MI. There are many other possibilities–think of them

> During your exam, discover your patient's worries (e.g. heart attack, lung cancer) and wants (e.g. diagnosis and treatment, pain relief), so that you can respond to his specific needs as soon as possible.

2. Your patient wants:
   a. You to perform a thorough physical exam focused on possible causes of the chest pain and he wants appropriate tests (at least an EKG) and imaging studies
   b. A plausible explanation of the cause of the chest pain.
   c. Confident reassurance from you that it is not a dangerous or rare etiology. Tell him--"The good news, it's not your heart" (or whatever you believe his real worry is)
   d. To know the prognosis, short term (effects on job, home life, marriage; how soon he will be back to normal) and long term (if recurrences are possible; how to prevent recurrences; if it will cause any disability)
   e. Treatment to stop the pain now and to prevent recurrences e.g. nitroglycerin
   f. A specialist referral (cardiologist, pulmonologist, gastroenterologist) if you are not confident of the diagnosis

E. Know the symptoms that differentiate the 4 common causes of new or episodic chest pain.

1. The commonest cause is chest wall pain, accounting for at least 40% of chest pain in the office.

> The causes of most chest pains in the office patient:
> 1. Chest wall pain–<u>new</u> onset; respirophasic but not pleuritic; focal tenderness
> 2. Angina pectoris–<u>episodic</u>; onset >30-40 y/o; pain is ischemic, not respirophasic
> 3. Panic attack–<u>episodic</u>; onset <30-40 y/o; typical symptoms of sympathetic hyperarousal
> 4. Nonspecific chest pain–onset <30-40 y/o; <u>episodic or chronic</u>; not respirophasic or ischemic or chest wall pain

   a. Characteristics of chest wall pain (see Section G.3 for specific entities).
      (1) It is a <u>new</u>, moderately severe chest pain, or it is less severe and episodic. It occurs in isolation, that is, there are no other significant symptoms suggesting disease of another organ system

viz cardiac, pulmonary, GI or systemic infection
- (2) Often the pain is respirophasic, that is, it is brought on, aggravated, or intensified by inspiration, similar to pleuritic pain The patient may point to a small area on the chest wall when asked to "Show me where the pain is," and pressing with your finger on that site should exactly reproduce the pain that the patient is complaining of, or movements of the arms or torso e.g. twisting, turning, stretching, may precipitate or aggravate the pain. Pleuritic pain should not be provoked or aggravated by palpation or these body movements
- b. What suggests it might not be chest wall pain
  - (1) Anytime there is an associated symptom or sign suggesting a dangerous cause (see Section B)
  - (2) If your pressing on the site of pain does not reproduce exactly the pain that the patient is complaining of, or movements of torso or arms do not provoke or aggravate the pain
  - (3) If the chest pain is accompanied by other significant symptoms or any one sign suggesting involvement of cardiac or pulmonary or GI systems
2. Common look-alikes and how each differs from musculoskeletal chest wall pain
  - a. Angina pectoris
    - (1) It is episodic chest pain and it begins commonly in a patient >40-50 y/o
    - (2) Try to make a positive diagnosis of angina pectoris. To be as close to 100% sensitivity in diagnosis, it is:
      - (a) Any pain (pressure, burning) or dysesthesia, and
      - (b) It is located anywhere from the ear lobes to the umbilicus, and
      - (c) The sensation or pain comes on (increases to a plateau over 20-30 seconds) only with, or reproducibly with, some cause of increased oxygen demand (exercise, frustration, anger, sex, large meal, cold air or cold wind, outdoors, early morning, walking uphill or up stairs, significant arm movements, lying down after a large meal, after a cigarette, high heat or humidity), and
      - (d) The discomfort or sensation lasts no more than 5-10 minutes (by a watch) after stopping the exercise, or whatever preceded or brought on the pain (except 5-10 min longer if emotion precipitated the pain)
    - (3) If your patient's story fits this scenario, and this is either the first episode, or the present episode is worsened in severity compared to the first (or others), or there is increased frequency of chest pain, or less exertion causes the same severity of pain, by definition it is "unstable" angina pectoris and he needs ambulance transport to the ED
    - (4) If your patient says "I have angina" and this is "another episode," don't be satisfied with another clinician's diagnosis of "stable angina pectoris" unless his description elicits all of the criteria listed above (Section E.2.a.2). If you need to confirm a diagnosis of "angina," the next time he anticipates he will do something that predictably brings on the pain:
      - (a) Have him stop the activity after the pain starts, and time precisely (minutes and seconds) how long it takes for the pain

Chapter 3 Chest Pain 43

   to disappear; then
   (b) Repeat the activity again and this time, after the pain starts, simultaneously stop the activity and take a nitroglycerin tablet sublingually and note the time in minutes and seconds until the pain is gone. Nitroglycerin takes 1-2 minutes to act, then it should significantly (by minutes) decrease the time needed for disappearance (no ongoing aching) of the pain, <u>if</u> it is "angina"
b. Panic attack
   (1) It is <u>episodic</u> chest pain and it begins in a patient <30-40 y/o
   (2) Panic attack has associated symptoms of anxiety preceding or concomitant with the chest pain and sympathetic hyperarousal symptoms, e.g. fear of death, free floating feeling, hyperventilation (SOB but <u>not</u> dyspnea), light-headedness, paresthesias, palpitations, sweating, trembling
   (3) Panic attacks occur frequently in patients with most psychiatric disorders, so make the psychiatric diagnosis in your patient and treat the psychological disorder:
      (a) Panic disorder–recurrent abrupt unexpected panic attacks; constant worry about losing control and the next panic attack; changes in behavior occur, e.g. agoraphobia, to avoid or control a future panic attack
      (b) GAD–almost constant anxiety and worry most of the day and night, about very unpleasant or disastrous events that might occur in the <u>future</u>
      (c) Somatization disorder–associated pain in a number of other organ systems besides chest pain, especially GI, CNS, GU, GYN, musculoskeletal systems
      (d) MD–anhedonia in its broadest sense, that is, an unexplained, decreased appetite for any one of his usual activities that he formerly greatly enjoyed e.g. gourmet food, hobbies, sex, music, work, hunting, sports; he also constantly worries, but about things that happened in the <u>past</u> i.e. guilt
c. Nonspecific chest pain
   (1) It is <u>episodic or chronic</u>, daily pain and it begins in a patient <40-50 y/o
   (2) Nonspecific means that the characteristics of the chest pain do not suggest either ischemic or pleuritic pain
   (3) Some characteristics that suggest it is nonspecific chest pain–the pain is:
      (a) Of abrupt onset and sudden disappearance
      (b) Not ischemic and lasts hours or days
      (c) Located precordial–often he points with one finger to the heart apex
      (d) Never exertional and the pain lasts seconds or more than 30 minutes or "all the time"
      (e) Relieved by activity (walking or running) or bending forward or by pressing over the site of pain
      (f) Precipitated or aggravated by postural change, e.g. lying recumbent on his side
      (g) Relieved almost <u>immediately</u> upon lying down or taking a nitroglycerin tablet
      (h) Described in vivid picturesque terms e.g. as "sharp," "knife-

44   WERNER'S OFFICE DIAGNOSIS

      like," "tingling," "electric shocks"
- (i) Localized by his voluntarily pointing with 1-2 fingers to the PMI or breast or axilla
- (j) Radiating down the lateral side of the forearm to the thumb
- (4) Caution: strongly against the diagnosis of nonspecific chest pain is any diffuse discomfort in the chest that the patient has great difficulty describing, or any symptom occurring only during an activity causing increased cardiac output, no matter what age

F. Use this summary for efficient diagnosis of one of the common causes. With the above information from Sections A-E in mind, here is the rapid approach to diagnosis of chest pain.

In the first minutes of your exam, be certain your patient is not now severely ill or by history was not in severe distress with chest pain earlier in the day. Almost never should such a severely ill patient come to your office instead of the ED, but if he does you must get him to the hospital immediately with no studies in the office. Once you are confident he is in no significant distress nor is he likely to be in distress soon, then proceed.

1. You already have determined:
   a. In Section A, by H&P, that it is chest pain, whether it is respirophasic or ischemic, and if it is related to cardiopulmonary or GI systems.
   b. In Section B, that there is no evidence in the H&P of any one dangerous cause of the chest pain.
   c. In Section C, that there is neither an easily diagnosed cardiopulmonary or GI cause nor a medication that is likely responsible for the chest pain.
2. From the focused H&P almost always you should quickly be confident of a working diagnosis. Confident final diagnosis is made only in followup the next few days, weeks, or months when the response to treatment or nontreatment is appropriate to your working diagnosis.
   a. Search assiduously for evidence of respirophasic chest pain:
      (1) If the chest pain is respirophasic (but not pleuritic) and you can reproduce the pain either by your pressing at a specific site or by his active movement of neck or arms or torso, it likely is either chest wall pain or referred pain.
      (2) If it is pleuritic in character, look for evidence of, and diagnose, one of the "5 Ps." If it is one of these respirophasic causes, tell him–"This does not mean you do not have heart disease, it means that this specific episode is not due to your heart."
   b. If the chest pain or dysesthesia is not respirophasic, and it is located anywhere between the earlobes and umbilicus; and it is brought on by any activity or emotion causing increased cardiac output; and it is relieved promptly in <5-10 minutes after stopping the activity, then it likely is angina pectoris. If this is the first episode of such chest pain, it is "unstable" and he promptly should be taken to the ED, but if it has occurred at other times, and it is unchanged in severity, it is "stable" angina pectoris.
   c. If the episodic chest pain has its onset in a patient <30-40 y/o and it is not angina pectoris, and there are symptoms of sympathetic hyperactivity that precede or coincide with the chest pain, diagnose a panic attack.

Chapter 3 Chest Pain

   d. If it is <u>new, nonpleuritic</u> chest pain in a patient <40-50 y/o, it does not meet any of the above criteria, and it has characteristics of "nonangina" chest pain, diagnose nonspecific chest pain.
3. Answer your patient's worries and wants that you determined early on during the exam (Section D). Have you done everything you can to help him?
4. You now have a working diagnosis, but only with followup can you be highly confident it is correct. In return visits you are always testing by H&P that your working diagnosis is correct.

G. Abandon your working diagnosis and look for an uncommon cause only if:

1. Any <u>one</u> dangerous symptom or sign (see above, Section B.) occurs in followup of hours, days, weeks, or months. Quickly obtain a consult or send your patient to the hospital as appropriate.

If your patient's symptoms do not respond as expected to your management, he may have an uncommon or rare cause listed in Section G.2 that you can diagnose and treat. Or you may want to refer your patient to a specialist.

2. Your patient's response to therapy is not as you expect or if the natural history of your working diagnosis does not occur. <u>Don't</u> spend time and money looking for one of the following causes until you are sure your patient doesn't have one of the 4 common causes of chest pain above. If he doesn't have one of them, it may be that the correct cause was a less common one listed below. These are important to recognize, because each has different treatment or prophylaxis. Almost all of these have new onset or episodic pleuritic pain. Except for the etiologies listed under lung disease, all the rest are causes of acute pericarditis (diagnosis by pericardial friction rub and EKG changes; think of pericarditis if pain improves on his leaning forward).
   a. Lung disease e.g. asbestosis, sarcoidosis, hypersensitivity pneumonitis, primary pulmonary hypertension, bronchopleural fistula, Wegener's granulomatosis, asthma, TB, neoplasm, empyema.
   b. Collagen vascular diseases–think of them if there are associated joint pains or rash: RA, scleroderma, SLE, spondyloarthropathies e.g. ankylosing spondylitis, Reiter's syndrome, IBD, Behcet's syndrome
   c. Infectious disease e.g. fungal, parasitic, coccidiomycosis, histoplasmosis, tularemia, tetanus, Lassa fever, leptospirosis
   d. Uremia, myxedema, sickle cell disease, neoplasm, FMF
3. Specific entities causing chest wall pain or referred pain to the chest. It is important to identify the etiology, because some can be treated with injection of an analgesic.
   a. Trauma including rib fracture–caution, you may not readily get a history of trauma in domestic violence
   b. Costosternal syndrome--tender over any of the costosternal joints; it commonly is called costochondritis; it may last a few days or become episodic; Tietze's syndrome is a type of costochondritis with firm, warm, tender swelling at one or more of the upper costochondral junctions
   c. Sternalis syndrome--think of it if there is bilateral anterior chest pain and tenderness of the sternalis muscle or area overlying the sternum
   d. Xiphodynia–tenderness localized to the xiphoid process on exam, but symptoms may present as generalized pain following a heavy meal or stooping or lifting movements
   e. Rib-tip or slipping rib syndrome–severe lancinating pain originating from the anterior ends of ribs 8-10; "hooking maneuver" is anterior traction by your flexed fingers at the lower ribs with the patient supine, and a clicking sensation may occur with the induced or intensified pain
   f. Sternoclavicular syndrome–it is a true joint, so it is susceptible to any form of arthritis; any movement of the joint e.g. shrugging the shoulders or elevating the

arms provokes the pain; warmth and swelling caused by arthritis may simulate Tietze's syndrome
   g. Fibromyalgia–characteristic multiple <u>bilateral</u> tender points include bilateral tenderness over the 2nd costochondral junctions
   h. Dermatomal pain distribution
      (1) Cervical disk osteoarthritis (spondylosis)--older patient; pain provoked by his movements of torso or neck; Spurling test–extend his neck, then laterally tilt (either to left or right) his head and press down gently on the top of his head to reproduce or aggravate the pain
      (2) Herpes zoster--thoracic involvement mostly young adult; chest pain may occur 1-2 weeks before onset of the rash; neither pain nor rash crosses the midline
      (3) Intercostal muscle cramp or intercostal neuritis with focal tenderness
   i. Breast disease--tender, localized lesion e.g. mass
   j. Precordial catch syndrome--sudden onset of brief respirophasic chest pain, usually in a young adult due to chronic poor posture
   k. Thoracic outlet syndrome–motor-sensory deficits in an ulnar nerve distribution
   l. Mondor's syndrome–painful superficial thrombophlebitis; palpable tender venous cord especially of the thoracoepigastric vein over the lateral chest wall
4. Symptoms <u>suggesting</u> an esophageal etiology of the chest pain
   a. Inconsistent and non-reproducible relationship of the chest pain to any activity causing increased cardiac output
   b. Pain is brought on just by change in posture e.g. stooping forward or lying recumbent, especially after a large meal
   c. Relief of pain by sitting up or by antacids, H_2 blocker, PPI
   d. Pain radiation most often to the back, rarely the arms
   e. Nocturnal chest pain <u>only</u>
   f. Timely relief of the pain does not occur with rest alone i.e. it lasts >10-15 minutes
   g. Pain continues as a "background aching" long after a specific episode
   h. Discomfort is localized to the retrosternal area i.e. no lateral extension
   i. Discomfort is provoked by swallowing
   j. History of regurgitation of fluids causing the pain
   (If he does not have at least one of the last 4 (g-j), then it is highly <u>unlikely</u> an esophageal etiology)

H. Use the glossary for precise thinking and accurate diagnosis.

1. **Adventitious** (Latin *adventicius* meaning "strange, extraneous.") Adventitious sounds are those not heard normally during lung auscultation; they are crackles, wheezes, rhonchi.
2. **Agoraphobia** (Greek *agora* meaning "market place" and *phobia,* "fear of.") It is inappropriate fear of losing control if the patient with panic disorder leaves his immediate well-controlled environment.
3. **Angina** pectoris (Latin word *angina* means "sore throat" e.g. Ludwig's angina; the Latin *angere* means "to choke or throttle" and *pectus,* "chest.") It is pain that causes a choking or suffocating sensation that takes his breath away, so the patient temporarily breathes faster.
4. **Cardiac** (Greek *kardia* meaning "heart," but also referring to structures nearby e.g. cardia of the stomach.)
5. **Costochondral** (Latin *costa* meaning "rib" and Greek word *chondros,* "cartilage.") *Costa* is the same word source for our words "coast" or "coastal."
6. **Decubitus** (Latin meaning "act of lying down" or just the horizontal position.)
7. **Diaphoresis** (Greek word meaning "profuse perspiration.")
8. **Dysesthesia** (Greek *dys* meaning "abnormal or unpleasant" and *aisthesis,* "perception.") It is an unpleasant abnormal sensation produced by either a usual stimulus or spontaneously.
9. **Dyspnea** (Greek *dys* meaning "difficult" and *pnoia,* "breath.") It is difficult or labored breathing such that the patient is <u>working</u> to breathe. All dyspnea is SOB, but all SOB is not dyspnea e.g. panic attack, pleurisy.
10. **Parietal** (Latin *paries* meaning "an encircling wall," as around a city). Ancients used the word *parietalis* to designate the wall of a body cavity, so parietal pleura lines or encircles the thoracic cavity, and visceral pleura lines the lung itself.
11. **Pleurisy** (French word meaning "pleuritis," which also is the Greek word). Ancients used *pleuritis* for any disease of the chest wall, and we now use it specifically for any inflammation of the pleura, which characteristically causes pleuritic chest pain, splinting, and an impulse to breathe slower; pleuritic pain is unaffected by palpation or body movement.

Chapter 3 Chest Pain

12. **Pleurodynia** (Greek word *pleura* meaning "rib" or "chest wall" and *odyno*, "pain.") Some use it for any chest wall pain, but more specifically, it is chest pain due to disease of the pleural membrane.
13. **Precordial** (Latin *pre* meaning "in front of" and *cor*, "heart.") It is the lower thoracic area directly over the heart.
14. **Pyrexia** (Greek word *pyrexis* meaning "feverish.")
15. **Pyrosis** (Greek word for "on fire.") Our current lay term is "heartburn."
16. **Respirophasic** (Latin *respirare* meaning "to breathe" and Greek *phasis*, "appearance.") It is anything, such as chest pain, that occurs with inspiration and consequent expansion of the chest wall; all pleuritic chest pain is respirophasic, but all respirophasic chest pain is not pleuritic e.g. chest wall pain; palpation or body movement may provoke chest wall pain but not pleuritic pain.
17. **Retrosternal** (Latin *retro* meaning "backward.") Anything located behind the sternum, as opposed to substernal, "under" the sternum, implying epigastric.
18. **Supine** (Latin *supinus* meaning "lying on the back, face upward.")

Chapter 4 Constipation
Questions on Constipation
A. Your patient complains "I'm always constipated." In her description of "constipation," to be certain it is constipation, you look for:
   1.
   2.
B. Over 50% of the elderly take OTC laxatives, because:

C. In a young "healthy" woman with new onset of constipation, there are 5 easily diagnosed causes (or even "spot"diagnoses):
   1.
   2.
   3.
   4.
   5.
D. IBS is very common, and it has a number of characteristics. It is a syndrome, and it is a clinical diagnosis based on positive history, absence of physical findings and no lab findings
   1. One symptom is absolutely necessary for a diagnosis of IBS:

   2. There are 2 other important criteria for the diagnosis of IBS:
      a.
      b.
E. The commonest cause of constipation seen in the office and its 3 major characteristics are:
   1.
      a.
      b.
      c.
F. The other 3 common causes of constipation and their differentiating characteristics are:
   1.
      a.
      b.
   2.
      a.
      b.
   3.
      a.
      b.

Chapter 4 Constipation   49
Answers on Constipation
A. Be certain the symptom is constipation
  1. Quantity and quality, as in everything else in life! Fewer than 3 bowel movements (BMs) per week <u>or</u> recently decreased frequency from her usual
  2. Stools have become more difficult to pass because they are harder or drier, and she may now be straining to pass the stools
B. Why so many of the elderly take OTC laxatives
  Various reasons but mostly from misunderstanding of what "normal" is for the person's age. Thus some people take laxatives even when they have daily stools that are easily passed. Others believe "normal" is a daily BM. Educate your patient as to what is normal
C. Quick diagnoses in a young, healthy woman with a new complaint of constipation
  1. Pregnancy
  2. Dysmenorrhea
  3. Eating disorders (bulimia, anorexia nervosa)
  4. Major depression (MD)
  5. Hypothyroidism
D. Necessary criteria for IBS
  1. Absolutely necessary for diagnosis of IBS is the presence of episodic abdominal pain unexplained by another cause
  2. Other important criteria are:
    a. Changed appearance and consistency of her stools with onset of the abdominal pain *viz* diarrhea <u>or</u> constipation, or alternating diarrhea and constipation
    b. Either partial or total relief of the abdominal pain with BMs
E. Commonest cause of constipation and its 3 characteristic features
  1. IBS
    a. Onset of the constipation in a man or woman <30-40 y/o
    b. Abdominal pain is the dominant symptom and BMs give partial or total relief of pain
    c. Pain and constipation (may alternate with diarrhea) are episodic
F. The other 3 common causes of constipation almost never have diarrhea or significant abdominal pain
  1. Functional constipation
    a. Onset in a man or woman usually >30 y/o
    b. Chronic, persistent constipation
  2. Slow-transit constipation
    a. Onset in a woman <30 y/o
    b. <u>Lifelong</u> hard dry stools
  3. Pelvic floor dysfunction
    a. Onset >30 y/o, mostly <u>multiparous</u> women
    b. Chronic constipation, she commonly needs digital manipulation to evacuate even normal consistency stools

Constipation

Differential diagnosis: the 4 common causes of constipation
1. IBS–onset man or woman <30-40 y/o; <u>episodic</u> abdominal <u>pain</u> is the dominant symptom; episodic diarrhea or constipation
2. Functional constipation–onset man or woman >30-40 y/o; dominant symptom is <u>chronic</u>, persistent constipation with minimal abdominal pain
3. Slow transit constipation–<u>lifelong</u> constipation in a woman; minimal abdominal pain
4. Pelvic floor dysfunction–persistent <u>chronic</u> constipation; onset in a multiparous woman >30-40 y/o

A. **Be certain of the symptom and its distinguishing characteristics.** Your patient's problem or chief complaint is "I'm always constipated"
  1. First be certain the problem is constipation and not pain or itching or bloating or increased flatus or some other symptom misperceived to be "constipation." For example, one-third of patients complaining of "constipation" think the term refers either to inability to defecate at will, or to <u>any</u> difficulty evacuating stool, even if it is loose stool. "What exactly do you mean when you say you are constipated?" You are looking for constipation, that is, the presence of at least two of the following seven symptoms
     a. Frequency of BMs ≤2 times/week
     b. Lumpy or hard inspissated stools
     c. Significant straining at stool
     d. Sensation of incomplete evacuation
     e. Sensation of some degree of anorectal blockage
     f. Manual maneuvers sometimes are needed to facilitate evacuation (digital pressure vagina, rectum, or perineum)
     g. Time needed for complete defecation is often >10 minutes
     Determine which of the above 7 symptoms is most distressing to her, especially whether her complaints relate more to the first 4 symptoms (suggesting a diagnosis of functional constipation) or the last 3 symptoms (suggesting rectal outlet delay) or symptoms that occur also between BMs e.g. abdominal pain, sensation of bloating, malaise, diarrhea (suggesting a diagnosis of IBS)
  2. If you determine her problem is constipation, then ask:
     a. "Exactly when did you become constipated" or "When was the last time you remember having normal BMs?" then "What has the pattern been since then?"–you want to determine if it is a new or an episodic or a chronic, persistent problem; and what age she started having constipation
     b. "If it were not for the constipation, would you be essentially well?" You want to know about other symptoms or problems associated with the constipation, especially any abdominal pain and the relationship of the BMs to abdominal pain

Chapter 4 Constipation

   c. "How have you been treating the constipation?" that is, with which specific agents, prescribed or OTC meds, and "Have you found anything that helps, even partially?"
   d. If it is episodic or chronic, persistent constipation, why is she consulting you now, what has changed?

Be certain:
1. The symptom is constipation, that is, straining to pass hard stools and frequency of stools is either decreased from usual or ≤ 2 BMs weekly
2. Whether it is either new or episodic or chronic, persistent constipation
3. Whether constipation or abdominal pain is the dominant symptom
4. Of the patient's age at <u>onset</u> of constipation

---

   3. Physical examination
      a. Observe, percuss and palpate the abdomen for masses or distention; auscultate for hyperactive or absent bowel sounds
      b. Do a DRE for a mass (impaction or tumor), hematochezia, occult blood; assess anal sphincter tone, both resting and with voluntary contraction

By now you should be confident it is constipation, whether it is new or episodic or chronic constipation, if there are significant associated symptoms present, and of the patient's age at onset of the constipation. In almost all instances you now have the information you need for diagnosis of the obvious causes (Section C) and the common causes (Section E). In the rare instance that your patient appears different clinically from the usual office patient with constipation, be certain (Section B) that she does not have a symptom or sign of a dangerous disease

B. Be confident it's not a dangerous disease.

1. Send immediately to the ED by ambulance if there is:
   a. Elderly patient with depressed level of consciousness, severe constipation, hypothermia, think of myxedema coma
   b. Constipation, occult blood and new abdominal pain in a patient >50 y/o, think of colorectal malignancy or acute diverticulitis
   c. New onset constipation associated with neurological symptoms, e.g. weakness and urinary retention, think of cauda equina syndrome, prostatic obstruction
2. Admit at once to the ED or hospital if there is:
   a. Obstipation, often with colicky pain and failure to pass gas, think of large bowel obstruction
   b. Any progressively worsening or rapid onset constipation with objective abdominal distention, think of bowel obstruction (neoplasm, fecal impaction) or anal sphincter lesion
   c. Constipation, objective abdominal distention and fever, especially in a patient with known ulcerative colitis, think of impending toxic megacolon
   d. History of constipation, now fever and lower abdominal pain, think of diverticulitis
   e. Rapid onset of constipation (or incontinence) and numbness in the "saddle" distribution, think of cauda equina syndrome
3. Admit to the hospital or have a specialist consult as soon as appropriate if there is:
   a. Episodic constipation, bloating and cramping abdominal pain, think of

intermittent pseudoobstruction.
  b. Constipation, anorexia, weight loss, think of colorectal cancer, Addison's disease, PMR

Be certain in the first minutes of your exam that there is no evidence of any <u>one</u> dangerous symptom or sign associated with the constipation:
1. New onset of constipation with melena or occult blood in stools
2. Rapid onset of constipation
3. Unexplained anemia or weight loss or fever
4. Hematochezia
5. Abdominal or rectal mass
6. Nocturnal pain awakens the patient

Any suggestion of a dangerous disease, send your patient to the ED.

---

  c. Constipation in a patient with a history of "spells" or paroxysms of symptoms and difficult to control HTN, think of pheochromocytoma or hyperventilation syndrome (Arch Int Med 57, 945, 1997)
  d. New onset constipation in a patient with either a family history of colon cancer or familial polyposis, or associated with rectal bleeding, anemia, or unexplained weight loss, think of colorectal malignancy
  e. New onset constipation alternating with diarrhea in a patient >50 y/o, think of colon malignancy
  f. Need to press on the perineum or posterior wall of the vagina for effective evacuation, think of rectocele (surgical) or pelvic floor dysfunction
  g. Episodic almost constant desire to defecate with prolonged straining and minimal results, think of rectal prolapse or solitary rectal ulcer syndrome (Br J Surg 85, 1246, 1998)
  h. Constipation and hematochezia, think of rectal malignancy, stercoral rectal ulcer, diverticulosis
  i. Constipation, but the dominant symptom is pain
    (1) Pain is localized to the rectum, think of ischemia, IBD, abscess, fissure, proctitis, solitary rectal ulcer
    (2) Sharp pain at the anus lasting for seconds or at most, minutes, think of proctalgia fugax (reassure her it is benign)
    (3) Dull, aching pain high in the rectum, recurring and lasting hours or days, think of levator ani syndrome

C. **Make a quick diagnosis if it's obvious.** Is it an easily diagnosed and treated condition or a medication side effect causing the constipation? In most patients you will be <u>highly</u> confident of a common cause of the symptom by now. If not, one or more of the following tests may exclude an organic disease and increase your confidence in your working diagnosis: CBC, glucose, electrolytes, Ca, Mg, creatinine, TSH, abdominal XR
  1. Spot diagnoses–almost always the constipation is an isolated GI symptom, although occasionally there is mild abdominal discomfort
    a. Young adults
      (1) Pregnancy–especially last trimester
      (2) Dysmenorrhea–cyclic constipation
      (3) Eating disorders–think of anorexia nervosa or bulimia in a young person who is underweight (BMI <20 or weight <100 for 5' and 4 lb for each inch, so <112 lb for 5'3", <124 lb for 5'6", <148 lb for 6'); diagnosis may be complicated by concomitant diuretic or laxative abuse or induced vomiting, or all three

Chapter 4 Constipation 53

together
- (4) MD–search for <u>any</u> evidence of anhedonia–i.e. loss of interest in her usual hobbies, work, sex, sports, entertainment
- b. Older adults
  - (1) Fecal impaction–often the complaint is "diarrhea" but impaction is apparent by DRE
  - (2) Dehydration–elderly have decreased thirst sensation; diuretic worsens dehydration
  - (3) Parkinsonism–resting tremor, bradykinesia, rigidity, gait problems

---

Diagnose and treat an easily diagnosed cause of constipation:
1. Spot diagnoses–in young people: pregnancy, dysmenorrhea, eating disorders (anorexia nervosa or bulimia), MD; in the elderly: fecal impaction, parkinsonism, dehydration
2. Metabolic diseases–hypothyroidism, diabetes mellitus, hypercalcemia
3. Medication side effects–onset of constipation soon after starting <u>any</u> new medication

---

2. Metabolic disease
   a. Hypothyroidism–it may be primary (high TSH, low free T4) or secondary hypothyroidism (TSH may be inappropriately normal or even <u>slightly</u> increased, low free T4)
   b. T1DM, poorly controlled for years, now has autonomic neuropathy; or recently diagnosed T2DM already may have autonomic neuropathy. If neuropathy is present, almost all will have complaints of constipation; if neuropathy has not yet occurred, about one-third still complain of constipation
   c. Hypercalcemia–any etiology e.g. hyperparathyroidism, sarcoidosis, bone malignancy
   d. Hypomagnesemia or hypokalemia of any etiology e.g. thiazide therapy for HTN; surreptitious diuretics, laxative abuse
   e. Uremia–abdominal pain, pseudoobstruction
3. Medication side effect–those listed below are major known possibilities for causing constipation, but any recently begun medication, followed in weeks by new constipation, should be suspect. Up to 5% of patients given placebo report new "constipation."
   a. Anticholinergics–TCAs especially amitriptyline and imipramine; phenothiazines e.g. chlorpromazine; antispasmodics e.g. Librax, belladonna; anti-parkinsonian agents e.g. amantadine, bromocriptine
   b. Antihypertensives e.g. CCBs (verapamil, diltiazem); diuretic e.g. furosemide; β-blockers e.g. propranolol; clonidine
   c. Opiate derivatives in analgesics or antidiarrheals e.g. loperamide, oxycodone, methadone, codeine; any narcotic can result in a "narcotic bowel syndrome," which can be treated with clonidine
   d. Antacids containing calcium or aluminum e.g. Tums or bismuth

e. Antihistamines–H1 receptor antagonists e.g. diphenhydramine; H2 receptor antagonists e.g. ranitidine; 5-HT3 receptor antagonists e.g. alosetron (used to treat IBS pain and diarrhea)
f. Sympathomimetics e.g. ephedrine, terbutaline, phenylpropanolamine
g. Antipsychotics e.g. clozapine, risperidone, olanzapine
h. Benzodiazepines e.g. alprazolam, estazolam
i. Anticonvulsants e.g. felbamate, carbamazepine, phenytoin
j. Hyperlipidemic agents esp. bile acid resins, statins
k. Antidepressants e.g. venlafaxine, nefazodone, lithium; some SSRIs *viz* fluvoxamine and paroxetine
l. Miscellaneous–laxative abuse, mineral supplements (iron, calcium), NSAIDs, acetazolamide, thalidomide, propafenone, barium sulfate, sucralfate, polystyrene resins, megestrol acetate, scopolamine

D. **Identify your patient's worries and wants.** Complaint of constipation occurs in up to 20% of people <60 y/o, and in more than 50% of people >65 y/o, and only few of these consult about it. During your interview and exam try to intuit or discover why your patient is here today, and not previously, for this problem. What is she worried about? Don't necessarily ask directly, but try to get some ideas from your patient's responses to questions about her perception of the constipation itself. You can't completely help your patient unless you know what she really worries about and wants from you. That's why she is here to see you--to satisfy her worries and wants! Here are only some of the possible worries and wants of your patient with constipation. You must discover her specific, unique ones
1. Common worries are:
   a. That the cause of the constipation is a dangerous etiology e.g. cancer, intestinal obstruction
   b. That the etiology is some rare disease e.g. botulinum toxin, heavy metal poisoning (lead, mercury), scleroderma
   c. What other fears or anxieties might be troubling your patient? For example, she may have had constipation at other times or for many years, and only now does she come for help. What has changed? Perhaps a friend or relative, who had similar chronic constipation, recently has been diagnosed with a colon cancer. There are many other possibilities–think of them

> During your exam, discover your patient's worries (cancer, "blockage") and wants (more frequent, softer stools), so that you can respond to her specific needs as soon as possible.

2. Your patient wants:
   a. You to perform a thorough physical exam focused on possible causes of the constipation, and she wants appropriate tests and imaging studies, even though you might determine they are not needed
   b. A plausible explanation of the cause of the constipation
   c. Confident reassurance from you that it is not a dangerous or rare etiology. Tell her--"The good news, it's not cancer" (or whatever you believe her real worry is)
   d. To know the prognosis, short term (effects on job, home life, marriage; how soon she will be back to normal) and long term (if recurrences are possible; how to prevent recurrences; if it will cause any disability)
   e. Treatment now to stop the constipation and to prevent recurrences
   f. A GI referral if she believes you are not confident of the diagnosis

E. **Know the symptoms that differentiate the 4 common causes of constipation.**
1. The commonest cause is IBS
   a. Characteristics of IBS
      (1) Abdominal pain (discomfort) is the dominant symptom, and it is

Chapter 4 Constipation 55

episodic pain
- (2) The abdominal pain always is in some way related to defecation, that is, there is a change in frequency or consistency of the BM (constipation or diarrhea) at the same time the pain begins, and the pain is relieved partially or totally with BMs
- (3) Onset of symptoms (not just constipation) is in a man or woman <30-40 y/o. Common associated findings with the pain and constipation are alternating diarrhea, sensation of bloating, and exacerbations of symptoms with menses or stress or postprandially
  b. What suggests it might not be IBS
  - (1) Anytime an associated symptom or sign suggests a dangerous cause (see Section B)
  - (2) If abdominal pain is neither the dominant symptom nor is the pain related in some way to defecation
  - (3) If the symptoms suggest the diagnosis of IBS, but the onset of these symptoms definitely began after age 50, never attribute it only to IBS, get a colonoscopy

---

The causes of most constipation in office patients:
1. IBS–onset man or woman <30-40 y/o; episodic abdominal pain is the dominant symptom; episodic diarrhea or constipation
2. Functional constipation–onset man or woman >30-40 y/o; dominant symptom is chronic, persistent constipation with minimal abdominal pain
3. Slow transit constipation–lifelong constipation in a woman; minimal abdominal pain
4. Pelvic floor dysfunction–persistent chronic constipation; onset in a multiparous woman >30-40 y/o

---

2. Common look-alikes causing constipation and how each differs from IBS
   a. Functional constipation
   - (1) It is recognized by the first 4 symptoms listed in Section A.1.a-d. She also may have "rectal outlet delay," if she has any of the 3 symptoms listed in Section A.1.e-g
   - (2) In patients 30-64 y/o, up to 30% have functional constipation or rectal outlet delay; the prevalence of constipation increases markedly in those >60 y/o, but ageing alone does not decrease the frequency of BMs
   - (3) There is minimal abdominal pain, but there may be subjective bloating and increased flatus
   - (4) Lifestyle factors are very important in causation, and treatment is to identify and reverse them; education is important in treatment
     - (a) Immobility (travel, illness, bedridden), low fluid intake (relative dehydration), low fiber diet
     - (b) "Cathartic colon" is very common due to stimulant laxative abuse; up to 50% of elderly take OTC laxatives

  (c) Diuretic abuse is common in eating disorders, especially bulimia
  (d) Voluntary stool retention is common (chronic deliberate suppression of the urge to defecate)
 (5) Treatment of functional constipation should emphasize increased daily physical exercise, pelvic muscle exercises, increased fluid intake (give a daily Rx of 8 large glasses of water), increased fiber (>10 gm/d). Only if necessary use bulk laxatives 1-3 times daily and add sorbitol or lactulose 15 ml daily, as needed for 3-4 BM/week. If there also is rectal outlet delay, use phosphate enemas for initial clearance of any impaction, then glycerine suppositories pc breakfast for 2-3 weeks prn to relieve symptoms. For hard, infrequent stool, add daily bulk laxative
b. Slow-transit constipation (STC) or "colonic inertia"
 (1) It is <u>lifelong</u> constipation in a <u>woman</u>. Common symptoms are due to slowed movement of contents through the colon toward the rectum (more water is reabsorbed causing inspissated feces). There are persistent infrequent BMs–($\leq$ 2/week) consisting of lumpy, hard stools
 (2) Because of the hard stools, there often is associated straining and sensations of incomplete evacuation or anorectal blockage. Neither diarrhea nor urgency ever occurs, and if there is any abdominal discomfort, it is mild and not the dominant symptom
c. Pelvic floor dysfunction (PFD) or "pelvic floor dyssynergia"
 (1) It accounts for 25% of patients referred to gastroenterologists for chronic constipation. Community prevalence in 30-64 y/o adults is 11%; most are <u>multiparous</u> women, and constipation began only after multiple childbirths
 (2) Any associated abdominal discomfort is minimal, and diarrhea does not occur
 (3) It is due to paradoxical contraction or failure of the pelvic floor muscles to relax appropriately during defecation. Symptoms alerting you that PFD might be present are: even normal consistency, soft or loose stools or enema fluid may be difficult to pass; prolonged excessive straining; frequent need for perineal or vaginal pressure, or even direct rectal digital manipulation to evacuate stools
 (4) Constipation due to this dysfunction is refractory to usual treatments of increased dietary fiber, laxatives, so refer to a specialist early

F. Use this summary for efficient diagnosis of a common cause. With the information from Sections A-E in mind, here is the rapid approach to diagnosis of the cause of constipation.

1. You already have determined:
 a. In Section A, by H&P, that it is constipation, and whether the constipation either is new or episodic or chronic, persistent constipation.
 b. In Section B, that there is no evidence in the H&P of any one dangerous cause of the constipation.
 c. In Section C, that there is neither an easily diagnosed condition nor a medication that is likely responsible for the constipation.

2. From the focused H&P almost always you should quickly be confident of a working diagnosis. Confident final diagnosis is made only in followup the next weeks, months, or years when the response to treatment or nontreatment is appropriate to your working diagnosis.
   a. If it is episodic constipation in a man or woman <30-40 y/o, and episodic abdominal pain is a dominant part of the problem, and the pain is partially or totally relieved by BMs, diagnose and treat IBS.
   b. If the constipation began only after multiple childbirths, and she often requires manual maneuvers for evacuation, it likely is PFD and probably is best to refer for a GI consult.
   c. If the constipation is not associated with significant abdominal pain diagnose either STC (woman, onset <30 y/o) or functional constipation (man or woman, onset >30-40 y/o), as appropriate, and empirically treat as for functional constipation (Section E.2.a.5). STC may respond to this regimen, but often it will not, so refer these patients early for GI consult.
3. Answer your patient's worries and wants that you determined early on during the exam (Section D). Have you done everything you can to help her?
4. You now have a working diagnosis, but only with followup, sometimes long term, can you be confident it is correct. In return visits you are always testing by questions and physical exam that your working diagnosis is correct.

G. Abandon your working diagnosis and look for an uncommon cause only if:

1. Any one dangerous symptom or sign (see above, Section B) occurs in followup of weeks, months, or years. Quickly obtain a GI consult or send the patient to the hospital as appropriate.

If your patient's symptoms do not respond as expected to your management, he may have an uncommon or rare cause listed in Section G.2 that you can diagnose and treat. Or you may want to refer your patient to a specialist.

2. Your patient's response to therapy is not as you expect or if the natural history of your working diagnosis does not occur.
   Don't spend time and money looking for one of the following etiologies until you are sure your patient doesn't have one of the 4 common causes of constipation above. Nevertheless, it may be she has an uncommon or rare cause of the constipation. These are important to identify, because each has a different treatment or prophylaxis. These are all classified as intestinal pseudoobstruction (as opposed to mechanical obstruction) and due to dysmotility. Symptoms are similar to obstruction–constipation, crampy pain, objective bloating.
   a. Neurologic or muscular causes
      (1) Parkinsonism–onset of the constipation probably begins early in the disease; rest tremor, bradykinesia, rigidity, gait difficulties
      (2) Hirschsprung's disease–usual onset is early childhood, but there may be symptom onset as a young adult if only a short segment of the distal rectum is aganglionic
      (3) MS--constipation precedes the diagnosis of MS in about one-half of patients with MS; severity of constipation correlates with duration of the MS diagnosis

(Gastroenterology 98, 1538, 1990)
- (4) Autonomic failure e.g. Shy-Drager syndrome, has orthostatic hypotension without appropriately increased pulse rate on standing
- (5) Neurofibromatosis–patches of cutaneous pigmentation
- (6) Myotonic muscular dystrophy--abnormal function of anal sphincters, eventually megacolon
- (7) Polymyositis or dermatomyositis–proximal muscle weakness, high CPK
- (8) Paraneoplastic visceral neuropathy e.g. lung small cell carcinoma and carcinoid tumors
- (9) Systemic sclerosis (scleroderma)–multisystem disease; Raynaud's phenomenon with normal ESR, high ANA

b. Endocrine-metabolic causes
- (1) Pheochromocytoma–occasionally (8%) there is adynamic ileus and constipation
- (2) AIP–may present like IBS with recurrent abdominal pain and constipation or diarrhea; unlike IBS, significant distention and vomiting

c. Infectious causes
- (1) Chagas' disease--duration and severity of the disease determines onset and severity of constipation, eventually megacolon
- (2) Chronic amebiasis–may develop toxic megacolon
- (3) Syphilis–late stages, tertiary disease
- (4) Lymphogranuloma venereum–late stages rectal stricture and obstipation

d. Idiopathic–no systemic disease; episodic pain, vomiting, distention

H. Use the glossary for precise thinking and accurate diagnosis.

1. **Anismus**–Recently made up word to describe spastic pelvic floor dysfunction *vis a vis* "vaginismus"; poor term but you will see it used in some literature.
2. **Borborygmi** (Greek word for "rubbing, growling bowels.") Likely, the word is an example of onomatopoeia, which means a word constructed of the sounds it represents.
3. **"Cathartic colon"** (Greek word meaning "cleansing or pure.") Excess use of laxatives (cathartics) may lead to hypofunctioning or slow transit colon, and thereby, worsening constipation.
4. **Colicky** (pain) (Greek *kolikos* meaning "related to the colon.") It describes intermittent severe crampy pain corresponding to smooth muscle peristalsis, usually small bowel.
5. **Constipation** (Latin word for "packing tightly.") Only in the 16th century was it applied to dilatory bowel function resulting in inspissated feces.
6. **Dyschezia** (Greek *dys* meaning "difficult or defective" and *chezia*, "stools or to defecate.") It is a generic term for any difficulty with defecation or passing stools.
7. **Dyssynergia** (Greek *dys* meaning "difficult or defective" and *synergy*, "coordination.") It represents disturbed coordination of any bodily function.
8. **Encopresis** (Greek *en* meaning "in" and *kopros*, "excrement.") It is fecal incontinence i.e. watery feces passed around a hard fecal impaction.
9. **Enema** (Greek meaning "to send into.") Injection of fluid into the rectum to stimulate defecation.
10. **Hematochezia** (Greek *hemo* meaning "blood" and *chezia*, "stool.") It is red blood in the stool.
11. **Inspissated** (Latin word for "condensed or thickened.") It is any dehydrated, hard substance e.g. stool.
12. **Laxative** (Latin word *laxare* meaning "to open or release.") It is any agent used to loosen or relax the bowel, allowing easier defecation.
13. **Melena** (Greek word for "black.") Present usage implies both black and tarry stools.
14. **Obstipation** (Latin *ob* meaning "in front of" and *stipation*, "to cram or stuff.") It is intractable constipation to the point of no BM, as with nearly complete obstruction.
15. **Purgative** (Latin word for "cleansing" as by cathartics or enema.) Note that cathartic (Greek) and purgative (Latin) mean the same thing. In the same way, the words "morals" (Latin) and "ethics" (Greek) mean the same thing--the character or custom of a people.
16. **Proctalgia fugax** (Greek *procto* meaning "anus" and a*lgia*, "pain" and *fugax*, "swift passing.") It is an intense, benign anal pain lasting seconds.
17. **Scybala** (Greek word meaning "dry hard mass of feces.") It is pronounced as "sĭb′ala."
18. **Stercoral** rectal ulcer (Latin *sterco* meaning "dung.") Chronic hard feces erode the rectal mucosa and cause an ulcer.
19. **Tenesmus** (Greek word *tenesmos* meant "straining at stool.") Now it implies ineffectual straining with a discomfort like incomplete evacuation or even spasm, and it suggests rectosigmoid spasm or disease.

CHAPTER 5 COUGH
Questions on Cough
A. In a patient complaining of cough, the most important information you find from the
   1. History is:
   2. Physical exam is:
B. Your immunocompetent patient <50 y/o has a <u>new</u> cough lasting <3-4 weeks. The 3 common causes are:
   1.
   2.
   3.
C. Your immunocompetent patient <50 y/o has a chronic cough (has been present >2-3 months). There are 4 common causes you quickly think of. Name the 4 causes and identify which ones you can exclude by history alone:
   1.
   2.
   3.
   4.
D. Your patient is a 37 y/o nonsmoker who has a new unexplained cough. Any <u>one</u> of the following two features on history or one on physical exam might make you consider pulmonary embolism (PE) as the cause:
   1. History:
   2. History:
   3. Physical exam:
E. Your 30 y/o patient recently had new onset cough with either a viral URI or influenza. She now has had the cough for a total of 6 weeks. There are 4 entities that might be responsible for the persistent or worsening cough:
   1.
   2.
   3.
   4.
F. Your 58 y/o long-time, heavy smoker patient has chronic cough ("chronic bronchitis") and tells you it is getting worse. For the tenth time, you tell him the only way to stop the cough is to stop smoking. Amazingly, he finally agrees to stop smoking. Even though the cough markedly is lessened after a month, he continues having cough. Besides congratulating him on stopping smoking, is there anything else to do?

Answers on Cough

A. Be certain of the symptom and whether it is either new onset or chronic cough.
   1. You first must determine if this is a new onset cough that began in the past 2-3 weeks; or whether it began with symptoms of an infection, which got better, but the cough has continued for another 4-5 weeks; or whether the cough is chronic and has been ongoing for >2-3 months. "When was the last time you did not have this cough?" or "When exactly did this cough begin?" "Were there other symptoms when the cough started?"
   2. On physical exam, first be certain there is nothing stimulating ENT cough receptors e.g. postnasal drip, pharyngeal erythema, tympanic membrane lesion; then auscultate the lungs for adventitious sounds, *viz* wheezing or crackles, suggesting possible dangerous cardiopulmonary disease
B. Common causes of a new cough
   1. Infection–almost all are viral etiologies of the respiratory tract, URI or acute tracheobronchitis
   2. Noninfectious causes–allergic rhinitis, GERD, laryngopharyngeal reflux
   3. Medication side effect e.g. ACEI, inhalant medications
C. Four common causes of chronic cough
   1. Chronic bronchitis –it is the only one excludable by history alone, the other 3 frequently are occult; each of the other etiologies requires either a therapeutic trial or a specific test
   2. Postnasal drip syndrome (PNDS)
   3. Cough variant asthma–"variant" means that the only symptom of the asthma is cough
   4. GERD
D. Think of PE anytime there is unexplained new onset cough
   1. History of any one of the following: either abrupt onset of unexplained dyspnea or abrupt onset of unexplained tachypnea or new onset of unexplained pleuritic chest pain
   2. History of any one risk factor for DVT e.g. morbid obesity (BMI >40), recent immobilization including long period of travel while sitting, pelvic or orthopedic surgery or trauma the last 3-4 months, ongoing pregnancy or postpartum, birth control pills and smoking, any previous history of DVT or PE
   3. Physical exam–any evidence of unilateral DVT *viz* unilateral pretibial pitting edema, leg pain, calf tenderness
E. Persistent cough following a respiratory infection
   1. Up to one-half of patients with a viral respiratory infection may have cough persisting 5-6 weeks after they recovered from the acute infection, but the cough usually is significantly less after 1-2 weeks, coinciding with relief of the other symptoms
   2. Pertussis–does not decrease in frequency or intensity, but it often worsens, may be vomiting associated with the cough
   3. Chlamydia
   4. Sinusitis
F. Persistent cough after stopping smoking
   The cough should stop completely, if it is due to chronic bronchitis alone. Look for a second etiology, especially lung cancer, or other causes of chronic cough (GERD, PNDS, asthma)

Cough

Differential diagnosis: the 3 common causes of <u>chronic</u> cough
1. Postnasal drip syndrome (PNDS)–frequent throat clearing; history of allergic rhinitis
2. Asthma–often occult; occasional wheezing by history
3. GERD–often occult; heartburn by history

(For recent onset cough, see Section G.3)

A. Be certain of the symptom and its distinguishing characteristics. Your patient's problem or chief complaint is "I have this nagging cough"

1. First, be certain the problem is cough and not another reflex or voluntary action e.g. throat clearing, regurgitation, hiccupping, or retching. Next, "Exactly, when did the coughing first begin?" or "When was the last time you can remember not having any cough?" If it began less than 3 weeks ago, it is new cough; if it began more than 2 months ago, it is chronic cough. If it began between 3-8 weeks ago, it may be either a new cough that will be self-limited, or one that will become chronic if not treated
2. "At the time the cough began, were there any other symptoms?" You are trying to determine if the cough was an isolated symptom or whether there were associated symptoms of an infection. "About how long did these other symptoms last?"
3. Are there symptoms suggesting chronic bronchitis (early morning cough), PNDS (throat clearing), asthma (subjective wheezing) or GERD (regurgitation, heartburn, hoarseness)?
4. Physical examination

Be certain:
1. The symptom is cough
2. Whether the cough is new onset cough or chronic cough (began > 6-8 weeks ago)
3. To identify symptoms associated with the cough, now and at its onset

(If the cough is new onset, see Section G.3 in the text for approach to diagnosis.)

    a. Look for evidence of systemic disease, especially fever (rectal temperature), weight loss (change in belt or clothes size) or cardiopulmonary disease (dyspnea, tachypnea, JVD, bilateral pretibial pitting edema)
    b. Inspect the ears (for hair, cerumen, foreign body against the tympanic membrane), nose, throat (mucus, erythema or cobblestoning of PNDS) and palpate for lymphadenectasis (cancer, TB, HIV)

    c. Auscultate for lung adventitious sounds, crackles (CHF, pneumonia, TB) or wheezes (asthma, COPD, CHF)
    d. Get a CXR only in those patients with a smoking history or if your patient is immunocompromised (malignancy, COPD, corticosteroid therapy, HIV-positive); or if he is significantly ill with fever, weight loss, dyspnea, hemoptysis, crackles, wheezes

By now you should be confident it is cough, whether it is new or chronic cough, and if there are significant associated symptoms present. In almost all instances you now have the information you need for diagnosis of the obvious causes (Section C) and the common causes (Section E). In the rare instance that your patient appears different clinically from the usual office patient with cough, be certain (Section B) that he does not have a symptom or sign of a dangerous disease

B. **Be confident it's not a dangerous disease.**
1. Send immediately to the ED by ambulance if there is:
    a. Cough associated with evidence of a catastrophic illness e.g. severe chest pain, dyspnea, hypotension, diaphoresis, pallor, mental status changes
    b. Unexplained chest pain or dyspnea associated with the cough, think of CHF, PE, pneumothorax; also bone fractures due to cough in a patient with MM, osteolytic metastases, severe osteoporosis
    c. Abrupt onset of cough in a patient in distress, think of pneumothorax, pneumomediastinum, AD, esophageal rupture, anaphylaxis, foreign body aspiration
    d. Elderly patient with new cough and associated tachypnea or changed mental status, think of pneumonia (fever may be absent)
    e. No obvious cause of new cough in a patient who has even <u>one</u> risk factor for DVT (recent immobility, recent pelvic trauma or orthopedic surgery, morbid obesity, past history DVT or PE), think of PE
    f. Unexplained cause of new cough in a patient who also has either abrupt onset of dyspnea <u>or</u> tachypnea <u>or</u> pleuritic chest pain, think of PE

Be certain in the first minutes of your exam that there is no evidence of any <u>one</u> dangerous symptom or sign associated with the cough:

1. New or different cough in a patient >50 y/o
2. Hemoptysis
3. Unexplained dyspnea <u>or</u> tachypnea <u>or</u> pleuritic chest pain
4. Unexplained weight loss
5. Inspiratory stridor
6. Mental status change
7. Any respiratory distress
8. Crackles or wheezes in a significantly ill patient

Any suggestion of a dangerous disease, send the patient to the ED.

---

    g. New cough and inspiratory stridor (auscultate over the larynx), think of foreign body aspiration, epiglottitis
2. Admit at once to the ED or hospital if there is:
    a. A rapidly progressing "flu-like" illness (fever, malaise, myalgias), think of the sepsis syndrome *viz*, hypotension (compared to his baseline BP), increased rate or depth of breathing, marked bandemia, thrombocytopenia
    b. New cough and bilateral wheezing, think of bronchial asthma, CHF, pneumonia
    c. New cough, fever, dyspnea and focal crackles, think of pneumonia, TB
    d. Evidence of significantly severe pneumonia in a sick patient--pleuritic chest pain, rigors (teeth chattering, patient shaking), along with dyspnea, tachypnea, and crackles

Chapter 5 Cough   63

   e. Unilateral localized wheezing, think of aspirated foreign body, lung carcinoma
   f. Thrombocytopenia associated with a nonspecific viral illness (fever, malaise, myalgias, cough), think of HPS, RMSF
   g. Nocturnal cough with new or increased nocturia, or new onset DOE, think of CHF, chronic interstitial pulmonary edema
3. Admit to the hospital or have a specialist consult as soon as appropriate if there is:
   a. A patient >50 y/o with new onset of nocturnal cough that awakens him, think of early CHF (in young patients, think of GERD, mild asthma, PNDS)
   b. Hemoptysis associated with new onset cough, think of acute bronchitis, pneumonia, PE, lung cancer, TB, bronchiectasis
   c. Unexplained new onset or different cough in a patient >50 y/o, think of lung malignancy, TB, CHF
   d. Unexplained cough and other significant respiratory symptoms e.g. dyspnea, think of HIV, TB
   e. New or chronic cough associated with weight loss, hemoptysis, fever, think of malignancy, TB, bronchiectasis, lung abscess
   f. Chronic cough with large amounts of purulent sputum (more than 2 tablespoons/d), think of bronchiectasis
   g. New cough or a chronic cough that changes in character in a cigarette smoker, think of lung cancer
   h. Dyspnea and inspiratory crackles, think of pulmonary edema, pneumonia, interstitial lung disease
   i. In a cigarette smoker with clubbing (hypertrophic osteoarthropathy) or hyponatremia (SIADH) or rash and muscle weakness (dermatomyositis), think of early lung cancer
   j. Cough worsened by exercise think of asthma, CHF
   k. Dry cough with deep inspiration and insidious worsening DOE, think of interstitial lung disease
   l. Diastolic murmur and worsening cough, think of mitral stenosis and early left ventricular failure
   m. New cough with URI, but it shows no evidence of diminishing after 2 weeks, with spasms of coughing, or there is post-tussive vomiting, think of pertussis
   n. Longtime cigarette smoker with worsening "chronic bronchitis" and the cough decreases, but does not cease when smoking is stopped, think of an underlying malignancy

C. **Make a quick diagnosis if it's obvious.** Is it an easily diagnosed condition or a medication that is responsible for the cough? In most patients you will be <u>highly</u> confident of a common cause of the symptom by now. If not, one or more of the following tests may exclude an organic disease and increase your confidence in your working diagnosis: WBC, CXR
1. Chronic bronchitis
   a. He expectorates phlegm as long as he is exposed to respiratory irritants e.g. cigarette smoke, pollution, dust, fumes. In smokers, the cough and expectorated phlegm may be greatest on awakening, and the cough ceases with his first cigarette

---

Recognize an easily diagnosed cause of chronic cough (*viz* chronic bronchitis) or <u>new</u> cough:
1. Recent respiratory tract infection
2. Noninfectious causes
3. Medication side effect, especially ACEI or inhalant medications

---

   b. Diagnosis is confirmed by the cough <u>ceasing</u> when exposure to the respiratory irritant is stopped. If he stops smoking, and the cough decreases but does not cease over a few weeks, be sure he doesn't

have lung cancer
2. Recent viral respiratory tract infection (dry cough may last 6-8 weeks)
   a. Up to 50% will have cough >2 weeks due to transient reactive airway disease, but the cough should be much less frequent and intense after 2 weeks
   b. Protracted severe cough longer than 2 weeks, think of pertussis or chlamydia infection or acute sinusitis
3. Noninfectious causes e.g. allergic rhinitis, GERD
4. Medications
   a. ACEI–class effect and not dose related; cough may persist for 3-4 weeks after stopping the medication
   b. Some angiotensin II receptor antagonists e.g. valsartan (J. Hypertension 17, 893, 1999) 3.6% incidence of cough vs placebo, 0.9%
   c. β-blockers, oral or ocular–may cause cough or worsen cough of variant asthma
   d. Any inhalant aerosol medication e.g. glucocorticoids or β-agonists for asthma
   e. Methotrexate–isolated chronic cough distinct from the cough due to methotrexate pneumonitis
   f. Allergic respiratory reactions–sulfonamides, piperazine, methoxsalen (PUVA)
   g. Therapies for comorbid conditions may make cough due to GERD resistant to therapy e.g. CCB, nitrates, progesterone

D. **Identify your patient's worries and wants.** Complaint of cough occurs in up to 20% of people < 60 y/o, and in more than 50% of people > 65 y/o, and only few of these consult about it. During your interview and exam, intuit or discover why your patient is here today and not previously for this problem. Don't ask directly, but try to get some ideas from your patient's responses to questions about his perception of the cough itself. You can't completely help him unless you know what he really worries about and wants from you. That's why he is here to see you--to satisfy his worries and wants! Here are only some of the possible worries and wants of your patient with cough. You must discover his specific ones

> Discover your patient's worries (cancer, HIV, infection) and wants (cough relief, antibiotic), so that you can respond to his specific needs as soon as possible.

1. Common worries:
   a. That the cause of the cough is a dangerous etiology e.g. cancer, TB, HIV
   b. That the etiology is some rare disease e.g. SARS, inhalation anthrax, HPS
   c. What other fears or anxieties might be troubling your patient? For example, he may have had cough for many years, and only now does he come for help. What has changed? Perhaps a friend or relative, who had similar chronic cough, recently has been diagnosed with lung cancer. There are many other possibilities–think of them
2. Your patient wants:
   a. You to perform a thorough physical exam focused on possible causes of the cough and he wants appropriate tests and imaging studies, at least a CXR
   b. A plausible explanation of the cause of the cough
   c. Confident reassurance from you that it is not a dangerous or rare etiology. Tell him--"The good news, it's not cancer " (or whatever you believe his real worry is)
   d. To know the prognosis, short term (effects on job, home life, marriage; how soon he will be back to normal) and long term (if recurrences are possible; how to

Chapter 5 Cough   65

prevent recurrences; if it will cause any disability)
e. Treatment to stop the cough now and to prevent recurrences
f. A specialist referral if he believes you are not confident of the diagnosis

E. Know the symptoms that differentiate the 3 common causes of chronic cough.
1. The commonest etiology is postnasal drip syndrome (PNDS)
   a. Characteristics of PNDS
      (1) Symptoms of postnasal drainage or frequent throat clearing or early predominant morning cough; may be history of allergic rhinitis
      (2) Signs of excessive nasal discharge and edematous nasal mucosa; much oropharyngeal mucus and cobblestone appearance to the oropharyngeal mucosa

---

The 3 causes of most chronic cough in immunocompetent patients:
1. Postnasal drip syndrome (PNDS)–frequent throat clearing; history of allergic rhinitis
2. Asthma–often occult; occasional wheezing by history
3. GERD–often occult; history of heartburn

---

   b. What suggests it might not be PNDS
      (1) Anytime an associated symptom or sign suggests a dangerous cause (see Section B)
      (2) If there is no improvement of the cough within 1-2 weeks using a first-generation antihistamine and decongestant; if it is only partially relieved by 3-4 weeks, either asthma or GERD, or both, may be additional causes needing treatment
2. Common look-alikes and how each differs from PNDS
   a. Asthma
      (1) Symptoms of episodic wheezing, dyspnea and cough, especially nocturnal awakening with one or more of these symptoms; or respiratory symptoms only with exercise, especially in cold weather
      (2) Bilateral diffuse wheezes auscultated during an acute episode
      (3) Cough-variant asthma is occult i.e. no sign or symptom of asthma except cough
   b. Gastroesophageal reflux disease (GERD)
      (1) Heartburn or pyrosis (retrosternal burning or discomfort), or a sour taste due to regurgitation of gastric contents, especially when supine; unexplained hoarseness; chronic pharyngitis
      (2) Cough is due only in part to aspiration of gastric juices; often it is due to a vagal mediated reflex which may explain resistance to treatment in some patients, even after months of aggressive PPI therapy

F. Use this summary for efficient diagnosis of a common cause. With the information from Sections A-E in mind, here is the rapid approach to diagnosis of the cause of chronic cough.
1. You already have determined:

a. In Section A, by H&P that it is chronic cough and whether it is new onset or chronic (>6-8 weeks).
   b. In Section B, that there is no evidence in the H&P of any one dangerous cause of the cough.
   c. In Section C, that there is no evidence in the H&P of chronic bronchitis, a recent respiratory infection, or a medication, especially ACEI or any inhaled medication, causing the cough.
2. From the focused H&P almost always you should quickly be confident of a working diagnosis. Confident final diagnosis is made only in followup the next few weeks or months when the response to treatment or nontreatment is appropriate to your working diagnosis.
   a. If your patient has symptoms suggesting any one of the 3 common etiologies of chronic cough, treat that cause. If he does not have suggestive symptoms, but he does have adventitious sounds on physical exam, get a CXR. Otherwise, approach management as follows, remembering that in many patients with chronic cough, it is due to two etiologies (in 53% of patients) or even all three combined (in 35% of patients).
   b. In all patients with chronic cough a therapeutic trial is the best approach, because, in <u>immunocompetent</u> patients, the 3 etiologies account for at least 90% of chronic cough. About 30% will have PNDS as total or partial cause of cough. A dosage bid of a first generation H_1- antagonist is important using either dexbrompheniramine 6 mg (NEJM <u>343</u>, 1715, 2000), or azatadine maleate 1 mg (Ann Int Med <u>119</u>, 977, 1993) and 120 mg sustained release pseudoephedrine. Symptomatic response should begin in a few days. If antihistamines are contraindicated (BPH, glaucoma), use intranasal ipratropium bromide.
   c. If there is only partial response to this antihistamine-decongestant therapy after 2-3 weeks, <u>add</u> a nasal corticosteroid preparation e.g. beclomethasone by MDI with spacer (four, 42 ng puffs, bid) and albuterol (two, 90 ng puffs, prn up to qid). Cough starts to improve in < 1 week but it may take >2 months to resolve completely if only the 2 etiologies are causative.
   d. If the cough is much improved, but there still remains some cough, get sinus films for chronic bacterial sinusitis and, if positive, treat with antibiotics for 2 weeks and oxymetazoline, 2 sprays bid for 5 days. If sinus films are negative, modify diet and lifestyle (stop cigarettes, alcohol, chocolate, spicy foods, peppermint, and lose weight), and begin an aggressive therapeutic trial for GERD using omeprazole and metoclopramide (NEJM <u>343</u>, 1715, 2000).
   e. Although failure of GERD to respond within 3 months to this regimen does not exclude GERD as the etiology of the cough, either you should refer the patient to a gastroenterologist or cough specialist, or try to diagnose an uncommon cause of the chronic cough (see below, Section G.2.)
3. Answer your patient's worries and wants that you determined early on during the exam (Section D). Have you done everything you can to help him?
4. You now have a working diagnosis, but only with followup can you be highly confident it is correct. In followup visits you are always testing by H&P that your working diagnosis is correct.

Chapter 5 Cough   67

G. Abandon your working diagnosis and look for an uncommon cause only if:

1. Any one dangerous symptom or sign (see above, Section B) occurs in followup of days, weeks, or months. Quickly obtain a consult or send your patient to the hospital as appropriate
2. The chronic cough does not respond to stopping smoking or to your therapeutic trials as you expect. Don't spend time and money looking for one of the following etiologies until you are sure your patient doesn't have one of the 3 common causes of chronic cough above. If he doesn't have one of those causes, it may be that the correct cause was one of the uncommon etiologies listed below. These are important to recognize, because each has different treatment or prophylaxis
   a. Nonasthmatic eosinophilic bronchitis is the cause of chronic cough in 13% of patients in a specialist referral practice (Am J Respir Crit Care Med 160, 406, 1999); there is negative methacholine challenge but it is corticosteroid responsive
   b. Chronic aspiration e.g. Zenker's diverticulum
   c. Lesion stimulating cough receptors at unusual sites--tympanic membrane (hair or impacted cerumen), larynx, esophagus or stomach, diaphragm, pleura, pericardium
   d. Interstitial lung disease--dominant early complaint is DOE followed by non-productive cough; bibasilar crackles
   e. Occult pulmonary bacterial infection–think of it if he has normal CXR and is clinically silent except for cough and minimal adventitious sounds (wheezes, crackles, ronchi) on physical exam; infection and cough may respond only to prolonged intravenous antibiotics (Am J Med 114, 602, 2003)
   f. Sarcoidosis–cough, dyspnea, lymphadenectasis on CXR (hilar, paratracheal)
   g. Air pollutants at home or workplace (Am J Resp Crit Care Med 156, S31, 1997)
   h. IBD (Medicine 72, 151, 1993)–responds to steroids
   i. Occupation e.g. flock worker's lung (Chest 117, 251, 2000)
   j. Psychogenic cough–make this a diagnosis of last resort; there are no characteristics for a positive diagnosis, but suspect it if it is a dry cough and it occurs only during the daytime

> If your patient's symptoms do not respond as expected to your management, he may have an uncommon or rare cause listed in Section G.2 that you can diagnose and treat. Or you may want to refer your patient to a specialist.

3. New onset cough requires a different approach to diagnosis. Generally, new cough began less than 3 weeks ago, but occasionally, it may have begun 4-8 weeks before you see him. Almost all new cough seen in the office is caused either by a respiratory infection (most are viral) or by inhaled irritants
   a. Infectious causes, productive cough
      (1) Viral URI often is called common cold or head cold or "coryza." It produces symptoms mainly affecting the head: nasal congestion or runny nose (rhinorrhea) dominates the picture, producing sneezing and coughing, increased lacrimation; headache may be "severe, pounding"; mild ST. Systemic symptoms of low grade fever, malaise, and myalgias may occur with any of the infectious causes of cough, including acute bronchitis and pneumonia, and a dry cough may last 2 months
      (2) Acute tracheobronchitis is often called a "chest cold" and may follow an URI. Large bronchi are predominantly infected; because these are the sites with the highest concentrations of cough receptors, cough and sputum production dominate the clinical picture, and dyspnea and crackles do not occur
      (3) Pneumonia affects the small terminal bronchioles and alveoli where oxygen transfer occurs. Thus only pneumonia, of these 3 infectious etiologies, alters lung function resulting in dyspnea. Because the pathological effects are at the alveoli, focal crackles heard late in inspiration is the key sign to diagnosis of early pneumonia (repeat–focal crackles, so you must listen over the whole area of lungs); crackles that disappear with voluntary cough are usually not pathological

(4) Acute sinusitis may occur with, or following, URI. Think of it with change from watery rhinorrhea to green sputum due to degenerated WBC's; facial pain and tenderness over the involved sinus (compared to control site pressure over the zygomatic arch)
(5) Influenza–epidemic period mostly late November-March, abrupt onset of cough and systemic symptoms that may dominate the clinical picture, viz high fever (up to 105°) and shivering, severe myalgias, dramatic malaise and toxic general appearance of the patient; cough is non-productive unless complicated by pneumonia, which then has prominent dyspnea
(6) Whooping cough (pertussis) may present acutely but almost always it is chronic. Think of pertussis with attacks of "whooping" or post-tussive vomiting; or cough following typical symptoms of URI, but it shows no sign of lessening even after 2 weeks
 b. Noninfectious causes, nonproductive or dry cough
(1) Medications, especially ACEI or β-blockers, commonly cause nocturnal cough; cough onset may be in the first week after starting the medication, or it may occur only months later; cough may last 3-4 weeks after ceasing the medication
(2) Bronchial asthma, similar to pneumonia, compromises lung function and causes dyspnea; the mechanism of pathology is bronchiolar spasm, hence bilateral expiratory wheezing, rather than inspiratory crackles (alveoli), as in pneumonia, is key to diagnosis of asthma
(3) Allergic rhinitis–itching eyes or nose, and rhinorrhea; no signs of infection e.g. no fever, pharyngitis, myalgias
(4) Sarcoidosis–cough, DOE, weight loss, arthralgias; lymphadenectasis is generalized, high ESR
(5) Psychogenic cough--does not awaken the patient i.e. not nocturnal, but often, neither chronic bronchitis nor GERD has nocturnal cough
4. Sepsis syndrome masquerading as a "flu-like" illness or "viral syndrome"; send immediately to the ED
 a. Symptoms of a "viral syndrome" are fever, malaise, myalgias, and other mild constitutional symptoms. No rash or other localizing signs
 b. Sepsis is defined as evidence of infection plus at least 2 of the following
(1) Fever above 100.4°F (38°C) or hypothermia below 98.8°F (36°C)
(2) Tachycardia--heart rate greater than 90 bpm
(3) Tachypnea–respiratory rate greater than 20/min
(4) Peripheral WBC–greater than 12,000 or less than 4000/mm^3 or greater than 10% bands
 c. Sepsis syndrome is sepsis plus evidence of impaired organ perfusion--altered mental status, oliguria, hypoxemia, lactic acidosis
 d. Some dangerous illnesses starting as a "viral syndrome" and progressing to sepsis syndrome are:
(1) RMSF
(2) Hantavirus pulmonary syndrome
(3) Infective endocarditis or SBE
(4) Tularemia
(5) Psittacosis
(6) Postsplenectomy infection
(7) Plague
(8) Staphylococcal septicemia

H. Use the glossary for precise thinking and accurate diagnosis.

1. **Adventitious** (Latin *adventicius* meaning "foreign, strange, extraneous.") Adventitious lung sounds are abnormal lung sounds *(viz* crackles, wheezes, rhonchi) suggesting lung or cardiac disease.
2. **Asthma** (Greek word for any "gasping or panting.") Later the Romans defined it as "sonorous wheezing."
3. **Bioaerosol** (Greek word *bios* meaning "life" and *aer,* "air.") Literally it is "life in air" and we use the term for airborne microorganisms, an indoor-released pollutant which may act to sensitize a susceptible host to allergic rhinitis.
4. **Catarrh** (Greek, *kata* meaning "down" and *rhein*, "to run or flow.") Formerly, it was any excess humor discharged from the body e.g. nasal catarrh. Now we call it rhinorrhea "flowing of the nose" or runny nose, or sometimes, incorrectly, rhinitis (meaning inflammatory nasal mucous membranes).
5. **Coryza** (Greek word meaning "a cold in the head" resulting in an acute catarrhal

condition of nasal mucous membrane i.e. runny nose.) Our "common cold" represents a "catarrhal disorder of the upper respiratory tract."
6. **Dyspnea** (Greek *dys* meaning "difficult or labored" and *pnoia,* "breathing.") It is not painful breathing, which would be pleuritic pain; dyspnea indicates that ordinary breathing now involves work, rather than the usual unawareness of breathing.
7. **Dysphagia** (Greek *dys* meaning "difficult" and *phagein,* "to eat.") It is difficulty performing the act of swallowing, not pain, which is odynophagia.
8. **Expectorate** (Latin *ex* meaning "from or out of" and *pectus*, "chest.") It is the act of expelling phlegm from the chest, and cough aids this process.
9. **Fracture** (Latin word *frangare* meaning "to break.") It is a breaking of any part e.g. bone, cartilage.
10. **Grippe** (French word meaning "a seizure or attack" especially for an acute febrile illness.) It was a common name for influenza, *la grippe,* or in English "the grip."
11. **Hemoptysis** (Greek *hemo*, "blood" and *ptysis*, "a spitting" of blood from any source.) More recently hemoptysis was restricted to coughing up blood originating from the respiratory tract only; in contrast, "blood tinged sputum," may be nonrespiratory tract in origin.
12. **Hiccup** English term derived by onomatopoeia, that is, an imitative word that when pronounced sounds like what it means.
13. **Inflammation** (Latin *inflammare* meaning "to set on fire.") The cardinal features of inflammation (rubor, color, tumor, dolor) suggested a smoldering fire.
14. **Influenza** (14th century Italian word meaning "influence" or "a visitation" by an epidemic disease.) This disease was thought due to "influence" by environmental forces e.g. planets or stars.
15. **Odynophagia** (Greek *odyne* meaning "pain" and *phagein,* "to eat.") It is painful swallowing.
16. **Paroxysm** (Greek word *para* meaning "during" and *oxys*, "sharp or acute.") It refers to an abrupt, accentuated attack of some symptoms occurring episodically.
17. **Pertussis** (Latin *per* indicating "intensity" and *tussis,* "cough.") It refers to the violent cough typical of "whooping cough."
18. **Phlegm** (Greek meaning "flame or heat.") Originally it was used to refer to any inflammation; later archaic humoral pathology (hot, dry, cold, wet system) oddly applied the word "phlegm" to any cold or moist humor e.g. mucus secreted by respiratory tract, and we continue this usage.
19. **Pneumonia** (Greek word *pneumonia* was a general word for "disease of the lungs," referring to Greek *pneumon* meaning "lung.") Now we restrict its usage to an infection causing inflammation of lung parenchyma (the essential or functional elements of the lung).
20. **Pneumonitis**–also inflammation of lung parenchyma, but this term usually is reserved for noninfectious causes e.g. aspiration, hypersensitivity or allergic, chemical pneumonitis.
21. **Protussive** (Latin *pro* meaning "before' and *tussive,* "cough.") It is an agent used to stimulate cough to determine sensitivity of cough receptors e.g. capsaicin.
22. **Purulent** (Latin *purulentus* meaning "consisting of, or containing, pus," which is from Greek *pyon* meaning "corrupt matter" exuding from sores.) Now we know the color reflects the intactness of WBCs; white early and intact WBCs; yellow, less intact; and green, mostly degenerating WBCs.
23. **Pyrosis** (word in Greek meaning "on fire or a burning.") Our lay term is "heartburn" for this retrosternal burning sensation due to regurgitation of stomach acid, i.e. GERD.
24. **Rale** (French verb *raler* meaning "to make a rattling sound in the throat.") Laennec invented the stethoscope and applied the term to various adventitious crackling sounds he heard when listening to a number of congestive cardiopulmonary diseases. Recently, the term rale has been changed arbitrarily to "crackle," so rale is no longer used.
25. **Reflux** (Latin *refluere* meaning "to flow back" in a gradual, effortless way). As does esophageal reflux.
26. **Regurgitation** (Latin *re* meaning "back" and *gurgitare* "to flood.") It implies a more forceful action than reflux e.g. flooding back in mitral regurgitation.
27. **Rhonchus** (Greek word meaning "a snoring sound.") It likely is derived by onomatopoeia. Rhonchi are louder and coarser than crackles, and rhonchi have no specific diagnostic meaning except "junky lungs."
28. **Singultus** (Latin word meaning "hiccup.")
29. **Stridor** (Latin for "shrill sound or harsh noise.") It is auscultated over the larynx, associated with respiratory distress, and always an emergency.
30. **Tachypnea** (Greek *tachy* meaning "rapid," and *pnoia*, "breathing.") It is a respiratory rate more than usual for that individual, or more than 20/min on average.

Chapter 6 Diarrhea
Questions on Diarrhea
A. In your patient with complaint of "I'm having diarrhea," the most important
   1. Question to ask is:
   2. Physical exam to perform is:
B. The commonest cause of diarrhea you will see in the office patient is:
   1. Its distinguishing characteristics are:
      a.
      b.
C. The other 2 common causes of diarrhea seen in the office and their distinguishing characteristics are:
   1.
      a.
      b.
   2.
      a.
      b.
D. Your patient is essentially well, but she "frequently has diarrhea." She cannot remember when the diarrhea began, and it is unassociated with abdominal pain or with other symptoms. She likely has a disorder called functional diarrhea and many of these patients believe the cause is:

E. Your new patient is a 24 y/o woman who just moved to Amarillo from Omaha, where she was diagnosed with "irritable bowel syndrome." Today she has "really severe abdominal pain and diarrhea." She has never had constipation, and having a BM has little effect on the abdominal pain. On exam there is no fever, bowel sounds are normally active. Rectal exam shows runny stool and mildly positive hemoccult test. What is your management?

F. The "brown bag test" is:

G. Your patient is 25 a y/o woman with chronic daily diarrhea. There are 3 major classes of chronic daily diarrhea. As a first step, how can you quickly approach this problem?

Chapter 6 Diarrhea 71

Answers on Diarrhea
A. Be certain of your patient's symptom and its distinguishing characteristics
   1. You must be absolutely certain it is diarrhea–"What exactly do you mean by the word, diarrhea?" And "How exactly are your stools different from usual?" You are looking for any change in quality or quantity of the stools from her usual

   Then you must know if this is new onset diarrhea or episodic diarrhea or chronic diarrhea. If episodic, it recently began but she has had one or more previous similar bouts of diarrhea, with varying periods of "normal" stools in between. If the diarrhea is present almost daily >1-2 months, it is chronic diarrhea
   2. Abdominal exam by auscultation and palpation, particularly listening for the hyperactive bowel sounds of gastroenteritis. Also DRE to obtain a stool specimen (for stool consistency, that is, if it is diarrhea), stool for occult blood and WBCs (either one suggests an inflammatory etiology of the diarrhea), rectal temperature >101°F (38.3°C) suggesting an infectious cause
B. The commonest cause of diarrhea in the office patient
   1. Infectious gastroenteritis (GE)
      a. New onset diarrhea
      b. Associated symptoms of infection–mild fever, myalgias, headache, nausea vomiting
      c. Hyperactive bowel sounds
C. The other 2 common causes of diarrhea have normal bowel sounds
   1. Irritable bowel syndrome (IBS)
      a. Episodic diarrhea (often alternating with constipation)
      b. Abdominal discomfort or pain is the dominant symptom, and the diarrhea (or constipation) follows or occurs concomitant with the pain; having a BM decreases or relieves the abdominal pain
   2. Functional diarrhea
      a. Episodic or daily diarrhea (it does not alternate with constipation)
      b. Abdominal pain is minimal or absent
D. Recognize the common perception that "food allergy" causes diarrhea

   Depending on a person's particular focus on her BMs, and the consistency of the stool, almost everybody occasionally has "diarrhea" or loose bowels. The person who tends to interpret serious illness in any changes in her bodily activities is the one likely to consult you about her "diarrhea." Know that up to 40% of the population thinks they have a "food allergy" (really a food intolerance) causing symptoms, especially "diarrhea." Many of these patients have either IBS or functional diarrhea
E. Be alert for dangerous symptoms or signs when diagnosing IBS. Signs of possible danger in this patient should leap out
   1. RBCs (hemoccult positive) or WBCs in the stool are never consistent with IBS. They suggest an inflammatory cause of the diarrhea, such as Crohn's disease or ulcerative colitis
   2. Other potentially dangerous symptoms are also present: she always has diarrhea (never constipation), and there has been lack of any relief of the abdominal pain with a BM. She needs a colonoscopy or GI consult, at minimum
F. Medications are a common cause of either new, episodic or chronic

diarrhea

Have her bring in for you to examine "everything that you swallow except food and drink." You especially want to know about medications prescribed by other clinicians, OTC medications, nutritional supplements, salt substitutes, illicit drugs. Almost <u>any</u> chemical, in the broadest sense of the term, can cause episodic diarrhea

G. Quick approach to chronic daily diarrhea

Obtain a stool sample by DRE

1. Test for occult blood and WBC for an <u>inflammatory</u> etiology
2. Test for fat globules by Sudan III stain for <u>steatorrhea</u>
3. If both tests are negative, the diarrhea likely is a <u>watery</u> diarrhea due to osmotic (maldigested carbohydrates, laxatives) or secretory causes. If diarrhea disappears with a 2-3 d fast, think of maldigested foods

Diarrhea

Differential diagnosis: the 3 common causes of diarrhea
1. Infectious gastroenteritis–<u>new</u> diarrhea; other symptoms of infection e.g. fever, headache
2. IBS–<u>episodic</u> diarrhea; associated abdominal pain
3. Functional diarrhea–<u>episodic</u> or daily diarrhea; no other symptoms

(For chronic daily diarrhea, see Section G.3 for diagnosis)

A. **Be certain of the symptom and its distinguishing characteristics.** Your patient's problem or chief complaint is "I'm having diarrhea." Be certain the problem is a change from her usual formed stools either to more frequent, loose stools than usual for her or to runny or watery BMs. Ask her "What do you mean by diarrhea?" Have her describe precisely what is new about her BMs, and don't let her use the word "diarrhea" in the description. Be sure it's not something else, such as rectal discharge, straining (tenesmus), incontinence (involuntary discharge), change in stool color or consistency, or just increased frequency with formed stools (hyperdefecation). Be sure she really has looked at the stool, previous to the onset of "diarrhea" as well as since it started, because many people are conditioned to avoid viewing their stool
1. Determine if it is new onset diarrhea. Ask her "When was the last time your stools were well-formed?" If they were always well-formed until the diarrhea started, then it is new onset diarrhea, suggesting almost always, either some change in food habits or a new medication or an infection. If she had one or more previous bouts of diarrhea like this one, and she was well in between bouts, she has episodic diarrhea. If the diarrhea has been occurring almost daily for at least 3-4 weeks, and she cannot identify the exact onset, it is likely chronic (See Section G.3 below for approach to chronic diarrhea)
2. Determine if the diarrhea is accompanied by either episodic abdominal pain (suggesting IBS) or significant GI symptoms suggesting ongoing infection (vomiting, crampy pain, fever) or if it is primarily an isolated symptom (other than minor constitutional symptoms) of the lower GI tract. For example, ask "If I could immediately make the diarrhea disappear, how close to normal would you be?" and let her explain what she is feeling. If she would be about normal without the diarrhea, then it is an isolated symptom
3. If the cause of the diarrhea is unlikely one of the 3 common causes (or it is chronic diarrhea), while listening to her description try to locate the part of the GI tract that is diseased
    a. Small intestine, proximal colon–pain is periumbilical or RLQ, minimal or no relief with defecation; large volume, watery stools; may be few in number of daily stools; diarrhea may closely follow meals

b. Lower colon or rectum–pain is lower abdomen or LLQ, and it often is relieved by a BM or enema; diarrhea is frequent (>6/day) and of low volume
   c. Rectum–suggested by the presence of urgency, tenesmus, incontinence

---

Be certain:
1. The symptom is diarrhea, that is, either unformed, watery stools or increased frequency of loose stools
2. Whether it is new diarrhea, episodic diarrhea or chronic, daily diarrhea (>3-4 weeks)
3. Whether there are associated symptoms of abdominal pain or infection e.g. fever, myalgias, headache

(If it is chronic, daily diarrhea, see Section G.3 for a diagnostic approach)

---

4. Physical examination
   a. Abdomen–listen for the hyperactive bowel sounds (not borborygmi) of GE and the absence of rushes of high-pitched tinkly sounds of obstruction; be sure there is no sign of a surgical abdomen including absent bowel sounds, local tenderness, rebound tenderness; get a rectal temperature and do a DRE for signs of localized disease, but especially to obtain stool to test for WBCs (or lactoferrin test), occult blood and fat (Sudan III); absence of both WBCs and blood helps to exclude inflammatory causes of diarrhea, and absence of fat globules excludes steatorrhea
   b. Systemic–overall appearance and mental status; vital signs, especially orthostatic hypotension, high fever, anemia, rash, arthralgias, weight loss

By now you should be confident the patient has diarrhea, whether it is new onset, episodic or chronic diarrhea, and if there are concomitant pertinent symptoms either of abdominal pain or infection. In almost all instances you now have the information you need for diagnosis of the obvious causes (Section C) and the common causes (Section E). In the rare instance that your patient appears different clinically from the usual office patient with diarrhea, be certain (Section B) that she does not have a symptom or sign of a dangerous disease.

B. Be confident it's not a dangerous disease.
1. Send immediately to the ED by ambulance if there is:
   a. Diarrhea, often bloody and abrupt onset, very severe persistent lower abdominal pain, think of ischemic colitis (in an elderly patient, or in a younger patient with known atherosclerotic disease or cocaine use) or partial obstruction e.g. intussusception in a younger patient
   b. Rapid onset of RLQ tenderness and pain, think of retrocecal appendicitis, *Y. enterocolitica*, acute diverticulitis (up to 15% are right-sided in Caucasians, and higher incidence in Asians), Crohn's disease
   c. History of recent diarrhea and high fever after foreign travel, and now abrupt abdominal pain and absent bowel sounds, think of intestinal perforation after typhoid fever
   d. History of mild chronic diarrhea, weight loss and now unexplained orthostatic

Chapter 6 Diarrhea 75

  hypotension, think of Addisonian crisis
  e. Toxic appearance, profuse bloody diarrhea, crampy pain, high fever and marked leukocytosis after recent antibiotics, think of severe form of pseudomembranous colitis
  f. Toxic patient with bloody diarrhea and megacolon, think of fulminant ulcerative colitis or EHEC 0157:H7
  g. Confusion with mild fever and relative tachycardia (inappropriately rapid heart rate relative to height of fever) and recent history of chronic "diarrhea," think of thyroid storm
  h. Rapid onset diarrhea associated with urticaria or angioedema, think of anaphylaxis
2. Admit at once to the ED or hospital if there is:
  a. Rapid onset of paresthesias, flushing, cramps <1 hr after eating, think of chemical effect e.g. histamine fish poisoning, paralytic shellfish poisoning, monosodium glutamate
  b. Dizziness or orthostatic hypotension in an elderly or debilitated patient with significant diarrhea, think of volume depletion
  c. Diarrhea and lymphadenectasis, think of lymphoma, Whipple's disease, HIV enteropathy
  d. Diarrhea, LLQ abdominal pain, fever, tachycardia, and perhaps signs of peritoneal irritation in an elderly patient, think of diverticulitis (20 % have onset <50 y/o)

Be certain in the first minutes of your exam that there is no evidence of any one dangerous symptom or sign associated with the diarrhea:
1. Toxic, very ill appearance
2. Confusion or prostration
3. Sudden onset severe, persistent abdominal pain
4. Bloody diarrhea
5. Orthostatic hypotension, fever >101°F (38.3°C)
6. Unexplained weight loss
7. Immunocompromised patient

Any suggestion of a dangerous disease, send your patient to the ED.

---

  e. Severe diarrhea ("pea soup"), high fever and relative bradycardia in a patient with recent foreign travel, think of typhoid fever (*S. typhi*)
  f. High fever, rigors, very ill appearance, think of sepsis complicating any bacterial cause of diarrhea
  g. Patient who gets diarrhea from eating sushi or raw oysters and then becomes extremely ill, think of *Vibrio* species causing fulminant liver failure
  h. Rapid onset of bloody diarrhea without signs of infection, think of IBD (young or in the 60's age group); in the elderly, think of ischemic bowel, acute mesenteric vascular thrombosis, diverticular bleeding, AV malformation, malignancy
  i. Signs of infection with many watery stools which then become bloody with severe cramping pain and vomiting, think of EHEC 0157:H7
  j. Diarrhea, hypersalivation, rhinorrhea, miosis in a person using pesticides, think of organophosphate poisoning
  k. Diarrhea, abdominal pain and symptoms of pneumonia, think of Legionnaires' disease
  l. Very severe headache, diarrhea and other GI symptoms suggesting acute GE, think of meningitis or RMSF (early stage)
  m. Recent infectious cause of diarrhea and now lower limb weakness, think of GBS secondary to *C. jejuni*
  n. Symptoms suggesting GE (nausea, vomiting, diarrhea) but also dyspnea and tachypnea, think of carbon monoxide poisoning; if GE occurs with diplopia, dysarthria, weakness, think of botulism
  o. Severe diarrhea and then anemia and anuria, think of HUS associated with shigellosis or EHEC 0157: H7
  p. Massive diarrhea (>3L/d) with dizziness and hypotension, think of pancreatic

cholera i.e. VIPoma
- q. Severe colicky abdominal pain, profuse diarrhea and "garlicky" breath, think of arsenic poisoning
- r. Rapid onset of severe watery diarrhea in a person with a bone marrow transplant, think of graft-versus-host disease

3. Admit to the hospital or have a specialist consult as soon as appropriate if there is:
   a. History of diarrhea, weight loss >3-4 kg, think of malignancy, fecal impaction, malnutrition, mesenteric ischemia, hyperthyroidism, uncontrolled DM, Addison's, HIV, malabsorption
   b. Rectal occult blood, tenesmus and a "mass" by DRE, think of rectal malignancy, proctitis
   c. Episodic diarrhea, abdominal pain and occult blood or hematochezia, think of IBD, diverticular disease
   d. Diarrhea and flushing think of carcinoid syndrome, MTC, mastocytosis
   e. Tenesmus, rectal pain, rectal discharge, think of severe proctitis
   f. Diarrhea in a patient with MD and new or increased dose of antidepressant medication, think of serotonin syndrome (SSRI, tricyclics), lithium toxicity
   g. Diarrhea and hyperadrenergic symptoms of tachycardia, restlessness, agitation, think of opioid withdrawal
   h. Fecal incontinence, think of fecal impaction due to neuromuscular disease, anorectal disease (rectal prolapse, fistula, neuropathy), dementia
   i. HIV positive patient with diarrhea that is negative for stool cultures and *C. difficile* toxin, or nonresponsive to treatment, think of unusual causes, so refer to gastroenterology

C. Make a quick diagnosis if it's obvious.

Is it an easily diagnosed condition or a medication causing the diarrhea? In most patients you will be <u>highly</u> confident of a common cause of the symptom by now. If not, one or more of the following tests may exclude an organic disease and increase your confidence in your working diagnosis: CBC, Chem 7, albumin, ESR, TSH, HIV; stool blood, WBCs, fat. Almost always with the following causes, the diarrhea is an isolated GI symptom, with only mild nausea, mild abdominal discomfort, flatus. The "diarrhea" is not the very frequent (>6/d), watery or runny stools, but the stools just may occur more often than usual and they are "looser." No physical signs except possibly with food allergy. Have her bring to you <u>everything</u> she puts in her mouth (including OTC drugs, nutritional supplements, illicit drugs), except for food (the "brown bag test.")

1. Foods

Diagnose and treat an easily diagnosed cause of <u>new or episodic</u> diarrhea due to noninfectious causes:

1. Dietary–vegetarian diet; food intolerances
2. Spot diagnoses–runners' diarrhea; antibiotic-associated mild diarrhea; after GI surgery; history of toxin ingestion (heavy metal, mushroom, fish); with migraine headache
3. Medications--temporal association of the diarrhea with starting the medication

---

   a. Change from an omnivore diet producing a single compact stool every 2-3 days, to a predominant herbivore-like, "healthy" diet of cereals, fruits, vegetables produces more frequent, bulky, "looser" stools
   b. Food intolerances are perceived by 20-40% of the adult

Chapter 6 Diarrhea

population and elimination of certain foods in 60% of patients with IBS results in marked symptom improvement. About 30 common food items (especially grains, dairy products, fruits, vegetables) are identified, but in the individual patient there are many more possibilities (J Human Nutr Diet $\underline{8}$, 159, 1995). Items not thought of as foods--heavy "social" alcohol use, large amounts of caffeine (coffee or tea), chocolate, nuts, preservatives, dietetic "sugar-free" candies and gums, fruit juices, soda, are common offenders. Thus almost any "food" can cause abdominal symptoms and diarrhea in the individual patient
  c. Food allergies are rare compared to frequency of food intolerance. Think of allergy if there is rapid onset of symptoms, usually in minutes but <2 hr after eating, especially milk, eggs, tree nuts, fish, shellfish, soybeans, wheat. Almost everybody with diarrhea thinks it is due to a food allergy
2. Medications: More than 700 medications are known to cause diarrhea as a side effect; also OTC drugs including nutritional (vitamin C, magnesium) and herbal therapy may cause diarrhea. Liquid medications often contain sorbitol as vehicle. Almost any medication can cause diarrhea in the individual patient, so any new medication or one with recently increased dosage may be causing the diarrhea. Heavy "social" alcohol intake causes loose stools, and cocaine use causes anorexia and diarrhea
3. Spot diagnoses
  a. Runners' diarrhea occurs in up to 40% of competitive runners. It may occur during or after running vigorously, and it occurs more frequently in runners beginning training or escalating their intensity of exercise. If there is gross or occult blood, be alert to ischemic colitis (Gut $\underline{28}$, 896, 1987), no matter how young the patient
  b. Antibiotic-associated diarrhea is a mild diarrhea but only in half of the patients is there an obvious connection to antibiotics. For treatment, she may need only oral cholestyramine, which binds the toxin
  c. Diarrhea occurs commonly after surgery of GI or biliary tracts, including: gastric surgery with, or without, vagotomy; small intestine resection, with or without proximal colon resection; ileostomy (after total colectomy), or cholecystectomy. It is a secretory type of diarrhea (large volume, watery stool) and worsens with eating. Trial of cholestyramine (for malabsorbed bile acids) and psyllium may improve fecal consistency

D. **Identify your patient's worries and wants.** Diarrhea occurs in everybody, and very few patients with diarrhea consult about it. During your interview and exam try to intuit or discover why your patient is here today, and not previously, for this problem. What is she worried about? Don't necessarily ask directly, but try to get some ideas from your patient's responses to questions about her perception of the diarrhea itself. You can't completely help your patient unless you know what she really worries about and wants from you. That's why she is here to see you--to satisfy her worries and wants! Here are only some of the possible worries and wants of your patient with diarrhea. You must discover her specific, unique ones.
  1. Common worries are:
    a. That the cause of the diarrhea is a dangerous etiology e.g. colon cancer, infection, IBD
    b. That the etiology is some rare disease, e.g. HIV, heavy metals

    c. What other fears or anxieties might be troubling your patient? For example, she may have had diarrhea at other times or for years, and only now does she come for help. What has changed? Perhaps a friend or relative, who had similar diarrhea, recently has been diagnosed with IBD. There are many other possibilities–think of them
2. Your patient wants:
    a. You to perform a thorough physical exam focused on possible causes of the diarrhea, and she wants appropriate tests and imaging studies, even though you might determine they are not needed

---

During your exam, discover your patient's worries (cancer, infection, IBD) and wants (antibiotic, antidiarrheal), so that you can respond to her specific needs as soon as possible.

---

    b. A plausible explanation of the cause of the diarrhea
    c. Confident reassurance from you that it is not a dangerous or rare etiology. Tell her-- "The good news, it's not ulcerative colitis" (or whatever you believe her real worry is)
    d. To know the prognosis, short term (effects on job, home life, marriage; how soon she will be back to normal) and long term (if recurrences are possible; how to prevent recurrences; if it will cause any disability)
    e. Treatment now to stop the diarrhea and to prevent recurrence
    f. A gastroenterology referral if she believes you are not confident of the diagnosis

E. Know the symptoms that differentiate the 3 common causes of diarrhea.
1. The commonest cause of new diarrhea is GE due to microbial

---

The etiologies causing most <u>new or episodic</u> diarrhea in the office patient are:
1. Infectious gastroenteritis–<u>new</u> diarrhea; other symptoms of infection e.g. fever, headache
2. IBS–<u>episodic</u> diarrhea; associated abdominal pain
3. Functional diarrhea–<u>episodic</u> or daily diarrhea; no other symptoms

---

agents
    a. Characteristics of infectious GE
      (1) The diarrhea is <u>new</u> onset (she was in her usual good health before this episode of illness)
      (2) There are associated symptoms of an infection–fever, nausea, vomiting, myalgias, headache, cramping abdominal pain
      (3) <u>Hyperactive bowel sounds</u> by auscultation
      (4) The infectious etiologies differ in the following:
        (a) Viral etiologies have no or minimal fever; no stool blood or WBC's; mild to moderate abdominal pain
        (b) Food poisoning by eating preformed enterotoxin also elicits no fever and no occult blood or WBC's in the stool; abdominal pain is rapid onset and may be severe, but the pain remains diffuse:
          (i) If symptoms begin 1-6 hours after eating some unusual food, think of *S. aureus* in dairy or meat products or *B. cereus* in

Chapter 6 Diarrhea   79

fried rice
- (ii) If symptoms occur later, i.e. 6-16 hours after eating, think of the diarrheic form of *B. cereus* (long incubation type) or *C. perfringens*, because their toxins are released in the ileum
- (c) If symptoms begin 1-3 days after eating contaminated food, think of bacterial etiologies. Often *Campylobacter* or *Yersinia* have stool positive for blood and fecal WBC's, but *Salmonella* and *Shigella* are positive <70% of the time. Reasons you might hospitalize or empirically treat a bacterial cause with oral quinolone, even though treatment shortens the illness by only 1-2 days: fever ≥102°F and pulse >110/minute with no relative bradycardia, orthostatic dizziness and hypotension, bloody diarrhea, severe abdominal pain, or HIV patient
- (d) Traveler's diarrhea ("turista") begins a few days after arrival in the foreign country and persists 2-5 days; typically there is no fever or clinical dysentery; if it persists >10-14 days, think of amebiasis, giardiasis or pseudomembranous colitis (if antibiotics were taken). If diarrhea persists weeks (chronic diarrhea), think of "post-dysentery IBS" or "post-dysentery lactase deficiency"

  b. What suggests it might not be GE
  - (1) Anytime there is an associated symptom or sign suggesting a dangerous cause (see above, Section B)
  - (2) If the diarrhea is episodic
  - (3) If an organ system other than the GI tract also is involved (not including constitutional symptoms of headache, myalgias, fever) e.g. rash, arthritis
2. Common look-alikes causing diarrhea and how each differs from GE
   a. IBS
   - (1) Episodic abdominal pain is the dominant symptom
   - (2) Some change in stool consistency is associated with the onset of pain, so there is episodic diarrhea or constipation
   - (3) Defecation provides some or almost total relief of the abdominal pain
   - (4) Although only the GI tract is involved episodically, the patient with IBS frequently is not asymptomatic between episodes; often there are chronic headaches or fibromyalgia or chronic dyspepsia or LBP or dysmenorrhea
   - (5) Never diagnose IBS without further investigations, if any one of the following is present:
     - (a) New onset of symptoms that suggest IBS, but the patient is >50 years old
     - (b) Nocturnal diarrhea, and especially if the patient soils the bedsheets
     - (c) Unexplained weight loss >3-4 kg, with or without anorexia
     - (d) Any evidence of systemic disease (anemia, high ESR, fever, unexplained weight loss, lymphadenectasis, low serum albumin)
     - (e) Occult blood or WBCs or fat in stools
   b. Functional diarrhea
   - (1) Functional diarrhea is either daily or episodic diarrhea like IBS

(2) Unlike IBS, there is no abdominal pain associated with the episodes of diarrhea

F. Use this summary for efficient diagnosis of a common cause.
With the above information from Sections A-E in mind, here is the rapid approach to diagnosis of the cause of diarrhea.
1. You already have determined:
   a. In Section A, by H&P, that it is diarrhea, and that the diarrhea is either new or episodic or chronic, daily diarrhea.
   b. In Section B, that there is no evidence in the H&P of any one dangerous cause of the diarrhea.
   c. In Section C, that there is not an easily diagnosed dietary cause, a spot diagnosis, or a medication that is likely responsible for the diarrhea.
2. From the focused H&P almost always you should quickly be confident of a working diagnosis. Confident final diagnosis is made only in followup the next few days, weeks or months when the response to treatment or nontreatment is appropriate to your working diagnosis.
   a. If the diarrhea is new, rapid onset and associated with vomiting and malaise, it most likely is due to an infectious agent. If there is significant fever (>101°F) and either hemoccult positive stool or WBC'S in the stool specimen, it likely is bacterial diarrhea; otherwise it likely is viral GE or food poisoning.
   b. If it is episodic diarrhea associated with abdominal pain, and BMs provide some relief of the pain, and the patient is essentially well between episodes, it is likely IBS.
   c. If it is either episodic or chronic daily diarrhea, and there are no associated symptoms, it is likely functional diarrhea.
3. Answer your patient's worries and wants that you determined early on during the exam (Section D). Have you done everything you can to help her?
4. You now have a working diagnosis, but only with followup can you be highly confident it is correct. In return visits you are always testing by H&P that your working diagnosis is correct.

G. Abandon your working diagnosis and look for an uncommon cause only if:
1. Any one dangerous symptom or sign (see above, Section B) occurs in the following days, weeks or months. Quickly obtain a specialist consult or send your patient to the hospital as appropriate
2. Your patient's response to therapy is not as you expect or if the natural history of your working diagnosis does not occur. Even without treatment, viral GE and "food poisoning" should be much better in a few days, and the usual traveler's diarrhea is better in a week

   Don't spend time and money looking for one of the following etiologies until you are sure your patient doesn't have one of the 3 common causes of her diarrhea above. Nevertheless, it may be that she has an uncommon or rare cause of the diarrhea that either is, or will become, chronic diarrhea. These are important to identify, because each has a different treatment or prophylaxis
3. Chronic diarrhea (occurring almost daily for >4 weeks)–approach to diagnosis
   a. First, determine exactly what therapy the patient has tried including OTC meds, especially antibiotics and antidiarrheal agents. If the diarrhea started with rapid onset as GE and the diarrhea has continued for weeks or months, think of:
      (1) Continuing GI infection e.g. *Giardia, Campylobacter, C. difficile*,

Chapter 6 Diarrhea 81

Cryptosporidium, amebiasis, Y. enterocolitica, Aeromones, some *E. coli*. If stool blood or WBCs, antibiotic trial (Gastroenterology 116, 1464, 1999)
- (2) "Postdysentery lactase deficiency" or "postdysentery IBS"
- (3) Antibiotic-associated diarrhea–Rx cholestyramine
- (4) Pseudomembranous colitis

> If your patient does not have a common cause of her diarrhea, she may have an uncommon cause that will, in time, become chronic diarrhea. These uncommon or rare etiologies are listed in Section G.3. You can diagnose and treat it, or you may want to refer your patient to a gastroenterologist.

- b. Be sure it is not a cause listed in Section C e.g. food intolerances or medication side-effects
- c. If all of the following findings are present in your patient, and there is no other obvious cause e.g. medications, it is likely she has either functional diarrhea or IBS (see Section E)
  - (1) Diarrhea has been episodic or daily for months without progressively worsening
  - (2) No hematochezia, occult blood or WBCs in a stool sample
  - (3) Not fatty stool by Sudan III stain
  - (4) No soiling of underwear or bedsheets and no nocturnal urgency to defecate that awakens her
  - (5) No unexplained weight loss or fever (get rectal temp tid at home for 1-2 days)
- d. If she has daily diarrhea, have her fast 48-72 hr. Continuing diarrhea suggests laxative abuse or factitious diarrhea. Cessation of diarrhea suggests maldigestion e.g. lactose, sorbitol
- e. If your patient does not fit exactly the above description, or you still have some uncertainty, e.g. she occasionally has a BM at night, but you can't be certain urgency caused it; obtain blood for CBC, ESR, electrolytes, calcium, magnesium, albumin, TSH, and also test stool for occult blood, WBCs and fat, now and at future exams
- f. If you still want assurance it is not a dangerous cause, get a 24-hour stool collection while she is on her usual diet. Often you will find the amount of "diarrhea" is <200-250 gm/d, which is further evidence of functional diarrhea or IBS or "nondiarrhea." If stool weight is >250-300 gm, obtain measurements of stool Na, K, osmolality, pH, Mg, PO_4, SO_4 (laxative screen)
- g. If the 24 hour collection shows loose, runny stool (>250-300 gm.), have your patient fast for 48-72 hours, collect stool the last 24 hr, and test for high urine ketones to confirm she did fast. Osmotic-caused diarrhea should stop or be markedly decreased with fasting. Though a few secretory diarrheas (those with previous GI surgery) also decrease with a fast, the dangerous ones do not *viz* IBD, tumors, chronic infections. If your patient has a secretory diarrhea, it may be best to refer her to a specialist or hospitalize for further workup
- h. Common causes of chronic diarrhea that you may recognize from the clinical presentation, and you may possibly give a treatment trial before extensive workup:
  - (1) There are two causes of "diarrhea" with weight loss but with usual or even increased food intake:
    - (a) Hyperthyroidism rarely has watery stools, but rather there is hyperdefecation, an increased frequency of formed stools, but stool weight is <200 gm/d. Suppressed serum TSH confirms hyperthyroidism, and the diarrhea will disappear with euthyroidism
    - (b) Malabsorption syndromes also may have diarrhea (really steatorrhea), but the stools are foul smelling, usually large and floating and greasy containing bits of food particles. Fecal fat $\geq$ 14 gm/day is highly specific for fat malabsorption caused by diseases of the pancreas or small intestine, e.g. celiac disease (antigluten and antiendomysial antibodies), altered bile salt metabolism. Give a therapeutic trial of gluten-free diet, cholestyramine, pancreatic enzyme replacement, as indicated
  - (2) Diarrhea is common after 5-10 years of DM. Other signs of neuropathy occur e.g. loss of Achilles DTRs, orthostatic hypotension, impotence. Diarrhea characteristically is postprandial, but it may be nocturnal, urgent and explosive,

and cause soiled bedsheets. If it is due to bacterial overgrowth, it is treatable with tetracycline; but usually various mechanisms are causative and therapeutic trials of a number of medications are tried. A common treatable cause in diabetics is the frequent consumption of "sugar-free" products (sorbitol).
(3) Two entities formerly were included under the rubric, IBS:
 (a) Lactase deficiency or lactose intolerance results in diarrhea when lactose-containing foods, meat or dairy products, are eaten, and the diarrhea occurs within 6 hours of eating. Mostly it occurs in people of African and Mediterranean origin. Also there is decreased lactase with ageing and there is transient lactase deficiency following GE; both circumstances can lead to confusion in diagnosis. Response to restriction of all milk and milk products is diagnostic and therapeutic
 (b) Giardiasis from wild animals or due to drinking contaminated water. Because symptoms may begin 1-3 weeks after the initial infection and last more than 6 months after the onset, an accurate history of possible causes may be difficult to elicit. There is bloating and excessive flatulence, and the diarrhea is foul-smelling, explosive, watery. Trial of metronidazole is curative
(4) Surreptitious laxative abuse may be used by your patient to lose weight or for secondary gain of attention. Gastroenterologists diagnose it as causative of 30% of chronic diarrhea that has negative workup by the referring physician. Often there are many other complaints including diarrhea, abdominal pain, fatigue, cyclic edema. Unexplained hypokalemia (use ≤ 4.0 mEq/L in the morning as lower limit of normal; diurnal rise up to 1 mEq/L in the afternoon) is an important finding suggesting laxative abuse
(5) Idiopathic chronic diarrhea accounts for another 50% of patients referred to gastroenterologists by physicians finding negative workup for chronic diarrhea. Extensive diagnostic workup is negative, but all patients resolve the diarrhea in 7-31 months, thus, an unidentified infectious etiology is postulated
(6) Microscopic colitis or collagenous colitis (Am.J.Gastroenterol. 84, 763, 1989) is a nonbloody, chronic, watery secretory diarrhea. The colon is endoscopically normal, but there is microscopic inflammation. It occurs in middle age and older, and it persists for months or years. Treatment is high dose bismuth subsalicylate for 8 weeks (Gastroenterology 114, 29, 1998)
(7) Chronic diarrhea caused by systemic disease
 (a) Inflammatory–abdominal pain, fever, stool blood and WBCs
  (i) Granulomatous inflammatory disease (sarcoidosis, Wegener's, secondary syphilis, Crohn's, TB, *Yersinia*)–abdominal pain, fever, diarrhea, stool blood
  (ii) PAN– abdominal pain, vomiting, GI bleeding
  (iii) Eosinophilic gastroenteritis–peripheral eosinophilia
  (iv) Chronic graft versus host disease–transplant patient
  (v) Cancer–chemotherapy, radiation therapy
 (b) Steatorrhea–weight loss, floating greasy difficult to flush stools, positive Sudan III for fat in stool sample
  (i) Chronic pancreatic or liver (cirrhosis) disease–alcoholic, cystic fibrosis, somatostatinoma
  (ii) Bacterial overgrowth occurs with any cause of decreased intestinal motility
  (iii) Celiac sprue–unexplained deficiencies of folate or iron, low albumin, rash of dermatitis herpetiformis has nocturnal scratching causing eczema
  (iv) Whipple's disease–middle aged white men, large joint arthralgias, fever, weight loss
  (v) Abetalipoproteinemia–low LDL cholesterol, diarrhea, acanthocytosis
 (c) Secretory diarrhea–watery, large volume diarrhea persists after fasting; think of these if no stool blood, WBCs or fat
  (i) GI tumors e.g. GI carcinoid, gastrinoma, VIPoma, villous adenoma
  (ii) MTC–thyroid nodule
  (iii) Systemic mastocytosis–urticaria
  (iv) Bile acid malabsorption–trial of cholestyramine
 (d) Dysmotility causes may mimic IBS
  (i) Bacterial overgrowth of any cause e.g. neuropathies (DM) or myopathies causing gut hypomotility; any causes of pseudoobstruction
  (ii) Carcinoid syndrome–flushing, wheezing, diarrhea
  (iii) Hyperthyroidism–weight loss without anorexia
 (e) Miscellaneous
  (i) Pellagra--4 D's are diarrhea, dermatitis, dementia, death; treat with niacin
  (ii) Seronegative spondyloarthropathies–diarrhea, crampy pain, LBP

Chapter 6 Diarrhea   83

(iii) Plummer-Vinson syndrome–diarrhea, dysphagia, iron-deficiency anemia
(iv) Henoch-Schonlein purpura–abdominal pain, diarrhea and vomiting may precede the purpuric rash
(v) Glucagonoma–hyperglycemia, weight loss, rash (annular erythema in the groin or buttocks, later bullae; migratory necrolytic erythema)

H. Use the glossary for precise thinking and accurate diagnosis.

1. **Albumin** (Latin *albus* meaning "white.") Egg white protein is termed "albumen," whereas albumin refers to a water soluble substance found in almost all animal and plant tissues.
2. **Anemia** (Greek *an* meaning "without" and *haima*, "blood.") Decreased numbers of RBCs.
3. **Anorexia** (Greek *an* meaning "lack of" and *orexis*, "appetite.") Appetite is from Latin *appetitio*, "a craving"; hunger is a drive, whereas appetite stimulates eating even after hunger is satisfied; hunger sustains life, but heightened appetite (culturally driven) results in obesity.
4. **Borborygmus** (Greek word meaning "rumbling bowel sounds.") It is a normal sign of hunger just before eating.
5. **Bowels** (Latin *botulus* meaning "sausage.")
6. **Diarrhea** (Greek word *diarrhoia* meaning "a flowing through.") Excessive watery evacuation from the bowel.
7. **Dysentery** (Latin *dys* meaning "disordered" and *enteron*, "intestine" or simply "any bowel complaint.") Now it implies infectious colitis meaning abdominal pain, tenesmus and diarrhea with stool blood and WBC's, and toxic presentation *viz* tachycardia, leukocytosis, dehydration, hypotension, mental status changes.
8. **Dysmenorrhea** (Greek *dys* meaning "disordered or abnormal" and *men*, "month" and *rhein*, "to flow.") Originally related to symptoms emanating from congested uterus, now it is any pain related to menses.
9. **Dyspepsia** (Greek *dys* meaning "difficult" and *pepsis*, "digestion.") Now it is synonymous with indigestion, i.e. upper abdominal discomfort, belching, feeling of fullness.
10. **Enteric** (Greek *enterikos* meaning "intestinal.") Related to the small intestine.
11. **Excrement** (Latin *ex* meaning "out" and *cernere*, "to sift or separate." A casting out of body wastes.
12. **Feces** (Latin *faecis* meaning "dregs or sediment.") Formerly the word referred only to dregs of fermentation; only in the 1600's do feces refer to "bowel dregs or excrement"; defecate is a "cleansing" of the dregs from the bowels, from *de* "down or remove."
13. **Fever** (Latin *fervere* meaning "to seethe or to steam.")
14. **Hematochezia** (Greek *haima* meaning "blood" and *chezein*, "to defecate.") Passing bright red blood in the stool.
15. **Incontinent** (Latin *in* meaning "not" and *continens*, "restrained.")   Loss of bladder or bowel control.
16. **Intussusception** (Latin *intus* meaning "within" and *suscipere*, "to take up.") A proximal segment of intestine is telescoped or "taken up" into a succeeding segment, causing a partial or total obstruction.
17. **Malabsorption** (Latin *mal* meaning "bad or faulty" and *absorbere*, "to suck up.") Digestion may be normal, but faulty transfer of digested materials into the blood.
18. **Maldigestion** (Latin *mal* meaning "bad or faulty" and *dis*, "apart" and *gerere*, "to carry.") Faulty conversion of food (large molecules) into smaller simpler substances that can be absorbed into the blood.
19. **Melena** (Greek word *melas* meaning "black.") Implied today is that it is black and tarry stool, not just black stool.
20. **Nausea** (Greek *nausia* meaning "seasickness.") A person who is about to vomit is "nauseated"; a person we find disagreeable or who makes us sick to be around, we call her "nauseous."
21. **Parasite** (Greek *para* meaning "at the side of" and *sitos*, "food.") Eating at the side of another, or at the same table; organism that feeds with its host.
22. **Pellagra** (Italian *pelle* meaning "skin" and *agra*, "rough.") Describing the dermatitis (erythema, pigmentation, hyperkeratosis) that occurs with diarrhea.
23. **Rigor** (Greek word *rhigos* meaning "shivering or shuddering from the cold or from horror.") Different from just chills, there is visible shaking or teeth-chattering.
24. **Steatorrhea** (Greek *steatos* meaning "fat" and *rhoia*, "a flow.") Excessive fat in feces, usually due to malabsorption.

25. **Stool** (Anglo-Saxon *stol* meaning "a seat.") When a firm support (stool) became used to sit on while having a bowel movement, "to defecate" became "to stool," and the product itself became "stool."
26. **Tenesmus** (Greek word *tenesmos* meaning "to stretch.") We use the word as the ancients did, "to strain at stool"; implied is that the straining is painful and ineffective, giving the feeling of incomplete evacuation.
27. **Vomit** (Latin *vomere* meaning "to throw up from the stomach.") Greek word for the same meaning is *emein*, leading to our words "emesis, emetic."

Chapter 7 Edema

Questions on Edema

A. In a patient with complaint of leg swelling, the most important
  1. Historical information is:
  2. Physical exam is:

B. In the hospital, bilateral leg edema has 3 common causes, that is, disease of one of 3 possible organs:

C. In contrast, in the office, the commonest cause of bilateral leg edema and its distinguishing characteristics are:
  1.
     a.
     b.
     c.

D. The other 2 common causes of bilateral leg edema in the office patient and their distinguishing characteristics:
  1.
     a.
     b.
     c.
  2.
     a.
     b.
     c.

E. Your next patient is an unscheduled 45 y/o man who is driving "straight through" from Minneapolis to Phoenix. He stopped in Amarillo about an hour ago to get gas and as he was filling the tank he "couldn't get my breath for a minute." He feels well now, but he thought he should get it checked out before driving farther. His physical exam is normal except for 2+ pitting edema in both legs. Will you merely reassure him that everything will be all right?

F. Your 60 y/o patient with history of rheumatoid arthritis and osteoarthritis has new rapid onset of unilateral leg edema. There has been chronically a bulge at the medial aspect of the popliteal fossa, and you are certain it is a Baker's cyst. You do not want to anticoagulate because Baker's cysts tend to bleed. In this patient at this moment, will you do anything besides observation?

Answers on Edema

A. Be certain of your patient's symptom and its distinguishing characteristics.
   1. History: You must know if it is new onset in the last few days or weeks or if it is episodic–most but not all days of the week, or if it is chronic, daily, persistent swelling.
   2. Exam: Examine both legs to determine if the swelling "pits" on fingertip pressure over the pretibial areas bilaterally or only unilaterally or it doesn't "pit." Immediately determine if it is new onset, unilateral swelling because dangerous diseases present in this manner and you want to identify them quickly. Bilateral chronic edema without another dangerous symptom or sign is not immediately worrisome.
B. Diseases of organs causing bilateral, pitting edema.
   Heart, liver, kidneys. Look for associated symptoms of heart disease e.g. JVD; get serum creatinine, albumin, protime, LFTs for kidney or liver disease.
C. The commonest cause of bilateral edema in the office patient.
   1. Idiopathic edema
      a. It is episodic, bilateral swelling, that is, it occurs on most days but not all days; the swelling is minimal (or much less) in the morning, and it is worst in the evening after upright posture all day. Other aggravating factors contributing to its episodic nature are hot weather, luteal phase of the menstrual cycle, high salt intake
      b. Idiopathic edema has only been described in women with onset between puberty and 45 y/o
      c. Generally, the edema is an isolated symptom
D. Two other common causes of bilateral edema in the office patient.
   1. Premenstrual syndrome (PMS)
      a. It is episodic, bilateral edema
      b. It occurs only cyclically, just before and during menses
      c. Other concomitant symptoms occur, that is, the edema is only one of a number of typical PMS symptoms–irritability, headaches, depression, breast tenderness
   2. Venous insufficiency
      a. It is chronic, daily edema. Depending on the specific etiology it may be unilateral (postphlebitic syndrome) or bilateral (varicose veins, morbid obesity)
      b. The edema may occur in either a man or woman
      c. Any concomitant symptoms result from the venous insufficiency e.g. leg pain, discoloration, rash
E. A major risk factor for DVT and symptoms of PE.
   Everything is not all right because almost certainly he just had a PE. Any time your patient has abrupt onset of unexplained dyspnea or abrupt onset of unexplained tachypnea or onset of unexplained pleuritic chest pain, then think of PE. If he also has any one risk factor, such as his ongoing prolonged immobilization while driving (causing the bilateral leg edema)–there is a high probability of PE. He should be started immediately on Lovenox and then any necessary diagnostic studies performed only later.
F. Always think of DVT if there is new onset, unilateral edema. About 10% of patients with Baker's cyst also have a DVT, so quickly get a duplex ultrasonography test of his legs.

Chapter 7 Edema

Edema

Differential diagnosis: the 3 common causes of leg edema
1. Idiopathic edema–<u>episodic</u>, bilateral leg edema in women; onset <45 y/o; no other associated symptoms
2. Premenstrual syndrome–<u>cyclic</u>, bilateral leg edema with menses; concomitant symptoms of PMS
3. Venous insufficiency–<u>chronic, daily</u> edema in a man or woman; either bilateral or unilateral; concomitant symptoms result from the leg swelling

A. **Be certain of the symptom and its distinguishing characteristics.** Your patient's problem or chief complaint is "I'm swollen all over" or "My legs are getting bigger"
   1. First, be certain the problem is ankle or foot edema, or at least pretibial edema. Be sure it is not lipidema (bilateral subcutaneous fat deposition of marked obesity, does not pit, and spares the feet); or lymphedema (early it may pit, but chronic it's non-pitting; note squaring of the toes and a dorsal hump on the foot; thickening of the skin produces a warty texture, magnifies skin creases and decreases your ability to pinch a fold of skin at the base of the second toe)
   2. Fewer than 30% of patients seen in the office with new onset leg edema will have an organic disease causing the edema, that is, more than 70% must be diagnosed clinically by H&P
   3. Ask your patient
      a. "Show me everywhere on your body where you have noticed swelling, and where it is now"
      b. "When does the swelling start and when is it the worst?"–time of day, time of month or time of year
      c. "How old were you when you first noticed this swelling?"
      d. "Are there other symptoms just before or during the time the swelling occurs?"
   4. Physical examination and laboratory
      a. To determine whether the swelling is "pitting," firmly (so the distal 20% of your nail beds are blanched) press over the pretibial or ankle area for 15-20 seconds. Grading of the severity of edema is 1-4+ or 1-6/6; equally important in grading is to determine how high up on the body the pitting edema occurs e.g. thigh, scrotum, abdomen, chest
      b. To estimate systemic venous pressure, determine if the external jugular veins are inappropriately dilated, that is, increased JVP. First, place your patient supine to be certain you can even visualize normally dilated veins, e.g. in obesity. If you can see the normally filled neck veins at 0°, then elevate her to a 45° angle at the waist, strip the right external jugular vein down to the clavicle using your right index finger and continue with pressure on the vein; then with the left index finger, strip the vein from the site of the right finger cephalad to the angle of the jaw, release the lower right finger pressure and determine if the jugular vein fills even

partially from below, suggesting increased systemic venous pressure and possibly CHF

> Be certain:
> 1. The symptom is pitting edema and bilateral
> 2. Whether it is either new edema or episodic edema or chronic, persistent edema
> 3. If it is cyclic edema
> 4. If there are any associated symptoms
>
> (If it is unilateral leg edema, see Section G.3 for approach to diagnosis.)

    c. If there is no, or only slight, elevation of the venous column with the above maneuver, keep your left index finger pressure at the jaw angle with the patient still supine at 45° angle, and now apply gentle, slow but firm pressure with your right hand to the periumbilical area and hold it for 10-30 seconds while the patient breathes quietly; resultant rise in the column of blood indicates abdominal-jugular reflux suggesting mildly increased venous pressure, consistent with mild CHF

    d. If there is any possibility of liver or kidney disease, get a urinalysis and obtain blood for serum creatinine, albumin, AST, ALT, bilirubin, electrolytes

By now you should be confident it is bilateral edema, whether it is new, episodic or chronic daily edema, and if there are associated significant clinical findings present with the edema. In almost all instances you now have the information you need for diagnosis of the obvious causes (Section C) and the common causes (Section E). In the rare instance that your patient appears different clinically from the usual office patient with edema, be certain (Section B) that she does not have a symptom or sign of a dangerous disease

B. **Be confident it's not a dangerous disease.**

1. Send immediately to the ED by ambulance if there is:
   a. Evidence of a catastrophic illness (very ill appearing patient in distress) present with edema e.g. syncope, hypotension, diaphoresis, pallor, pain, dyspnea
   b. Abrupt onset of pleuritic chest pain and dyspnea, think of PE, pneumothorax
   c. Abrupt onset of dyspnea and facial edema, think of angioedema (auscultate for inspiratory stridor over the larynx)
   d. Abrupt onset of dyspnea, think of pulmonary edema, PE, angioedema
   e. Edema and unexplained dyspnea with some relief by sitting, think of pulmonary edema, pericardial effusion (cardiac tamponade), constrictive pericarditis, severe ascites
   f. Rapid onset edema, headache, and venous engorgement of the face, chest, and arms, with distended nonpulsatile JVD, think of SVC obstruction
2. Admit at once to the ED or hospital if there is:
   a. An ill-appearing patient with dyspnea and bilateral inspiratory crackles, think of CHF, pneumonia
   b. New onset unilateral edema, think of DVT, bacterial cellulitis
   c. Edema with localized pain, tenderness, redness, think of bacterial cellulitis, thrombophlebitis, lymphangitis
   d. Rapid onset of edema, usually painful and unilateral, think of DVT, cellulitis, compartment syndrome, lymphangitis
   e. Sudden severe pain in an extremity followed by edema, think of compartment syndrome, muscle rupture e.g. gastrocnemius

Chapter 7 Edema

    f. New onset severe headache, fever, rash, myalgias, edema, think of RMSF, Kawasaki syndrome
3. Admit to the hospital or have a specialist consult as soon as possible if there is:
    a. New onset of swelling of the whole leg suggesting proximal obstruction, think of malignancy, relapsed malignancy or secondary to past cancer surgery or radiotherapy
    b. New onset of whole leg swelling in a person recently traveling to an endemic area of the world, think of filariasis
    c. Tenderness or redness of or near the leg swelling, think of thrombophlebitis, lymphangitis, cellulitis

---

Be certain in the first minutes of your exam that there is no evidence of any <u>one</u> dangerous symptom or sign associated with the edema:
1. Ill-appearing patient in distress
2. Severe dyspnea
3. Inspiratory stridor and facial edema
4. New onset unilateral leg edema
5. Leg erythema and pain

Any suggestion of a dangerous disease, send the patient to the ED.

---

    d. Unilateral leg swelling and LBP "radiating to the thigh," think of pelvic malignancy
    e. Pain and tenderness in a swollen extremity, think of thrombophlebitis, cellulitis, lymphangitis, RSD, inflamed lymphedema, musculoskeletal disorder, peripheral nerve injury
    f. Pain and swelling on the medial aspect of the popliteal space, think of Baker's cyst (it may extend distally and mimic a DVT; caution: don't anticoagulate a Baker's cyst)
    g. Edema limited to the face, neck, upper arm, think of obstructed SVC by tumor or aortic arch aneurysm
    h. Upper body vesicle, then painless black eschar with surrounding localized non-pitting edema, think of cutaneous anthrax
    i. Gradual onset of dyspnea and bilateral edema, no crackles but there is a loud S2, think of pulmonary hypertension

C. **Make a quick diagnosis if it's obvious.** Is it an easily diagnosed condition or a medication that is responsible for the edema. In most patients you will be <u>highly</u> confident of a common cause of the symptom by now. If not, one or more of the following tests may exclude an organic disease and increase your confidence in your working diagnosis: CBC, UA, creatinine, LFTs, albumin, protime, TSH
1. Disease of heart, liver or kidneys
    a. Congestive heart failure (CHF)
        (1) Patient usually >45 y/o or with a history of heart disease, and the pitting edema is bilaterally symmetrical in the legs
        (2) Earliest symptoms of CHF are new onset of unexplained fatigue, DOE, and new onset or worsening nocturia. With more severe failure, there is dyspnea at rest, often with orthopnea, bibasilar inspiratory crackles, and paroxysmal nocturnal dyspnea
        (3) Increased CVP is suggested by an increased JVP; a sign of milder CHF is positive abdominal-jugular reflux
        (4) Be alert for, and treat quickly, those conditions that may precipitate overt CHF (which until now was mild and occult): anemia, fever, infection, pregnancy, hyperthyroidism,

uncontrolled HTN, new cardiac ischemia, PE, also <u>anything</u> increasing cardiac output e.g. excesses of exertion, diet, fluids
  b. Liver disease

Recognize any easily diagnosed cause of bilateral leg edema:
1. Known or occult disease of the heart, liver, kidneys, thyroid
2. Spot diagnosis–pregnancy, toxemia of pregnancy, morbid obesity, prolonged dependent legs, trauma, malnutrition
3. Medication side effect

---

   (1) Often there is a history of alcohol abuse, along with current signs of liver disease *viz* jaundice, spider angiomata, gynecomastia, collateral venous channels, small, soft testes
   (2) Dyspnea occurs only if ascites is severe; different from CHF, JVP is not increased
   (3) Edema is due to decreased hepatic vein outflow and marked hypoalbuminemia, usually <2.5 gm/dL
  c. Renal disease
   (1) Often there is history of DM or HTN, and the edema usually is due to nephrotic syndrome with marked proteinuria (>3.5 gm/d) and low serum albumin (<2.5 gm/dL)
   (2) If the edema is rapid onset, it likely results from acute glomerulonephritis, and there is hematuria, proteinuria, urine RBC's and RBC casts
  d. Hypo-or hyperthyroidism, anemia
 2. Spot diagnoses
  a. Pregnancy–usually last trimester
  b. Preeclampsia–pregnancy with concomitant complications of systemic HTN, proteinuria, edema
  c. Morbid obesity is BMI >40 kg/m^2 (quick calculation–morbid obesity is >200 lb for 5 feet tall, then 8 lb/inch; thus a 5'6" person is morbidly obese > 250 lb, and a 6 foot tall person is morbidly obese > 300 lb)
  d. Prolonged dependent legs e.g. transoceanic flights, paralyzed limb
  e. Starvation or malnutrition with associated weight loss, cachexia
 3. Medications
  a. Antihypertensives e.g. CCBs (nifedipine, felodipine, amlodipine), α-adrenergic blockers, hydralazine, methyldopa, minoxidil, clonidine
  b. Anti-inflammatory agents e.g. all NSAIDS, prednisone, indomethacin
  c. Steroids e.g. estrogen, oral contraceptives, testosterone, anabolic-androgenic steroids, progesterone
  d. Other medications e.g. lithium, fludrocortisone, chlorpropamide, phenothiazines, insulin, growth hormone, cyclosporine, glitazones, any sodium-retaining drug

D. **Identify your patient's worries and wants.** Fluid retention ≥0.9 kg (2 lb) occurs in more than 70% of premenopausal women, and most obese people, and only few of these consult about it. During your interview and exam try to intuit or discover why your patient is here today, and not previously, for this problem. What has changed? Don't ask directly, but try to get some ideas from her

Chapter 7 Edema

responses to questions about the fluid retention and edema itself. You can't completely help your patient unless you know what she really worries about and wants from you. That's why she is here to see you--to satisfy her worries and wants! Here are only some of the possible worries and wants of your patient with edema. You must discover her specific ones

> During your exam, discover your patient's worries (e.g. heart failure, malignancy) and wants (e.g. reassurance, diuretic), so that you can respond to her specific needs as soon as possible.

1. Common worries are:
   a. That the cause of the edema is a dangerous etiology e.g. "blood clot," malignancy, CHF
   b. That the etiology is some rare disease e.g.–RSD, cat scratch fever
   c. What other fears or anxieties might be troubling your patient? For example, she may have had bilateral edema for many years, and only now does she come for help. What has changed? Perhaps a friend or relative, who had similar chronic edema, recently has been diagnosed with CHF? There are many other possibilities–think of them
2. Your patient wants:
   a. You to perform a thorough physical exam focused on possible causes of the edema and she wants appropriate tests and imaging studies
   b. A plausible explanation of the cause of the edema
   c. Confident reassurance from you that it is not a dangerous or rare etiology. Tell her–"The good news, it's not a blood clot" (or whatever you believe her real worry is)
   d. To know the prognosis, short term (effects on job, home life, marriage; how soon she will be back to normal) and long term (if recurrences are possible; how to prevent recurrences; if it will cause any disability)
   e. Treatment to stop the edema now and to prevent recurrences e.g. diuretics
   f. A specialist referral if she believes you are not confident of the diagnosis

E. Know the symptoms that differentiate the 3 common causes of edema.

1. The commonest cause is idiopathic edema, accounting for at least 80% of all new onset bilateral edema in women seen in the office
   a. Characteristics of idiopathic edema
      (1) It is bilateral edema occurring only in <u>women</u> after onset of puberty and before age 45 y/o
      (2) The edema has diurnal periodicity being worst at the end of the day, and sometimes absent on awakening in the morning
      (3) Aggravating factors are more prolonged upright posture or sitting, hot weather, and during the luteal phase, just before or during menses, high salt diet, and certain medications
      (4) On awakening she may note edema in the eyelids, face and fingers, but not at these sites late in the evening after being ambulatory all day. At the end of the day, it is worst in the feet, ankles, legs, abdomen and sometimes breasts
      (5) See Section G.4 for identifying "orthostatic edema"
   b. What suggests it might not be idiopathic edema
      (1) Anytime there is an associated symptom or sign suggesting a dangerous cause (see Section B)
      (2) If the edema is cyclic, that is, it <u>only</u> occurs just before or during menses
      (3) If the eyelid edema is worse in the morning but continues throughout the day, think of myxedema, exophthalmos, allergies, or a local cause in the eyes or face

> Most causes of leg edema in the office patient:
> 1. Idiopathic edema–<u>episodic</u>, bilateral leg edema in women; onset <45 y/o; no other symptoms
> 2. Premenstrual syndrome–<u>cyclic</u>, bilateral leg edema with menses; concomitant symptoms of PMS
> 3. Venous insufficiency–<u>chronic, daily</u> edema in a man or woman; either bilateral or unilateral; concomitant symptoms are due to the leg swelling

      (4) If edema occurs only in the legs and never is noticeable in the eyelids or fingers, think of venous or lymphatic obstruction or other local causes in the legs
      (5) If there is no demonstrable objective pitting edema over the pretibial area or feet at 4-8 pm after a typical day of upright activity. Very importantly, lack of objective leg edema on exam earlier in the day, e.g. in the morning or at noon, is <u>not</u> evidence against idiopathic edema
      (6) If there is <u>any</u> other pertinent physical sign besides pitting edema e.g. JVD
  2. Common look-alikes and how each differs from idiopathic edema
    a. Premenstrual syndrome (PMS)
      (1) Bilateral edema occurs cyclically, that is, only before or during early menses; concomitant PMS symptoms of headache, irritability, depression, breast tenderness
      (2) The patient with cyclic complaints only during the luteal (premenstrual) phase may have mild idiopathic edema during the rest of the month, and the edema is aggravated in the premenstrual time The same tests for orthostatic edema might be done (see Section G.4)
    b. Venous insufficiency
      (1) In a recent study venous insufficiency was the initial diagnosis in 70% of patients as the etiology of new onset bilateral edema, but it was the final diagnosis in only 22%, that is, venous insufficiency probably is very over-diagnosed in the office (Am J Med <u>105</u>, 192, 1998)
      (2) Varicose veins or venous thromboses often precede venous insufficiency, but only 20% of patients with postphlebitic syndrome causing edema can recall an episode of DVT.
      (3) It may be either unilateral or bilateral asymmetrical pitting edema. With chronicity there often is golden brown skin discoloration (hemosiderin) or rash, and trauma <u>readily</u> causes venous stasis ulcers

F. Use this summary for efficient diagnosis of a common cause. With the information from Sections A-E in mind, here is the rapid approach to diagnosis of bilateral leg edema.
  1. You already have determined:
    a. In Section A, by H&P that it is bilateral leg edema and it is pitting

Chapter 7 Edema

edema. (If it is unilateral edema, see below, Section G.3).
   b. In Section B, that there is no evidence in the H&P of a dangerous cause of the edema.
   c. In Section C, that there is not an easily diagnosed cause of the edema–neither physical disease, a spot diagnosis, nor a medication side effect.
2. From the focused H&P almost always you should quickly be confident of a working diagnosis. Confident final diagnosis is made only in followup the next days, weeks, or months when the response to treatment or nontreatment is appropriate to your working diagnosis.
   a. If there is evidence for diurnal worsening of bilateral edema later in the day, most days when she is ambulatory, in an otherwise healthy woman, it likely is idiopathic edema
   b. If the bilateral leg edema occurs only near the time of menses and there are associated typical symptoms, it likely is edema associated with premenstrual syndrome (PMS)
   c. If there is chronic, persistent unilateral or bilateral leg edema associated with signs of venous stasis and cutaneous pigmentation, it likely is due to venous insufficiency
3. Answer your patient's worries and wants that you determined early on during the exam (Section D). Have you done everything you can to help her?
4. You now have a working diagnosis, but only with followup can you be confident it is correct. In return visits you are always testing by H&P that your working diagnosis is correct.

G. Abandon your working diagnosis and look for an uncommon cause only if:

1. Any <u>one</u> dangerous symptom or sign (see above, Section B) occurs in followup of weeks, months, or years. Quickly obtain a consult or send the patient to the hospital as appropriate
2. The edema does not respond to treatment as you expect or the natural history of your working diagnosis does not occur. Idiopathic edema does not worsen, and orthostatic edema (the 80% with abnormal water excretion, see Section G.4) should get much better with treatment. Morning weight can be reduced by up to 9 lb and mean weight gain during the day can be decreased toward normal of <1.5 lb. There should be significant symptomatic response and diminished evening edema

> If your patient's symptoms do not respond as expected to your management, he may have an uncommon or rare cause listed in Section G.2 that you can diagnose and treat. Or, you may want to refer your patient to a specialist.

<u>Don't</u> spend time and money looking for one of the following causes until you are sure your patient doesn't have one of the 3 common causes above. Nevertheless, it may be that she has an uncommon or rare cause of the edema. These are important to recognize because each has a different treatment or prophylaxis
   a. Myxedema--get a serum free T4 level and TSH; even subclinical hypothyroidism may aggravate the idiopathic edema (serum TSH >2.0 with normal range fT4)
   b. Syndromes of glucocorticoid excess e.g. Cushing's syndrome--get 24 hr urine for cortisol, total protein and creatinine clearance if suggested by signs or symptoms
   c. Syndromes of mineralocorticoid excess e.g. Conn's syndrome–obtain 24 hr urine aldosterone, plasma renin and aldosterone

d. Nutritional deficiency e.g. beriberi, scurvy, marasmus, kwashiorkor–evidence of malnutrition e.g. alcoholic, homeless, food faddists
e. Anorexia nervosa–suspect clinically by BMI <20.
f. Cardiac valve disease--mitral stenosis, tricuspid regurgitation
g. Eosinophilic fasciitis–rapid onset of pain, extreme tenderness, and pitting edema of upper or lower extremities, often following strenuous exercise
h. Right atrial myxoma–mimics tricuspid regurgitation
i. Whipple's disease--edema, diarrhea, weight loss, arthralgias in middle-aged white men
j. Pulmonary hypertension–symptoms suggesting CHF (fatigue, progressively worsening DOE, bilateral edema) but loud S2 on exam and no crackles
k. Autonomic insufficiency–orthostatic hypotension, erectile dysfunction
l. Scleroderma (early stage)–pitting edema feet and dorsum hands
m. Hyperbradykininism–orthostatic decreased SBP (low pulse pressure), tachycardia, supine flushing, purplish discolored legs on standing
n. Capillary leak syndrome–episodic, rapid onset edema associated with profound hypotension
o. Factitious edema–unusual or changing clinical presentation; diagnosis of exclusion only

3. Unilateral leg edema requires a different approach to diagnosis. Ask "Have you ever had this swelling before now?" and "Exactly when did this swelling begin?"
   a. New onset unilateral swelling, think of:
      (1) Deep venous thrombosis (DVT)--unless you are very confident it is not a DVT, get an ultrasound study of the legs immediately
      (2) Bacterial cellulitis–localized plaque with pain, tenderness, redness and increased warmth over the area of swelling
      (3) Erythema nodosum–raised red, smooth areas usually below the knees; may be fever, pain in joints and muscles, malaise
      (4) Either popliteal (Baker's) cyst or ruptured head of the gastrocnemius muscle may mimic DVT; the latter occurs suddenly during exercise, with tearing or severe pain in the calf and only 1-2 days later, ankle swelling; again, any question that it could be DVT, Doppler ultrasound should be done
      (5) Osteomyelitis may be difficult to distinguish by plain films from early Charcot's joint; each can cause unilateral edema
      (6) Compartment syndrome–sudden severe pain, then induration and edema
      (7) Retroperitoneal fibrosis–unilateral or bilateral edema
   b. Chronic unilateral swelling, think of:
      (1) Venous insufficiency (see above, Section E.2.b)--If this swelling has begun recently for the first time, get a Doppler ultrasound study. Get the study more urgently if there is any one risk factor for DVT (any past history of DVT or PE; morbid obesity; recent immobilization, even prolonged sedentary travel; pelvic or hip surgery or trauma in the past 3 months)
      (2) Lymphedema (see above, A.1.)–Usually it is painless and non-pitting, and it may precede signs of malignancy, which is responsible for the obstructed lymphatics; get pelvic CT scan and in men, PSA; other causes are infection or scarring from previous surgery or radiation therapy
      (3) RSD (complex regional pain syndrome) is a clinical diagnosis, that is, no specific test. It has 3 clinical aspects or stages, each lasting variable times up to 3-6 months:
         (a) An initiating event or trauma followed by Stage I, burning pain and edema in the extremity, especially when the extremity is dependent
         (b) State II, "dystrophic" stage with change from edema to induration, cool hyperhidrotic skin and cyanosis
         (c) Stage III, "atrophic" stage with proximal spread of the pain and irreversible tissue damage; thin, shiny skin, wasted digits, Dupuytren's contractures

4. Evidence consistent with diagnosis of idiopathic edema is the following:
   a. Obtain 3-4 weeks of body weights daily after voiding, both on arising in the morning and just before bedtime after daily upright activities. Weights must be in the nude and NPO in the morning before weighing. Do not alert her to your predominant interest in diurnal weight differences. Also have her record times of menses, significant changes in activity (shopping, travel, naps, illness with bed rest), medications, water intake, dietary, environmental (heat) changes. Mean weight gains from morning to bedtime ≥0.7 kg (1.5 lb) along with the typical history strongly suggests idiopathic edema is the etiology
   b. About 80% of patients with idiopathic edema can be further identified as "orthostatic edema." This is important because specific therapy may become available. Each day she comes to the office NPO, and between 0730-0900 hr she

Chapter 7 Edema 95

drinks un-iced tap water (20 ml/kg) at a maximum of 1500 ml over 15-20 minutes. On day 1 she remains supine throughout the 4 hr test, and day 2 she is up walking slowly or standing during the 4 hr test. All urine is collected during the 4 hr, and the bladder is emptied at the end of 4 hr each day for urine total volume excreted.
  (1) Failure to excrete >55% of the water load in the upright position, along with excretion >65% supine is typical of orthostatic edema
  (2) Abnormally low excretion rates on both days suggest an alternative diagnosis e.g. cardiac or renal disease, SIADH

H. Use the glossary for precise thinking and accurate diagnosis.

1. **Anascara** (Greek *hydrops ana sarka* meant "fluid throughout the flesh.") We still use the term for generalized massive edema.
2. **Angioedema** (Greek *angeion* meaning "vessel" and *oidema*, "swelling.") It is localized swelling due to vasodilatation and increased capillary permeability in the dermis or subcutaneous tissues.
3. **Anthrax** (word in Greek for "coal.") The skin lesion of anthrax is a carbuncle (Latin *carbo* for "coal") with a hard black center surrounded by a red rim, and it resembles a hot coal or charcoal.
4. **Ascites** (Greek *askos* meaning "pouch or sack" for carrying wine.) It is fluid-filled abdomen resembling such a partially full leather bag.
5. **Beriberi** (word in Singhalese for "extremely weak" due to thiamine deficiency.) It is a "disease of progress" in that the processing to obtain white rice required the husk containing thiamine be removed.
6. **Dropsy** (Greek *hydrops* meaning "fluid.") Then the French used *hydropsie* as a generic term for accumulated excess fluid in any tissue or body cavity, or more specifically for the edema of CHF. The term is no longer medically useful, but you may occasionally hear it used, especially by an older patient.
7. **Dyspnea** (Greek *dys* meaning "difficult' and *pnoia*, "breathing.") It is difficult or labored breathing in any position.
8. **Edema** (Greek *oidema* meaning "a swelling.") It is a generic term for any tumorous condition, but now we restrict the term to tissue swelling due to accumulation of fluid in the interstitial spaces.
9. **Hydrothorax** (Greek *hydro* meaning "water" and *thorax,* "chest.") It is a collection of watery fluid in the pleural cavity, which is more commonly called pleural effusion.
10. **Idiopathic** (Greek *idios* meaning "personal or one's own" and *pathos*, "suffering or disease.") Formerly it identified a disease peculiar to that one individual, in that the disease arose from within him, rather than from a cause outside of him. Now the word often is used to describe a disease or sign of unknown causation.
11. **Interstitial** (fluid) (Latin *inter* meaning "between, among" and *sistere*, "to put or to place.") It is fluid occupying space between the cells of a tissue.
12. **Kwashiorkor** (from Ghana meaning "red boy," referring to red hair and lightened skin.) It indicates very severe malnutrition with serum albumin <2.5 gm/dL and wasted abdominal muscles causing a potbelly due to ascites.
13. **Lymphedema** (Latin *lympha* meaning "water" and Greek *oidema*, "swelling.,") It is swelling of an extremity due to accumulated watery fluid caused by obstruction of lymph channels.
14. **Marasmus** (Greek *marairein* meaning "to waste away.") It now refers to severe protein-calorie malnutrition with serum albumin >2.5 gm/dL. It is less severe than kwashiorkor.
15. **Nephrosis** (Greek *nephros* meaning "kidney.") It refers to any disease of kidneys, especially degenerative lesions of renal tubules leading to albuminuria, hypoalbuminemia, edema.
16. **Orthopnea** (Greek *ortho* meaning "straight or erect" and *pnoia*, "breathing.") It commonly refers to CHF, when upright posture allows easier breathing and the supine position causes rapid onset of dyspnea.
17. **Paroxysmal** (nocturnal dyspnea) (Greek *paroxysmos* meaning "a sudden recurrence of symptoms.") It refers to abrupt awakening after a few hours sleep and it is due to pulmonary edema causing severe dyspnea.
18. **Platypnea** (Greek *platy* meaning "flat" and *pnoia*, "breathing.") It is easier breathing in the recumbent position, and more difficult breathing in the upright position.
19. **Preeclampsia** (Latin *pre* meaning "before or preceding" and *eklampein*, "a sudden shining or flashing.") Originally the flashing referred to scintillating flashing lights seen just before any type of seizure or eclampsia. Later it referred to the hypertension, edema, proteinuria (renal impairment), that came before (preeclampsia) the more severe eclampsia.
20. **Pregnant** (Latin *pre* meaning "before" and *natus*, "birth.") A woman's condition before giving birth.

Chapter 8 Fatigue

Questions on Fatigue

A. In a patient who complains "I'm weak all over," the most important
   1. Finding in the history is:
   2. First physical exam test is:
B. If your patient is certain her "weakness" began "the week before Thanksgiving," 6 weeks ago, in any workup you must:

C. List some characteristics you listen for while she is telling you about her "weakness," to tell you it is chronic fatigue:
   1.
   2.
   3.
D. You now are confident it is chronic fatigue and there is no symptom or sign suggesting an organic or dangerous disease. The commonest cause of <u>chronic</u> fatigue and its distinguishing characteristics are:
   1.
      a.
      b.
E. The other 3 common causes of <u>chronic</u> fatigue are:
   1.
   2.
   3.
F. What is problematic about the following statement?
"If you want to know whether a certain medication causes fatigue, just look it up in the PDR."

G. How do you differentiate chronic fatigue syndrome (CFS) from other causes of chronic fatigue, and which is commoner?

H. In physical exam testing for fibromyalgia, where are the "control points"?

Chapter 8 Fatigue

Answers on Fatigue
A. Be certain that the symptom is fatigue
  1. Precisely what it is she cannot do because of her "weakness." If she identifies a specific action requiring a single muscle or muscle group, then she likely has weakness, and not fatigue. Weakness points to a neurological or muscular disease, whereas fatigue suggests a syndrome e.g. fibromyalgia. But if she volunteers "I just feel ill" or "I'm not myself, something is wrong," be concerned that it is malaise suggesting an occult disease
  2. If there is any suggestion it is weakness (and not fatigue) perform strength testing in appropriate muscles or muscle groups. If it is fatigue, there will be no abnormal sign on exam
B. Implications of a new onset "fatigue"
  It is an organic disease until proven otherwise. Certainty that fatigue began <1-2 months ago dictates a dedicated search for an organic disease etiology. In most instances, however, an obvious cause e.g. infection can be found by history. You must be alert, as always, for any one sign of a dangerous disease
C. Typical characteristics of chronic fatigue
  1. The "weakness" definitely did not begin recently i.e. it has been present months, and usually years, and it has not been progressively worsening
  2. She awakens just as tired as she was when she went to bed
  3. She always is tired, just lying around, so her tiredness is not related to physical or mental effort
D. The commonest cause of chronic fatigue
  1. Fibromyalgia
     a. Generalized pain is an equally important symptom
     b. Physical exam finding of bilateral symmetrical tender points at typical locations (upper back, posterior neck-hairline, upper anterior chest, greater trochanters)
E. The other 3 common causes of chronic fatigue
  1. Psychiatric disorders *viz* MD, GAD, somatization disorder
  2. Chronic fatigue syndrome (CFS)
  3. Idiopathic chronic fatigue
F. Limitations of the PDR (Physician's Desk Reference) to determine if a medication causes fatigue (or any new symptom)
  Any medication can cause new onset fatigue. In clinical trials of new drugs, new onset fatigue in patients taking placebo occurs in up to 25% of patients. Moreover, any drug can cause almost any new symptom in your individual patient. Thus onset of a new symptom, such as fatigue, within 2-3 weeks of starting a new medication suggests the medication may be responsible
G. Recognize the low prevalence of CFS
  CFS is uncommon. CFS accounts only for about 1% of all chronic fatigue, and prevalence of chronic fatigue in the general population might be up to 40%. Idiopathic chronic fatigue and fibromyalgia are very common diagnoses in patients with chronic fatigue
H. Know and test the control points in any patient with chronic pain
  Control points are areas where pressing with your thumb, at increasing pressure, can not elicit pain. Sites commonly used are the patient's thumbnail and center of the forehead. In any patient complaining of pain, firm pressure at these sites can provide you with some idea of your individual patient's "pain sensitivity." You then can evaluate better whether the problem is either too much pain or your patient's heightened sensitivity to mild pain

Fatigue

Differential diagnosis: the 4 common causes of chronic fatigue
1. Fibromyalgia–bilateral tender points; generalized pain
2. Psychiatric disorder:
   a. MD–anhedonia, depressed mood
   b. GAD–constant worrying about a future catastrophe
   c. Somatization disorder–multiple system pains
3. CFS–profound exhaustion, ST, tender lymph nodes
4. Idiopathic chronic fatigue–patients not meeting CFS criteria

A. **Be certain of the symptom and its distinguishing characteristics.** Your patient's problem or chief complaint is "I'm weak all over." Ask her–"Tell me exactly what you mean by that." Let her tell you at length exactly what she has been feeling, and don't let her use the words "tired" or "weak" in her description. Sometimes it really is sleepiness or SOB or "sadness" and not fatigue. Get clearly in your mind precisely what is going on in her daily life, especially regarding her usual activities at home, at work, and on weekends (it takes you only minutes if you listen carefully). "What exactly does the fatigue or tiredness keep you from doing?" and "When did it begin, that is, when was the last time you had lots of energy?" If she cannot remember when the fatigue began, then it almost certainly is chronic fatigue with insidious onset. Most important–"How are you sleeping?" and "Everybody has pains–show me everywhere you hurt"

1. As soon as possible in talking with her, be certain that her problem is not weakness. Weakness commonly is regional and not generalized. When a person is weak, she is unable to do certain physical movements or use a certain muscle group, many times, or at all, compared to previously. For example, if there is muscle weakness, she may volunteer "I can't comb my hair" or "I can't lift the baby (or groceries)" or "I can't get out of a chair or climb stairs." That suggests weakness and indicates, almost always, organic disease due to a neural or muscular lesion. If her story suggests weakness, immediately test the likely involved muscle groups for strength, but recognize that patients with fatigue commonly do not expend much effort in your strength tests, so your judgment is very important. Also, a patient with pain in the involved limb may have antalgic weakness, that is, the pain prevents full effort

2. Be alert while listening to her narrative of her problem for her volunteering "I feel ill (or sick)" or "I just don't feel well." This suggests malaise, which is a clue that an underlying occult disease may be present. For the same reason, be alert for the patient whose stamina, or capacity for hard work has recently significantly decreased

3. If she does not have weakness or malaise, she likely has fatigue. Characteristics to look for in her description of her daily life

Chapter 8 Fatigue

suggesting the typical patient with chronic fatigue:
  a. The problem has been present more than a few months, and it may fluctuate in severity but it is not worsening
  b. She lacks ambition or desire to "do anything"
  c. She goes to bed at night tired, and awakens in the morning just as tired

---

Be certain:
1. The symptom is fatigue (tiredness or lack of energy) and not either muscle weakness or malaise
2. Whether it is either new fatigue (present <1-2 months) or chronic daily fatigue
3. If the onset of fatigue was either rapid or insidious
4. Whether the fatigue is generalized or regional
5. If there are significant concomitant symptoms

---

  d. She feels tired just lying in bed or sitting or before beginning any activity, that is, her fatigue or tiredness is not related to any physical or mental effort
4. If she has not volunteered it, ask her "How has the fatigue affected your daily life?" You must grasp how much the fatigue has changed her "appetite" for sex, hobbies, sports, food, job–whatever it is that she really enjoyed in the past, before the fatigue began. Also, most patients with fatigue are chronically sleep deprived, and sleep disorders are common. Ask: "What is your usual bedtime?", "What time do you get up from sleep?" and "How many times do you get up at night?" Very importantly "What time of day do you usually take a nap?" Naps lead to disturbed night sleep, and they are a common cause of fatigue
5. Physical examination
  a. Look for symptoms and signs of undiagnosed organic diseases, especially cardiopulmonary, thyroid, liver, renal, DM, HIV infection, anemia, electrolyte disorder
  b. If it is new onset fatigue (<1-2 months) always get rectal temperatures at home tid for a few days. Patients who don't get you such readings, let you know that the fatigue really is not much of a problem to them, whereas detection of fever may convert the problem to a possible, dangerous, treatable FUO
  c. Tender points characteristic of fibromyalgia are bilateral and generalized, that is, not just regional or unilateral
  d. Search thoroughly for tender lymph nodes of CFS, and be especially thorough in searching for lymphadenectasis suggesting organic disease. Also, get a rectal temperature in the office, remembering the diurnal increase (<1°F) in the afternoon

By now you should be confident your patient has fatigue and not weakness or malaise, whether it is new onset or chronic fatigue, and if there are concomitant important symptoms, especially pain. In almost all instances you now have the information you need for diagnosis of the obvious causes (Section C) and the common causes (Section E). In the rare instance that your patient appears different clinically from the usual office patient with fatigue, be certain (Section B) that she does not

have a symptom or sign of a dangerous disease.
B. Be confident it's not a dangerous disease.
1. Send immediately to the ED by ambulance if there is:
   a. Severe fatigue, confusion, bradycardia, hypothermia, think of myxedema coma.
   b. Elderly patient with new onset atrial fibrillation and confusion, think of apathetic hyperthyroidism, possible thyroid storm
   c. Chronic fatigue, weight loss, confusion, orthostatic hypotension, think of Addison's disease or crisis, severe hypercalcemia
   d. Chronic fatigue and now pallor and acute chest pain, think of cardiac ischemia due to anemia
   e. New onset fatigue, mild fever in an elderly confused patient, think of meningitis, pneumonia, urosepsis

---

Be certain in the first minutes of your exam, that there is no evidence of any one dangerous symptom or sign associated with the fatigue:

1. Rapid onset fatigue in a patient >50 y/o
2. Any one mental status change
3. Any one focal neurological sign
4. New cardiac murmur
5. Unexplained night sweats or fever or weight loss
6. Lymphadenectasis or rash or high ESR

Any suggestion of a dangerous disease, send your patient to the ED.

---

2. Admit at once to the ED or hospital if there is:
   a. Recent onset of fatigue and personality change, and now difficulty speaking, think of an encephalitis, e.g. HIV, WNV
   b. Fatigue, fever, heart murmur, high ESR, think of SBE, atrial myxoma
   c. Recent onset of fatigue, fever and "gastroenteritis" in an asplenic patient, think of early sepsis
   d. Chronic fatigue and now fever and localized back pain, think of spinal epidural abscess
   e. Episodic fatigue and simultaneous headache only in the winter, think of carbon monoxide poisoning
3. Admit to the hospital or have a specialist consult as soon as appropriate if there is:
   a. Fatigue, anorexia and weight loss, high ESR, think of malignancy, Addison's disease, PMR, TA, SBE
   b. New onset of fatigue and nocturia in a patient with known CAD, think of CHF, undiagnosed T2DM
   c. Muscle fatigue recurring with exercise and recovering with rest, think of MG
   d. Fatigue and unexplained rash, think of SLE
   e. Fatigue and somnolence, think of myxedema coma, narcolepsy, OSA, MD, illicit drugs, medications
   f. Characteristics of fatigue suggesting an organic disease causation: new onset; fatigue relieved by sleep; no morning fatigue, fatigue only later in the day; progressively worsening fatigue over weeks

C. Make a quick diagnosis if it's obvious.
Is it an easily diagnosed cause or a medication that is responsible for the fatigue? In most patients you will be highly confident of a common cause of the symptom by now. If not, one or more of the following tests may exclude an organic disease and increase your confidence in your working diagnosis: CBC, ESR, HIV, β-hCG, creatinine, albumin, UA, glucose, electrolytes, Ca, Mg, TSH, LFTs

1. New onset (<1-2 months) fatigue
   a. Recent or ongoing infection–almost any self-limited viral infection can cause fatigue lasting 1-2 months; also be alert for symptoms of IM, HIV, HBV, HCV, SBE, Lyme disease

Chapter 8 Fatigue 101

   b. Undiagnosed common organic diseases of heart, lung, liver, kidney, thyroid; almost always diagnosis should be evident from your H&P (and lab, only if indicated)
2. Sleep disorders–
   a. OSA– loud snoring, frequent awakenings, significant obesity (20% of OSA patients are not obese).
   b. RLS– dysesthesias in the legs (sometimes arms also) causing an uncontrollable urge to move the affected limbs; occurs especially at night or with inactivity; very common and treatable by dopaminergic drugs
   c. Substance abuse–alcohol, caffeine, illicit drugs
   d. Medications–hypnotics, tranquilizers, diuretics

Recognize any easily diagnosed cause of fatigue:
1. <u>New onset</u> (<1-2 months) fatigue–recent infection, pregnancy, or previously undiagnosed organic disease (HIV, hepatitis, heart, lungs, liver, kidney, thyroid, uncontrolled DM) shown by abnormal signs on physical exam or lab
2. <u>Chronic</u>
   a. Sleep disorders (OSA, insomnia, narcolepsy, RLS)
   b. The patient's style of living (high stress, substance abuse); morbid obesity
   c. PMS–associated cyclic symptoms
   d. Medication side effect

---

3. Lifestyle factors–There are multiple daily demands, most self-imposed, on the typical individual in our culture. From an evolutionary perspective, our bodies and minds are simply not suited for many of these demands, and it's a wonder there aren't more complaints of fatigue than the reported 30-40% prevalence. From Section A, you should already have a clear picture of her daily life, and the demands she makes on her body, so you can judge the contribution that lifestyle factors might play in her fatigue, and you can treat appropriately. Although illicit drugs are always identified as one cause of fatigue, the overwhelming majority of people with chronic fatigue in our society abuse either or both of the following legal substances:
   a. Obesity–excess food intake is a substance abuse (abstinence from food results in immediate withdrawal symptoms)
   b. Daily "social" alcohol intake almost always is more than she admits, and it is a common cause or contributor to many symptoms, especially sleep problems, fatigue, GI symptoms of dyspepsia and diarrhea
4. Miscellaneous–pregnancy, PMS or menopause commonly have associated fatigue.
5. Medications
   a. Almost any medication can cause fatigue, for example, 25% of people taking placebo in a drug trial complained of new fatigue. So any medication that was started or increased in dosage near the time of onset of the fatigue should be suspect for causing fatigue

in your patient. Insist the patient bring everything she puts into her mouth except food–the "brown bag test." Let her know that includes vitamins and herbs and "natural remedies" that she might consider to be food. Recognize that she may be reluctant to reveal some of them to you
- b. Common medications known to cause fatigue:
  (1) Glucocorticoids
  (2) Antihypertensives (β-blockers, clonidine, reserpine, methyldopa)
  (3) Most sedatives and tranquilizers (even those to treat anxiety)
  (4) Antihistamines e.g. diphenhydramine, chlorpheniramine
  (5) Antidepressants especially amitriptyline, doxepin, trazodone
  (6) Anticholinergics
  (7) See below, Section G.3.c.(6) for drugs causing depression, and then concomitant fatigue

D. **Identify your patient's worries and wants.** Chronic fatigue occurs in 25-40% of 40 y/o "healthy" people, and few people with symptoms of fatigue consult about it. During your interview and exam try to intuit or discover why your patient is here today for her fatigue. If it is chronic fatigue, why has she waited until now? What has changed? Don't ask directly, but try to get some ideas from your patient's responses to questions about her perception of the fatigue itself. You can't completely help your patient unless you know what she really worries about and wants from you. That's why she is here to see you--to satisfy her worries and wants! Here are only some of the possible worries and wants of your patient with fatigue, you must discover her specific ones.

During your exam, discover your patient's worries (e.g. cancer, infection) and wants (e.g. reassurance, antibiotic), so that you can respond to her specific needs as soon as possible.

---

1. Common worries are:
   a. That the cause of the fatigue is a dangerous etiology e.g. cancer, chronic infection (TB, HIV, hepatitis, syphilis)
   b. That the etiology is some rare disease, e.g. WNV, SARS, multiple chemical sensitivity, Lyme disease
   c. What other fears or anxieties might be troubling your patient? For example, she may have had fatigue at other times, and only with this fatigue does she come for help. What has changed? Perhaps a friend or relative, who had similar chronic fatigue, recently has been diagnosed with colon cancer. There are many other possibilities–think of them
2. Your patient wants:
   a. You to perform a thorough physical exam focused on possible causes of the fatigue and she wants appropriate tests and imaging studies, e.g. testing for "chronic mono" or "hypoglycemia" or "systemic yeast infection" or "thyroid," whatever her friend or newspaper article has said might be responsible for her fatigue
   b. A plausible explanation of the cause of the fatigue
   c. Confident reassurance from you that it is not a dangerous or rare etiology. Tell her, "The good news, it's not cancer" (or whatever you believe her real worry is)
   d. To know the prognosis, short term (effects on job, home life, marriage; how soon she will be back to normal) and long term (if recurrences are possible; how to prevent recurrences; if it will cause any disability)
   e. Treatment to relieve symptoms and stop the fatigue now, and to prevent recurrences
   f. A specialist referral if she believes you are not confident of the diagnosis

E. **Know the symptoms that differentiate the 4 common causes of fatigue.**
1. The commonest cause is fibromyalgia
   a. Characteristics of fibromyalgia

(1) All patients have chronic <u>widespread</u> musculoskeletal aching and stiffness
(2) Insidious onset of symptoms in a patient <50 y/o
(3) <u>Tender points (bilateral)</u> are an essential feature for diagnosis

---

Common disorders causing <u>chronic daily</u> fatigue in the office patient:
1. Fibromyalgia–bilateral tender points; generalized pain
2. Psychiatric disorder:
   a. MD–anhedonia, depressed mood
   b. GAD–constant worrying about a future catastrophe
   c. Somatization disorder–multiple system pain
3. CFS–profound exhaustion, ST, tender lymph nodes
4. Idiopathic chronic fatigue– patients not meeting CFS criteria

---

    b. What suggests it might not be fibromyalgia
      (1) Anytime there is any one associated symptom or sign suggesting a dangerous cause (see above, Section B)
      (2) If characteristic bilateral tender points are absent on your exam
2. Common look-alikes causing fatigue and how each differs from fibromyalgia
    a. Psychiatric disorders. Not uncommonly, fibromyalgia occurs along with a psychiatric disorder, so both conditions must be treated
      (1) MD
        (a) Anhedonia almost always is present. That is, she no longer has her usual "appetites" for one or more previously enjoyable activities–food, sex, hobby, work, music, sports. She enjoys the activity much less or not at all, and this is very different from the past, before she had fatigue.
        (b) Depressed mood and worry about past actions (guilt)
      (2) GAD
        (a) She especially has trouble falling asleep at night, commonly because she lies awake worrying about <u>future</u> catastrophic events that could occur, but are extremely unlikely to occur; this characteristic worrying dominates most of her waking day also
        (b) She may feel much stress and anxiety just due to her everyday life, an inner turmoil, and she can't deal with everyday problems effectively, as others do or as she did in the past
      (3) Somatization disorder
        (a) She has now, or has a history of, multi-organ pain e.g. headache, backache, joint, muscle, abdomen, rectum
        (b) Commonly she has one or more GI and GU symptoms e.g. nausea, bloating, food intolerance, sexual indifference, decreased libido, change in menses, and at least one symptom suggesting neurological disease
    b. CFS
      (1) Chronic fatigue (>6 months), that is, profound exhaustion dominates the clinical picture. Frequently there is history of infection preceding onset of the fatigue; onset was sudden, and she can often date the onset. Fibromyalgia and depression may

occur concomitant with CFS.
  - (2) If there are at least 4 of the following symptoms present for 6 months and since the fatigue began, then diagnose CFS: impaired concentration or short term memory loss, ST, tender cervical or axillary lymph nodes, myalgias, multijoint arthralgias, new type of headache, unrefreshing sleep, postexertional fatigue lasting >24 hr
  c. Idiopathic chronic fatigue–If your patient does not meet criteria for either CFS or fibromyalgia, diagnose idiopathic chronic fatigue. Treatment is symptomatic for either diagnosis, including treatment for concomitant MD or GAD

F. Use this summary for efficient diagnosis of a common cause.
With the information in mind from Sections A-E, here is the rapid approach to diagnosis of fatigue.
  1. You already have determined:
     a. In Section A, by H&P, that she has generalized fatigue and not weakness or malaise.
     b. In Section B, that there is no evidence in the H&P of a dangerous cause of the fatigue.
     c. In Section C, that there is not an obvious cause of her fatigue– neither physical disease, style of living, nor medication.
  2. From the focused H&P almost always you should quickly be confident of a working diagnosis. Confident final diagnosis is made only in followup the next weeks, months, or even years when the response to treatment or nontreatment is appropriate to your working diagnosis.
     a. If there is chronic fatigue with widespread aching pains and <u>bilateral</u> tender points on exam, diagnose fibromyalgia; if tender points are not present but there is history of sudden onset of profound fatigue following an "infection" and there are other characteristic symptoms, diagnose CFS; or if criteria are insufficient for CFS, diagnose idiopathic chronic fatigue
     b. If there is evidence of anhedonia unassociated with any single objective sign of physical illness, the likely cause is MD; diagnose and treat appropriately.
     c. If the patient is the "worry wart" in the family, has difficulty falling asleep at night, especially because she worries about future possible but highly unlikely catastrophic events, the diagnosis likely is GAD
     d. If in addition to her chronic fatigue, she has now or in the past, had multisystem pains, plus GI, GU, and neurological symptoms, she likely has somatization disorder
  3. Answer your patient's worries and wants that you determined early on during the exam (Section D). Have you done everything you can to help her?
  4. You now have a working diagnosis, but only with followup, sometimes long term, can you be confident it is correct. In return visits you are always testing by H&P that your working diagnosis is correct.

G. Abandon your working diagnosis and look for an uncommon cause only if:
  1. Any one dangerous symptom or sign (see above, Section B) occurs in followup of

Chapter 8 Fatigue 105

weeks, months, or years. Quickly obtain a consult or send your patient to the hospital as appropriate.
2. The cause of the fatigue does not respond to treatment as you expect or the natural history of your working diagnosis does not occur. The common etiologies, MD and

> If your patient's symptoms do not respond as expected to your management, he may have an uncommon or rare cause listed in Section G.2 that you can diagnose and treat. Or, you may want to refer your patient to a specialist.

GAD, should respond to SSRI antidepressant medications, although response may take a few months. Somatization disorder, however, may be resistant to most therapies and require referral. Fibromyalgia may respond to an exercise program and a TCA. If a different "fatigue" occurs after adequate treatment and relief of the original fatigue, be sure it is not psychiatric weakness or malaise, and proceed as appropriate.

Don't spend time and money looking for one of the following etiologies until you are sure your patient doesn't have one of the common causes of fatigue. Nevertheless, it may be that she has an uncommon or rare cause of the fatigue. These are important to recognize because each is an organic disease and has specific treatment.
  a. Endocrine diseases: Cushing's, Addison's, Conn's syndrome (hyperaldosteronism), pheochromocytoma, prolactinoma
  b. Liver diseases--chronic active hepatitis, primary biliary cirrhosis, sclerosing cholangitis, intrahepatic malignancy, abscess, recurrent intrahepatic cholestasis
  c. Heart diseases– cardiomyopathy, coarctation of aorta, pulmonic stenosis, mitral stenosis, ASD, constrictive pericarditis
  d. Neurological diseases– parkinsonism, MS, demyelination disorders
  e. Chronic infection--malaria, Lyme disease
  f. Nutritional deficiency
  g. Autoimmune disorders–SLE, MG, RA
  h. Sarcoidosis–lymphadenectasis, dry cough, DOE, anorexia, weight loss, high ESR
  i. MM–malaise, bone pain (especially on movement), anemia, patient >40 y/o, history of infections
3. "Depression" may be due to one or more of the following mental disorders
  a. Major depression (MD)
  b. Bipolar disorder–additional manic episodes
  c. Other depressive conditions
     (1) Uncomplicated bereavement
     (2) Dysthymic disorder–prolonged depressed mood (>2 yr) but less severe than MD
     (3) Cyclothymic disorder--chronic mood swings >2 yr but less severe than bipolar
     (4) Adjustment disorder with depressed mood–maladaptive reaction to stress; tearfulness and depressed mood
     (5) Borderline personality disorder
     (6) Depression secondary to medication or drugs
        (a) Depression–alcohol, cocaine, illicit drug withdrawal, glucocorticoids, benzodiazepines, oral contraceptives, tamoxifen, interferon, digitalis intoxication, naltrexone
        (b) Mania-hypomania–glucocorticoids, amphetamines, cocaine, other recreational drugs, antidepressants, anabolic-androgenic steroids, L-dopa, L-thyroxine

H. Use the glossary for precise thinking and accurate diagnosis.

1. **Anhedonia** (Greek *an* meaning "without" and *hedone*, "pleasure.") Loss of enjoyment in activities that formerly gave pleasure e.g. hobby, eating, sex, movies, sports, music.
2. **Antalgic** (weakness) (Greek *anti* meaning "against or counteracting" and *algia*, "pain.") She changes her usual movements so as to avoid pain in that limb e.g. posture, gait, hand grip
3. **Appetite** (Latin *appetere* meaning "to desire or crave" for something.) Appetite is not a basic drive for survival, as is hunger. Once hunger is satisfied with small amounts of food, any further eating is directed by appetite, so there can be hunger without appetite; also there is still appetite without hunger as we all have

experienced after eating many *hors d'oeuvres*; anyone near starvation will eat a maggot-laden piece of meat to satisfy hunger, but she will have no appetite for it. Obesity results when food intake, directed by appetite, continues unabated long after hunger has been satisfied.
4. **Anxiety** (Latin *anxietas* meaning "worry.") It still means worry today, as it did for the Romans, but it now implies nonspecific worrying. Useful worry about a specific problem can be helpful in solving it.
5. **Apathetic** (Greek *apatheia* meaning "lack of feeling or emotion.") It resembles the affect of depression. Remember that *pathi* or *pati* from Greek means "feel" or "suffer" and is also the root word of "patient"--one who suffers, in contrast to "client" meaning one who is dependent on a patron, e.g. lawyer or car dealer.
6. **Asthenia** (Greek *a* meaning "lacking or without' and *stheno*, "strength.") Now the connotation is an equivalence with fatigue or tiredness.
7. **Diabetes** (mellitus, insipidus) (Greek *dia* meaning "through" and *banein*, "to run or pass" so resembling a siphon). *Mellitus* is Latin for "sweetened with honey'; *insipidus* is Latin for "tasteless."
8. **Dysesthesia** (Greek *dys* meaning "uncomfortable" and *aisthesis*, "perception.") It is an unpleasant, abnormal sensation produced by a normal (or no) stimulus.
9. **Ergolytic** (drugs) (Greek *ergon* meaning "work" and *lysis*, "dissolution.") It is a drug inhibiting the ability to do work.
10. **Fatigue** (French *fatigatio*, a state of increasing discomfort and decreasing efficiency resulting from prolonged, excessive exertion, i.e. "fatigued" muscle.) This continues to be the physiological meaning, but clinically, the term fatigue has come to be synonymous with lacking energy or tiredness unrelated to physical activity.
11. **Hypnotic** (Greek *hypnos* meaning "sleep.") It is an agent helping to induce sleep.
12. **Idiopathic** (Greek *idios* meaning "one's own" or unique to that person and *pathos*, "disease.") Originally the term suggested a "disease" originating within that person, as opposed to outside, like trauma or infection. Now we use it to denote a symptom of unknown cause.
13. **Illicit** (Latin *il* meaning "not" and *licitus*, "permitted" so not permitted or unlawful.) The word "license," also derived from *licitus*, permits you to practice medicine or nursing.
14. **Lymphadenectasis** (Latin *lymph* meaning "water" --originally from Greek *nymph* for young girl, or goddess of water–and Greek *aden*, "gland," and *ektasis*, "distention.") It means simply, enlarged lymph nodes.
15. **Lymphadenitis** (Latin *lymph* meaning "water" and Greek *aden*, "gland" and *itis*, "inflammation.") Generally it is a reaction to nearby infection, and it is a pathology term.
16. **Lymphadenopathy** (Latin *lymph* meaning "water" and Greek *aden*, "gland" and *pathos,* "disease.") It is a term in pathology meaning diseased lymph nodes; most palpable lymph nodes are not diseased, but functioning normally.
17. **Lymphodynia** (Latin *lymph* meaning "water" and Greek *odyne,* "pain.") Its literal meaning really has no meaning, but some use it to mean painful lymph nodes.
18. **Malaise** (Old French *mal* meaning "bad or ill" and *aise*, "ease," so literally "ill at ease.") It is a vague feeling of bodily discomfort suggesting occult disease.
19. **Narcolepsy** (Greek *narke* meaning "numbness" or state of stupor and *lepsis*, "a taking hold.") It is recurrent uncontrollable brief episodes of sleep.
20. **Neurasthenia** (Greek *neur* meaning "nerve" and *astheneia*, "debility," or "without strength.") Formerly it referred to chronic mental and physical fatigue, supposedly caused by exhaustion of the nervous system. Throughout medical history different terms represented what we now call "fatigue": asthenia, lassitude, lethargy, post-viral syndrome, chronic mono, hypoglycemia syndrome, etc.
21. **Somatization** (Greek *somatos* (*soma*) meaning "body," as distinguished from the mind.) The concept is that a mental disturbance reveals or expresses itself in bodily or somatic symptoms, but not objective signs.
22. **Somnolence** (Latin *somnolentia* meaning "sleepiness.") Now it refers to excessive daytime drowsiness.
23. **Stamina** (Latin word meaning "continuing vigor or strength" even after a considerable period of exertion) We use it similarly today.

Chapter 9 Headache

Questions on Headache

A. In a patient with complaint of headache, it is most important that you find
  1. In the history:
  2. In the physical exam:

B. The commonest cause of headache seen in the office patient and its two major distinguishing characteristics are:
  1.
   a.
   b.

C. The other two common etiologies of headache seen in the office, and their distinguishing characteristics are:
  1.
   a.
   b.
  2.
   a.
   b.

D. Your 30 y/o patient formerly had a migraine headache once every 2-3 months. Ten years later, she now has a headache every day. The kind of headache she most likely has now :

E. You notice that your next patient is an attractive, well-dressed young woman who coughs as she enters your next examining room. Your nurse notes that the patient says she has "the worst headache of her life."
  1. The first thing you do is:
  2. The likely cause of her "worst ever" headache is:
  3. The characteristics on exam that you look for to confirm your initial suspicion are:

F. Your patient is a healthy 75 y/o woman with her first tension-type headache. Your management is:

G. Your 37 y/o patient has headache that is "there all the time," that is, chronic, daily headache. Whenever you hear this complaint, frequently there is associated:

Answers on Headache
A. Be certain of your patient's symptom and its distinguishing characteristics
   1. Whether it is either new headache or episodic headache, and whether its onset to peak severity is abrupt, rapid (minutes) or gradual (hours-days)
   2. Ask the patient to touch her chin to her chest in order to determine she does not have nuchal pain or rigidity, suggesting meningitis or brain hemorrhage. You quickly should palpate the head and neck region to be certain it is a usual "headache" and that there is no significant localized tenderness suggesting facial pain, neck myofascial pain, TMJ pain, referred pain
B. Commonest cause of headache and its distinguishing characteristics
   1. Tension-type headache (TTH)
      a. Episodic headache
      b. The headache occurs in isolation, that is without other symptoms suggesting either a noncephalic infection or a migraine
C. The other two common causes of headache and their characteristics
   1. Migraine
      a. Episodic headache (rarely, a patient may present with the first migraine)
      b. Any one of the following symptoms: either photophobia or phonophobia or nausea and vomiting or head and body movements aggravating the headache
   2. Infection (such as common cold or other causes of fever)
      a. New onset headache
      b. Other symptoms associated with the infection–myalgias, cough, rhinorrhea, sneezing, low grade fever, arthralgias, diarrhea
D. Chronic daily headache is very common
   Chronic daily headache or "rebound headache" commonly is due to analgesic abuse. Patients are difficult to treat, because it requires stopping the offending analgesics, and starting a TCA
E. A patient with a catastrophic disease e.g. SAH, does not walk into your office
   1. Open the door, ask how she is feeling, note that she is not in distress; she is sitting, reading a magazine
   2. Localized viral infection e.g. common cold, acute bronchitis
   3. Look for other systemic symptoms of a viral infection *viz* rhinorrhea, low-grade fever, myalgias
F. Clues to an organic, or even dangerous, cause of headache
   Note that it is a new or different headache in a patient >50 y/o, a clue to the possibility of a dangerous disease. If she is well otherwise, with no dangerous symptoms and normal neurological exam, the minimal test is ESR for TA
G. Chronic daily headache commonly is associated with a psychological disorder, either MD, GAD, somatization disorder, panic disorder. Whether the disorder is primary or not is often difficult to determine, but it makes little difference therapeutically, because you need to treat the psychological problem as well as the headache

Headache

Differential diagnosis: the 3 common causes of headache
1. Tension-type headache (TTH)–episodic; no other significant symptoms with the HA
2. Migraine–episodic; photophobia or phonophobia or GI symptoms (anorexia, nausea, vomiting) or disabled by the pain
3. Localized infection–new onset headache; concomitant symptoms of the infection e.g. URI, GE

(For chronic daily headache, see Section G.3)

A. Be certain of the symptom and its distinguishing characteristics. Your patient's problem or chief complaint is "My head hurts" or "I have a headache"

1. First, be certain the problem is pain originating inside her head. Have your patient show you the site of pain, where it begins and where it radiates. "Show me everywhere it hurts." Don't ask her to point with one finger, but if she does, it may suggest some localized cause, such as facial pain (neuralgia or sinusitis) or ear pain (TMJ) or eye pain or myofascial neck pain. Always inspect and palpate these areas to elicit tenderness, which would divert you from further workup of the usual "headache"
2. Assuming no localized tenderness, determine whether the headache is new, episodic, or chronic. Ask her "How many different kinds of headache do you get?" and "Now we want to talk about this specific headache you are having"
   a. Ask her, "When is the first time you had a headache anything like this one, even though it might have been much less severe?" and "How often do you get this specific headache?" By now you should be confident it is headache, and it is either new or episodic or chronic, daily headache
   b. "Think back to the first time you had this specific headache. Was there anything unusual you remember that preceded the headache? Tell me about that first episode." Now, "Describe how this particular headache typically occurs–what brings it on, how you treat it." Very importantly, "From the moment the headache begins, about how long until it becomes as severe as it is gets?" and, "What other symptoms precede or accompany the headache?"
   c. If your patient's headache occurs on most days of the a month, by definition she has chronic daily headache and a different approach is needed (see below, Section G.3)
3. Physical examination–In every patient complaining of headache, always do the following:
   a. Palpate the head and face for tenderness suggesting neuralgia, acute sinusitis, or TA; palpate the neck both for lymphadenectasis and for a TrP suggesting myofascial pain syndrome, and for typical areas of bilateral tender points of fibromyalgia
   b. Ask her to touch her chin to her chest to detect meningismus; if in question about interpretation, perform a Kernig maneuver
   c. Note vital signs, especially look for diastolic BP >110, fever

>101°F, and appropriate pulse rate (for relative bardycardia–fever of 102°F should have a pulse rate of about 110 bpm; 103°F, 120 bpm; 104°F, 130 bpm; 105°F, 140 bpm. A large deviation from the expected rate suggests a cause of relative bradycardia)

Be certain:
1. The symptom is headache and not localized facial pain or referred pain
2. Whether it is either new onset headache or episodic headache (If it is a chronic daily headache, see Section G.3)
3. Whether its onset to peak severity was abrupt, rapid (<1 hour) or gradual
4. If there are associated symptoms of an infection (fever, myalgias, diarrhea, rhinorrhea, cough) or photophobia, phonophobia, nausea, vomiting

d. Do funduscopy looking for a normal pulsating vein at the edge of the cup on the disc and a normal cup/disc ratio <0.5; and for papilledema; also be alert for photophobia or nystagmus when visualizing the fundus

By now you should be confident it is headache, whether it is new, episodic or chronic daily headache, and if there are significant associated symptoms with the headache. In almost all instances you now have the information you need for diagnosis of the obvious causes (Section C) and the common causes (Section E). In the rare instance that your patient appears different clinically from the usual office patient with headache, be certain (Section B) that she does not have a symptom or sign of a dangerous disease.

B. Be confident it's not a dangerous disease.
1. Send immediately to the ED by ambulance if there is:
   a. Evidence of catastrophic illness e.g. unbearable pain, hypotension, diaphoresis, pallor
   b. Abrupt onset of a new severe headache that incapacitates the patient (even if meningismus or nuchal rigidity are absent), think of brain hemorrhage, meningitis, encephalitis
   c. Abrupt onset of headache with syncope or dizziness, think of cerebellar hemorrhage, basilar migraine
   d. Altered consciousness or confusion or any one focal neurological deficit, think of intracranial hemorrhage, meningitis, stroke, encephalitis, sepsis
   e. Stiff or painful neck on flexion or rectal temperature >101°F, think of brain hemorrhage, meningitis
   f. Abrupt onset of severe neck and head pain with a focal neurological sign, think of carotid artery dissection
   g. Abrupt onset of severe, explosive headache ("thunderclap headache"), think of SAH, cervicocephalic arterial dissection, cerebral venous sinus thrombosis
   h. Ill patient with fever and rash, think of meningococcemia, RMSF, sepsis syndrome, infective endocarditis, toxic shock syndrome, Stevens-Johnson syndrome
2. Admit at once to the ED or hospital if there is:
   a. BP > 200/120 with associated mental changes and retinopathy (flame hemorrhages, exudates, papilledema), think of emergent (malignant) HTN, pheochromocytoma
   b. Unilateral abrupt loss of vision or diplopia with headache; in a patient >50 y/o, think of TA or emboli from the ipsilateral carotid; in a younger person think of pseudotumor cerebri, complicated migraine, optic neuritis; any age, think of

Chapter 9 Headache 111

      pituitary hemorrhage
- c. New or episodic headache with symptoms suggesting acute GE (headache, vomiting, diarrhea), but no concomitant abdominal pain or hyperperistaltic bowel sounds, think of carbon monoxide poisoning
- d. Symptoms suggesting acute GE, but high fever and gradual onset of a very severe headache, think of RMSF, bacterial meningitis
- e. The "worst headache ever," think of SAH, meningitis, RMSF (but in the office almost always it is headache due either to new migraine or noncephalic infection)
- f. Abrupt onset of severe headache concomitant with any exertion or Valsalva maneuver (cough, sneeze, coitus, straining at stool), think of SAH, tumor, Chiari malformation
- g. Abrupt onset of unilateral eye pain and decreased ipsilateral visual acuity, think of acute glaucoma

---

Be certain in the first minutes of your exam that there is no evidence of any <u>one</u> dangerous symptom or sign associated with the headache:
1. Abrupt onset of a severely painful new headache
2. Any altered consciousness or confusion
3. Nuchal rigidity or pain on flexion
4. Any <u>one</u> focal neurological sign
5. New or different headache in a patient >50 y/o
6. Emergent hypertension, BP >220/120
7. Diplopia or amaurosis fugax
8. Rash or fever >101°F (38.3°C)

Any suggestion of a dangerous disease, send your patient to the ED.

---

3. Admit to the hospital or have a specialist consult as soon as appropriate if there is:
   - a. A new headache that has been constant since onset (syndrome of "new daily persistent headache"), think of SAH, post-trauma, chronic meningitis, low CSF volume, raised CSF pressure (J Neurol Neurosurg Psych 72 (Suppl II), 2, 2002)
   - b. Headache that is persistent and unilateral (always the same side) or progressively worsening headache at any age, MRI must be done to exclude any mass lesion
   - c. Papilledema or loss of venous pulsation on the optic disc, think of increased intracranial pressure due to brain tumor, subdural hematoma, pseudotumor cerebri
   - d. New onset of severe orbital pain and headache with decreased ipsilateral visual acuity: if >50 y/o, think of TA, acute glaucoma; if <40-50 y/o, think of retrobulbar (optic) neuritis, migraine, cluster headache
   - e. A new or different headache in an HIV-positive patient, think of CNS opportunistic infection
   - f. A new headache in a patient with coincident, progressive dementia or with any possible history of preceding head trauma, think subdural hematoma
   - g. Onset of a new or different headache in a patient >50 y/o, always get a sed rate for TA; pain is not deep, but superficial, and it may be located holocephalic, or any unilateral site e.g. temporal or occipital
   - h. Episodic headache associated with "spells" of spontaneous sweating, pallor (<u>not</u> flushing), palpitations, think of pheochromocytoma
   - i. Unilateral persistent headache, ipsilateral tinnitus, decreased hearing, imbalance or vertigo, think of acoustic neurinoma
   - j. Nocturnal or early morning headache, think of brain tumor, OSA, severe COPD, hypercarbia of any cause
   - k. New headache with secondary amenorrhea, galactorrhea, sublibido, erectile dysfunction, or visual field deficit (bitemporal hemanopsia), think of pituitary tumor
   - l. Persistent fever and headache, think of CNS tumor, chronic meningo-encephalitis, relapsing fever, rat-bite fever, brucellosis, malaria, brain abscess (get rectal temp tid)
   - m. New or different headache following trauma, think of subdural or epidural hematoma

n. Persistent fever, headache and relative bradycardia, think of leptospirosis, psittacosis, central fever, typhoid fever, malaria

C. **Make a quick diagnosis if it's obvious.** Is it an easily diagnosed cause or a medication that is responsible for the headache? In most patients you will be <u>highly</u> confident of a common cause of the symptom by now. If not, one or more of the following tests may exclude an organic disease and increase your confidence in your working diagnosis: ESR, WBC
1. Spot diagnoses
   a. Post-lumbar puncture headache is provoked by sitting or standing, and entirely relieved by recumbency; onset is 2-14 days after LP, and rarely it may persist for months
   b. Post-traumatic headache occurs 1-2 days following <u>any</u> head trauma and may persist for years; you need a CT to exclude subdural hematoma; if associated symptoms (unilateral facial sweating, dilated pupil, tender at carotid bifurcation) occur, this is dysautonomic cephalgia and it is treated with propranolol
   c. "Ice pick" headache (idiopathic stabbing headache) has jabbing pain lasting seconds in the orbit or parietal area; prompt prophylactic response to indomethacin 50 mg. tid
   d. Headache after eating certain foods

Recognize any easily diagnosed cause of headache–many are <u>new</u> headaches:

1. Spot diagnosis–post-lumbar puncture, post-trauma, "ice pick" headache, myofascial pain, GYN causes, acute sinusitis, fibromyalgia, ingestion of food products e.g. nitrates
2. Medication side effect

---

   (1) Monosodium glutamate–"Chinese restaurant syndrome" occurs 20-30 minutes after eating Chinese food with symptoms of headache, facial flushing and sweating, paresthesias, pain or discomfort in chest and abdomen, dizziness
   (2) Nitrates, nitrites– A "hot dog headache" with facial flushing soon after eating meats cured with these substances (hot dogs, sausage, bacon)
   (3) Aspartame–artificial sweetener (soft drinks, desserts, prepared foods) is a migraine trigger
   (4) Alcohol may have headache 30-45 min after ingestion, and it is a trigger for migraine and cluster headaches
   e. Myofascial pain syndrome–<u>unilateral</u> focal painful site (TrP) in muscle (e.g. posterior cervical muscles, sternocleidomastoid); pain or spasm prevents normal ROM; treated with injection of the TrP, then preventive therapy by exercises
   f. GYN causes are all cyclic headaches or related to menses
   (1) Premenstrual migraine occurs from 7-2 days before menses
   (2) Menstrual migraine occurs from 2 days before to 3 days after onset of menses and at no other times
   (3) Menstrual-related migraine occurs during menses and also at other times
   (4) TTH increases in frequency 1 day before to 2 days after onset of menses

Chapter 9 Headache 113

   (5) During pregnancy migraine commonly decreases or disappears, but in 10% there is new onset migraine
   (6) In some patients, menopause exacerbates migraine
   g. Acute sinusitis causes headache, but chronic sinusitis is rarely a cause of headache. Attribute a new headache to bacterial sinusitis only if there are symptoms lasting >7 days (fever, purulent or sanguinopurulent nasal discharge, maxillary tooth pain), and there is focal unilateral tenderness over the infected sinus (compared to no tenderness over the ipsilateral zygomatic arch as control site where you press with your thumb at gradually increasing pressure)

   h. Fibromyalgia–generalized aches and pains along with headache; find <u>bilateral</u> tender points at typical sites e.g. back of the neck, back, chest
2. Medications–up to 5% of people given placebo in drug studies complain of a new or different headache, so <u>any new</u> medication can be responsible for your patient's new headache. In addition, any <u>one</u> medication may cause new headache in an individual patient, even though the medication is not included in lists of drugs causing headache. Look for a temporal relationship between a new headache beginning after starting a new medication. Below is a list of medications that "cause" headache in drug trials at rates greater than placebo
   a. Vasodilators–nitroglycerin, isosorbide dinitrate, hydralazine, dipyridamole
   b. Vasoconstrictors–bromocriptine, dopamine; sympathomimetics (pseudoephedrine, dextroamphetamine)
   c. Antihypertensives–captopril, atenolol, metoprolol, propranolol, reserpine, prazosin, minoxidil, clonidine, losartan, methyldopa, hydralazine
   d. Antiemetics–domperidone, metoclopramide
   e. NSAIDs–indomethacin, diclofenac, piroxicam
   f. Antidepressants–SSRIs, trazodone
   g. Triptans–after extended daily use; class effect
   h. β-agonists– terbutaline
   i. H2-receptor antagonists–cimetidine, ranitidine
   j. PPI– class effect
   k. CCB– nifedipine, verapamil
   l. Antiepileptic drugs–gabapentin, lamotrigine, tiagabine, barbiturates
   m. Hormones–contraceptives, danazol, estrogens, clomiphene, growth hormone, progestens e.g. Norplant-Z
   n. Anxiolytics–lorazepam, buspirone, zolpidem, hydoxyzine, benzodiazepines
   o. Antibiotics–trimethoprim-sulfamethoxazole, griseofulvin, itraconazole, tetracyclines
   p. Miscellaneous–all <u>trans</u> retinoic acid, cilostazol, interferon, sibutramine, sildenafil, amiodarone, rosiglitazone, thalidomide, azelastine, budesonide, cocaine, dipyridamole, atorvastatin, nicotinic acid (including Niaspan), aminophylline, theophylline, digoxin, quinidine, erythropoietin
   q. Withdrawal headaches due to glucocorticoids, clonidine, propranolol, vasodilators (caffeine, alcohol, ergots, amphetamines, methysergide)

D. **Identify your patient's worries and wants.** Headache occurs annually in 90% of people, and only a few of these consult about it. During your interview and exam, try to intuit or discover why your patient is here today, and not previously, for this problem. Don't necessarily ask directly, but try to get some ideas from your patient's responses to questions about the headache itself. You can't completely help your patient unless you know what she really worries about and wants from you. That's why she is here to see you--to satisfy her worries and wants! Here are only some of the possible worries and wants of your patient with headache. You must discover her specific ones

During your exam, discover your patient's worries (brain tumor, stroke) and wants (pain relief, assurance the headache is benign), so that you can respond to her specific needs as soon as possible.

1. Common worries are:
   a. That the cause of the headache is a dangerous etiology e.g. brain tumor, stroke, severe systemic HTN, ruptured cerebral vessel, meningitis
   b. That the etiology is some rare disease e.g. WNV encephalitis, toxic chemicals
   c. What other fears or anxieties might be troubling your patient? For example, she may have had TTH for many years, and only now does she come for help. What has changed? Perhaps a friend or relative, who had similar episodic headaches, recently has been diagnosed with a brain tumor. Many other possibilities exist, so think of them
2. Your patient wants:
   a. You to perform a thorough physical exam focused on possible causes of the headache and she wants appropriate tests and imaging studies
   b. A plausible explanation of the cause of the headache
   c. Confident reassurance from you that it is not a dangerous or rare etiology. Tell her--"The good news, it's not a brain tumor" (or whatever you believe her real worry is)
   d. To know the prognosis, short term (effects on job, home life, marriage; how soon she will be back to normal) and long term (if recurrences are possible; how to prevent recurrences; if it will cause any disability)
   e. Treatment to stop the headache now and to prevent recurrences e.g. propranolol for migraines
   f. A specialist referral (neurologist) if she believes you are not confident of the diagnosis

E. Know the symptoms that differentiate the 3 common causes of headache.

1. The commonest cause is tension-type headache (TTH)
   a. Characteristics of TTH
      (1) Episodic headache
      (2) It occurs in isolation, that is, no other significant associated symptoms are present that repeatedly occur with the headache, unless the headache is just one feature of another disorder, e.g. MD, GAD, somatization disorder, fibromyalgia
      (3) TTH is never disabling, and the usual analgesics (aspirin or acetaminophen) relieve the headache for at least a few hours
   b. What suggests it might not be TTH
      (1) Anytime there is one associated symptom or sign suggesting a dangerous cause (see above, Section B)
      (2) If the headache is new and accompanied by systemic symptoms of a localized infection; or there is photophobia or phonophobia or GI (anorexia, nausea or vomiting) or worsening of the headache by head movements; or the headache disables her
      (3) If it definitely is a new or different headache in an HIV-positive patient or in a patient >50 y/o, never attribute it to TTH without further studies e.g. ESR, imaging studies
2. Common look-alikes and how each differs from TTH

a. Migraine
   (1) It also is episodic and it has gradual onset (<1-2 hours) to peak severity

> Common causes of most headaches in the office patient are:
> 1. Tension-type headache (TTH)–<u>episodic</u>; no other significant symptoms with the HA
> 2. Migraine–<u>episodic</u>; photophobia or phonophobia or GI symptoms (anorexia, nausea, vomiting) or disabled by the pain
> 3. Localized infection–<u>new onset</u> headache; concomitant symptoms of the infection e.g. URI, GE

   (2) Two major types of migraine headaches exist: "migraine with aura" (formerly called classic migraine) is less common, and it is recognized by visual (flashing lights, scotomata) or sensory (unilateral paresthesias) phenomena preceding or accompanying the headache. "Migraine without aura" (formerly called common migraine) accounts for the overwhelming majority of patients with migraine. Although migraine is described as very painful and often throbbing, starts unilaterally and may then affect the whole head, and begins on one side or the other at different times, none of these characteristics helps you separate it from TTH
   (3) What <u>does</u> differentiate migraine from TTH? Migraine does not occur in isolation from other symptoms. One or more of the following presents with the headache–sensitivity to light (photophobia) <u>or</u> sensitivity to loud sounds (phonophobia) <u>or</u> sensitivity to movements (especially moving the head), <u>or</u> GI of anorexia or nausea or vomiting
   (4) Again, different from TTH, migraine headaches at onset do not occur daily, and only rarely, even weekly; commonly they occur monthly, or even less often
   (5) Different from TTH, the patient with migraine is <u>disabled</u> from the pain–she does <u>not</u> work through it. Rather, she seeks a dark, quiet room to sleep (to avoid lights, sounds, movements), after which the headache often is relieved within 24 hours
b. Headache associated with localized infection
   (1) It is a <u>new</u> headache, not an episodic headache like tension-type headache or migraine. In winter, these may account for up to 30% of headaches in the office
   (2) It always is accompanied by some other symptoms of a localized infection (sneezing, rhinorrhea, myalgias, sore throat, cough, fever, diarrhea, abdominal pain, vomiting, dysuria) e.g. URI, acute bronchitis, GE, UTI
   (3) There may even be photophobia, nausea and vomiting as seen with migraine, or the headache may be so severe that she says "This is the worst headache I've ever had," and it may be a throbbing pain over the whole head, suggesting migraine or something even worse. But the important differentiating points are the systemic symptoms of a localized infection that accompany the headache

F. **Use this summary for efficient diagnosis of a common cause.** With the information from Sections A-E in mind, here is the rapid approach to diagnosis of a new or episodic headache.
1. You already have determined:
   a. In Section A, by H&P, that it is headache and not localized pain or referred pain.
   b. In Section B, that there is no evidence in the H&P of any one dangerous cause of the headache.
   c. In Section C, that there is neither an easily diagnosed cause nor a medication that is likely responsible for the headache.
2. From the focused H&P almost always you should quickly be confident of a working diagnosis. Confident final diagnosis is made only in followup the next few days or weeks when the response to treatment or nontreatment is appropriate to your working diagnosis.
   a. If it is a <u>new</u> headache, look for associated systemic symptoms of an infection, such as myalgias, sneezing, coughing, fever, sore throat, rhinitis, dysuria, diarrhea, vomiting. If such symptoms are present, almost always the diagnosis is headache secondary to an acute infection.
   b. If it is an <u>episodic</u> headache and there is either photophobia <u>or</u> phonophobia <u>or</u> gastrointestinal symptoms (anorexia, nausea, vomiting) <u>or</u> aggravation of headache on head movements, then the diagnosis most likely is migraine headache.
   c. If it is an <u>episodic</u> headache and it occurs in isolation, that is, there are no symptoms suggesting either localized infection or migraine, then the patient most likely has TTH.
3. Answer your patient's worries and wants that you determined early on during the exam (Section D). Have you done everything you can to help her?
4. You now have a working diagnosis, but only with followup can you be highly confident it is correct. In return visits you are always testing by H&P that your working diagnosis is correct.

G. **Abandon your working diagnosis and look for an uncommon or rare cause only if:**
1. Any <u>one</u> dangerous symptom or sign (see above, Section B) occurs in the following days, weeks, or months. Quickly obtain a neurology consult or send the patient to the hospital as appropriate
2. The headache does not respond to treatment as you expect or the natural history of your working diagnosis does not occur. Patients with each of the three common causes (TTH, migraine, localized infection) should be "well" or back to their usual health when the headache is absent. Headache associated with infection should get better at about the same time the other systemic symptoms fade. The patient with migraine should be well when the headache is gone, almost always in 24-36 hours. Although the patient with TTH may get frequent headaches, the headache should be relieved with aspirin or acetaminophen (1000 mg every 4-6 hr) and the patient otherwise well when the headache is absent

If your patient's symptoms do not respond as expected to your management, he may have an uncommon or rare cause listed in Section G.2 that you can diagnose and treat. Or you may want to refer your patient to a specialist.

Chapter 9 Headache 117

Don't spend time and money looking for one of the following etiologies until you are sure your patient doesn't have one of the 3 common causes of episodic or new headache above. If she doesn't have one of those causes, it may be that the correct cause was one of the uncommon etiologies listed below. These are important to recognize, because each has different treatment or prophylaxis.
  a. Headaches associated with autonomic symptoms *viz* lacrimation, nasal congestion, rhinorrhea, conjunctival injection, ptosis (Brain 120, 193, 1997):
     (1) Cluster headache is uncommon, perhaps one for every 500 patients with TTH. They are episodic, with rapid onset to peak severity in <15 minutes; they are excruciatingly painful ("sharp, ice-pick"), occur mostly in men with onset <50 y/o, most last <3 hours, may occur 1-3 times daily, may recur in "clusters" for 4-6 weeks, and then remit for months or years. The pain lasts such a short time that the patient rarely is seen in the office or the ED during the attack. The pain is strictly unilateral and especially periocular. Whereas the patient with migraine refuses to move about because it aggravates the pain, the cluster patient cannot sit still. Correct diagnosis is important because there is effective treatment (oxygen) as well as preventive therapy (verapamil)
     (2) Paroxysmal hemicrania may be episodic or chronic headaches, last <1 hour and they are treatable with indomethacin
     (3) Short lasting unilateral neuralgiform headaches with conjunctival injection and tearing (SUNCT) syndrome has unilateral orbital or temporal pain lasting <2 min; no known specific treatment
     (4) Hemicrania continua is a unilateral headache that is "there all the time" and it frequently is associated with idiopathic ("ice pick") stabbing headaches; prompt response to indomethacin
  b. Orthostatic headaches occur with POTS (no orthostatic hypotension, but pulse rate on standing increases >30 bpm and absolute pulse rate is >120 bpm; Neurology 61, 980, 2003)
  c. Hypnic headache occurs only at night. It is a benign headache with onset almost always only in elderly patients. The patient awakens with a pulsating headache that lasts <1-2 hr. It may recur that night and then occurs at about the same time most nights. Lithium at bedtime can prevent it
  d. Cervicogenic headache–In a patient >50 y/o, a new or different headache with characteristics that suggest a TTH may be due to OA (spondylosis) of the cervical spine. Pain radiates from C_{1-3} vertebrae to the occipital and parietal regions as a dull ache, usually unilaterally. Don't think of cervicogenic headache if it has been gradually worsening, wakes her at night or has other danger signs. Most patients >50 y/o have cervical spine changes on imaging, so positive radiological findings are not helpful, i.e. many false positives. Some respond to treatment with physical therapy exercises or steroid injections
  e. Carotodynia–not truly headache, but it may be confused with headache; pain is unilateral at the upper anterior neck and there is tenderness over the ipsilateral carotid or on swallowing
  f. Systemic diseases with associated headache:
     (1) Cardiovascular–during an attack of angina pectoris ("cardiac cephalgia," Neurology 49, 813, 1997), after carotid endarterectomy, severe aortic insufficiency, chronic CHF
     (2) Pulmonary–sarcoidosis (granulomatous meningitis), any cause of hypercapnia, e.g. COPD, OSA, polycythemia, high altitude, any cause of hypoxia
     (3) Kidney–CRF, during or following dialysis, anemia
     (4) Endocrine–hypoglycemia, hypercalcemia, prolactinoma, "empty sella" syndrome
     (5) Immune-mediated disorders (collagen-vascular)–vasculitis, SLE, scleroderma, PAN, Wegener's granulomatosis
3. Chronic daily headache (CDH)–approach to diagnosis of its cause. CDH means she has headache on most days of the month for the previous few months. Often the headache is described as being "there all the time"
  a. First, be certain she does not have a dangerous cause (see Section B) including "new daily persistent headache" (see above, Section B.3.a), which demands vigorous workup for secondary causes
  b. The majority of CDH are chronic TTH or chronic ("transformed") migraine, and most become CDH because of analgesic abuse. Any analgesic taken multiple times daily in anticipation of a headache can be causative. Patients frequently take the analgesic first thing in the morning and regularly through the day before they have a headache. The "rebound" headache occurs a few hours after taking the analgesic, that is, when the analgesic "wears off"
  c. Any one of the above causes of headache in Section G.2 may be a cause of CDH. A convenient classification of CDH is the following (Neurology 47, 871, 1996):

(1) Primary CDH
  (a) Headache duration >4 hours
    (i) Chronic migraine–70-80% of all CDH; as the migraine becomes more frequent, i.e. daily, the intensity of the characteristic symptoms of photophobia, phonophobia, vomiting, decrease or disappear. Except for the history of migraine, or occasional migraine, the daily headache becomes indistinguishable from chronic TTH
    (ii) Chronic TTH
    (iii) New daily persistent headache (See Section B.3.a)
    (iv) Hemicrania continua
  (b) Headache duration <4 hours
    (i) Cluster headache
    (ii) Paroxysmal hemicrania
    (iii) Hypnic headache
    (iv) Idiopathic stabbing headache
(2) Secondary CDH
  (a) Post-traumatic headaches
  (b) Cervical spine disorders
  (c) Intracranial disease–vascular and nonvascular
  (d) Extracranial disease–TMJ, sinus infection
d. Anytime problems with sleeping are prominent in a patient with CDH think of OSA (30% are not obese; headache often occurs on awakening)
e. CDH often is associated with a psychological disorder, even though it may not be causing the headache. Still, treat the psychological problem along with headache therapy
  (1) MD–look especially for associated anhedonia, that is, unexplained decreased "appetite" for any one of her formerly pleasurable activities (food, drink, sex, hobbies, job, sports, music). Helpful to find is associated depressed mood, early morning insomnia, mood swings, negativism, but if she does not have anhedonia as described above, MD is unlikely
  (2) GAD–she worries almost constantly about some future event that could happen, but it is highly unlikely; she just can't stop worrying about it, and the worrying interferes with her daily functioning
  (3) Somatization disorder--she has pain in a number of other organ systems along with headache
4. New or different headache in a patient >50 y/o
  a. In 3% of all patients who get migraines, onset of the migraine will be >50 y/o. For either TTH or cluster headache, the percentage of late onset headaches is 10%
  b. Even though the following causes of headache are uncommon, the incidence in patients >50 y/o increases markedly
    (1) Dangerous diseases–TA, acute glaucoma, exploding head syndrome, cerebrovascular disease, cardiac cephalgia, intracranial mass lesions (tumors, hematomas, infections)
    (2) Medication side effects, cervicogenic headache, hypnic headache, systemic diseases (see Section G.2.f)

H. Use the glossary for precise thinking and accurate diagnosis.

1. **Amaurosis fugax** (Greek *amaurosis* meaning "dark" or "obscure" and *fugax*, "swift.") Rapid onset, but transient total or partial blindness in one eye
2. **Analgesic** (Greek *an* meaning "without" and *algesis*, "sense of pain.") A medication that suppresses pain perception.
3. **Anorexia** (Greek *an* meaning "lack of" and *orexis*, "appetite.") Literally, lack of appetite; same meaning today, just as in Hippocrates' time.
4. **Aura** (Latin word meaning "a breeze or wind.") Now used as a premonitory sign of changes to come, as a heightening breeze signals a change in the weather; aura of migraine headache.
5. **Carotidynia** or carotodynia (Greek *karotis* meaning "deep sleep" and *odyne*, "pain.") Ancients noted that deep pressure on the carotid artery, and not other arteries, produced "deep sleep."
6. **Cephalgia** (Greek *kephale* meaning "head" and *algos*, "pain.") Another word for headache; as is cephalodynia (Greek *odyne*, "pain.")
7. **Cervicogenic** (Greek *cervix* meaning "neck" of anything (including body, uterus, bladder) and *gennan*, "to produce.") Headache produced by neck pathology
8. **Diaphoresis**--ancient Greek writers used the same term for "profuse sweating"
9. **Glaucoma** (Greek *glaukoma* meaning a "silvery swelling or tumor.") Ancients applied the term to a group of degenerative eye diseases, all causing a dense lens opacity or cataract; later distinction between cataracts and degeneration inside the

Chapter 9 Headache   119

    eye due to high intraocular pressure.
10. **Hemicrania** (Greek *hemi* meaning "half" and *kranion,* "skull.") A headache affecting one side of the head, but a different side at different times, in the particular case of migraine.
11. **Hypercapnia** (Greek *hyper* meaning "above, excessive" and *kapnos*, "smoke.") It refers to excess carbon dioxide in blood; a synonym is hypercarbia.
12. **Hypnic** (Greek *hypnos* meaning "sleep.") Anything that induced, or pertaining to, sleep.
13. **Meningismus** (Greek *meninx* meaning "membrane" especially meninges.) Now it refers to symptoms and signs of meningeal irritation with an acute febrile illness, but not actual infection of the meninges, which would be "meningitis."
14. **Migraine** (Greek word for "hemicrania.") It was Latinized to *migraena,* and later to French, *migraine.*
15. **Miosis** (Greek *meiosis* meaning "a lessening.") Lessening of anything, including the size of the pupil, or pupillary constriction.
16. **Neuralgia,** trigeminal (Greek *neur* meaning "nerve" and *algia,* "pain.") Paroxysms of severe, stabbing pain along the distribution of the involved nerve.
17. **Nuchal** (Arabic *nukha* meaning "back of the neck.")
18. **Paresthesias** (Greek *para* meaning "along with" and *aisthesis*, "perception.") An abnormal feeling, such as numbness or tingling, in addition to normal perception
19. **Paroxysmal** (Greek *paroxysmos* meaning "abrupt or rapid onset.") Applied to symptoms that occur as a group and that occur episodically.
20. **Phonophobia** (Greek *phone* meaning "voice" and *phobos*, "fear.") Avoidance of loud sounds that aggravate the pain of migraine headache.
21. **Photophobia** (Greek *phos* meaning "light" and *phobos*, "fear.") Painful sensitivity to the usual intensity of light.
22. **Pleiocytosis,** pleocytosis (Greek *pleon* meaning "more, excessive" and *cytosis*, "cells.") CSF containing more than 5 mononuclear cells or any RBC or PMN.
23. **Protean** (Greek sea god, *Proteus*, who could change his appearance at will.) We use the term for any disease with many varied appearances clinically, e.g. syphilis, AIDS, connective tissue diseases. In contrast to pronunciation of the word "protein," all the syllables in "protean" are pronounced.
24. **Ptosis** (Greek word meaning "a falling.") Now it refers only to a drooping eyelid.
25. **Scotomata,** plural of scotoma (Greek *skotos* meaning "darkness or gloom.") It is a blind spot or focal area of decreased acuity in the visual field.
26. **Stroke** (derived from the Greek word *apoplexia* meaning "seized by being struck down" by the gods as punishment.) Stroked or struck down persists in our English usage–we've just dropped the gods.
27. **Teichopsia** (Greek *teichos* meaning "city wall," like a crenellated fortress, and *opsis*, "vision.") Now it refers to a scintillating scotoma or flashing lights resembling jagged lines.

120 WERNER'S OFFICE DIAGNOSIS

CHAPTER 10 JOINT PAIN

Questions on Joint Pain

A. In a patient with complaint of "My joints hurt when I move," the most important:
1. Historical factor to determine is:
2. Factors to determine by physical exam are:

B. In the office patient, the commonest cause of joint pain and its 2 distinguishing characteristics are:
1.
   a.
   b.

C. The other 2 common causes of "joint pain" and their distinguishing characteristics are:
1.
   a.
   b.
2.
   a.
   b.

D. Your 45 y/o patient with a diagnosis of RA telephones to tell you she has a "severe flare" in her right knee. It is late Friday afternoon, so you do you tell her to increase her dose of medication and schedule her for an office visit early Monday morning? Or?

E. The following patients had in common a complaint of "joint pain" as well as pain on active ROM much greater than on passive ROM. Each differed, however, in the site of <u>focal</u> tenderness on palpation. The likely etiology for the following sites of tenderness are:
1. Lower medial knee
2. Left hip
3. Right buttock, especially when sitting
4. Right shoulder (he can't abduct >45°)

F. The two locations of bursitis that are especially prone to become a "septic bursitis" are:
1.
2.

G. If your patient complains "My joints hurt when I move," but there is no articular or periarticular evidence of disease on exam, you immediately think of 2 common causes, and your approach to diagnosis is to
1. Think of:
2. Distinguish them by:

Chapter 10 Joint Pain   121

Answers on Joint Pain

A. Be certain of your patient's symptom and its distinguishing characteristics
   1. "Show me which joints have been hurting." Anatomical location of the affected joints (or "non-joints," if it is bursitis or tendinitis or fibromyalgia), along with age, immediately helps you differentiate OA from RA. If he points with 1 finger to one or more joints, ask "Do you mean it is painful just at that point?" If it is at a single point on the joint, you think of tendinitis or bursitis, but if the whole joint is hurting, it likely is intra-articular disease. This is what you want to know–is the pain arising from intra-articular disease or not?
   2. "Show me what it is that brings on the pain." That is, you are testing for active ROM, which should provoke pain caused by either intra-articular disease or periarticular disease (tendinitis, bursitis, myalgia). Next, you want him totally relaxed, so you can passively move the joint through appropriate ROM. Sometimes having him supine helps him relax. Marked reduction of the complained-of pain on passive ROM (compared to active ROM) suggest a peri-articular etiology, whereas approximately equal pain on active ROM and passive ROM suggests intra-articular disease. Examine the whole circumference of the involved joints for evidence of synovitis, i.e. synovium that is swollen, boggy, tender, warm, pink (not red)
B. The commonest cause of joint pain
   1. Osteoarthritis (OA)
      a. Intra-articular disease i.e. active ROM pain is about the same intensity as with passive ROM
      b. No sign of synovitis
C. The other 2 common causes of "joint pain"
   1. Inflammatory arthritis, most commonly rheumatoid arthritis (RA)
      a. Intra-articular disease
      b. Signs of synovitis in the whole circumference of the involved joints i.e. warmth, swelling, tender, pink
   2. Periarticular disease (tendinitis, bursitis)
      a. Not intra-articular disease i.e. passive ROM much less or no pain compared to active ROM
      b. Point tenderness at the involved periarticular area
D. Recognize 2 clues to a dangerous joint disease
   1. The knee is a common site for septic arthritis, and it is an unusual site for uncomplicated RA
   2. It is a "monoarthritis," alerting you to the possibility of a septic joint. You must examine and do arthrocentesis of her right knee joint now
E. Common locations of bursitis and tendinitis
   1. Pes anserine bursitis
   2. Left trochanteric bursitis
   3. Right ischial tuberosity bursitis (weaver's or "internet" bursitis)
   4. Tendinitis of the right shoulder rotator cuff
F. Sites of bursitis that commonly become infected
   1. Prepatellar bursitis–tenderness on kneeling on the involved side
   2. Olecranon bursitis at the extensor tissue of the elbow
G. Both fibromyalgia and myofascial pain syndrome are common causes of "joint pain"
   Fibromyalgia has body pain in more than one region and tenderness to palpation in these regions. Bilateral tender points at specific sites are

diagnostic. Myofascial pain has trigger points (TrP) that may cause referred pain when the TrP is pressed on. So myofascial pain is never generalized, only <u>focal</u> or in a single region (neck, head, chest or limb). A TrP can be injected with an analgesic to give immediate pain relief. Fibromyalgia is generalized pain, so the only time an injection helps is in patients who also have a TrP of concomitant myofascial pain syndrome. The two conditions often occur together

Chapter 10 Joint Pain

Joint Pain

> **Differential diagnosis: the 2 common causes of chronic joint pain**
> 1. OA–onset of pain in a patient >50 y/o, no sign of synovitis
> 2. RA–onset of pain usually in a patient <50 y/o, signs of synovitis, morning stiffness >30-45 min; typical joints inflamed

A. **Be certain of the symptom and its distinguishing characteristics.** Your patient's problem or chief complaint is "My joints hurt when I move"
  1. First, be certain the problem is joint pain caused by movement, and not some other discomfort, such as joint stiffness or muscle pain. Determine whether it is new pain (onset <6 weeks ago) or it is chronic pain, and whether it is focal or regional pain
  2. Ask him to "Show me where it hurts" and "Show me what kind of movements provoke the pain." If joint "stiffness" also is complained of, ask him "From the moment you get out of bed, how long until your joints get as good as they are going to get for the day?" If uncertain, have him time it; >30-45 minutes suggests an inflammatory arthritis if synovitis is present
  3. Physical examination
     a. Is the pain due to intra-articular disease or periarticular disease?
        (1) Intra-articular disease should elicit about equal intensity of pain whether the patient moves the joint (active ROM) or you move the joint (passive ROM)
        (2) Periarticular disease should cause relatively much more pain on active ROM than passive ROM
     b. Is there evidence of inflammation?

> Be certain:
> 1. Whether the symptom either is intra-articular pain i.e. originating <u>in</u> the joint, or it is periarticular pain, originating <u>near</u> the joint
> 2. Whether the involved joint shows signs of inflammation (synovitis) around the whole joint or only at a single site near the joint
> 3. Whether the pain is new (began <6 weeks ago) or chronic, daily pain
> 4. What the distribution or pattern of diseased joints is
> 5. If it is not joint pain, but rather musculoskeletal pain, generalized or focal

        (1) If there is inflammation of a joint, i.e. synovitis, the joint is swollen, pink, warm and the synovium is boggy and tender around the <u>whole circumference</u> of the joint
        (2) If the joint <u>is</u> inflamed there will be <u>restricted ROM</u> especially

on extension, which decreases joint volume; the joint usually is held in a flexed position if inflamed
  - (3) If there is periarticular inflammation (bursitis, tendinitis), the tenderness and warmth are localized to a site of inflammation, i.e. a known bursa or tendon insertion
  c. If the pain source is neither intra-articular or periarticular, and not inflammatory, are there tender points of fibromyalgia or TrP of regional myofascial pain at typical sites e.g. neck, back, shoulders? Palpate everywhere he has pain or might have tenderness
  d. Is there any evidence of systemic disease, especially fever (get a rectal temperature), weight loss (change in belt or pants size), cutaneous lesions (rash, nodules, petechiae, ulcers)?

By now you should be confident it is intra-articular pain, whether it is new or chronic pain, if there is evidence of synovitis, or if there are regional areas of tenderness. In almost all instances you now have the information you need for diagnosis of the obvious causes (Section C) and the common causes (Section E). In the rare instance that your patient appears different clinically from the usual office patient with joint pain, be certain (Section B) that he does not have a symptom or sign of a dangerous disease.

B. Be confident it's not a dangerous disease.

1. Send immediately to the ED by ambulance if there is:
  a. History of trauma and focal tenderness, think of fracture
  b. Gait difficulty (hemi- or paraparesis), paresthesias in feet and hands, progressive weakness, hyperreflexia, think of spondylitic myelopathy (spastic paraparesis)
  c. Known RA or ankylosing spondylitis and signs of cervical myelopathy (quadriparesis, paresthesias), think of atlantoaxial subluxation

---

Be certain in the first minutes of your exam that there is no evidence of any <u>one</u> dangerous symptom or sign associated with the joint pain:

1. Rapid onset, severe pain in 1-3 joints
2. Unexplained fever >101°F (38.3°C) with any synovitis
3. Spastic paraparesis (leg weakness)
4. Migratory polyarthritis
5. New murmur or dysrhythmia
6. Amaurosis fugax
7. Anemia or unexplained weight loss or high ESR

Any suggestion of a dangerous disease, send the patient to the ED.

---

  d. Patient with RA with new onset dyspnea and stridor, think of cricoarytenoid joint inflammation
2. Admit at once to the ED or hospital if there is:
  a. A single (or 2-3), hot, swollen, red, very painful joint, think of septic arthritis, osteomyelitis, gout, pseudogout, palindromic rheumatism
  b. Patient with chronic polyarthritis, e.g. RA, now has rapid onset of a "flare" in one joint, think of septic arthritis
  c. Cardiac murmur, arthralgias, fever, think of infective endocarditis, atrial myxoma, rheumatic fever
  d. Migratory polyarthritis or a changing pattern over days of mono-or pauciarticular arthritis, think of gonococcal arthritis, SBE, meningococcal arthritis, brucellosis, acute rheumatic fever, viral arthritis
  e. New onset mono- or oligoarthritis associated with cardiac dysrhythmia, think of Lyme disease, acute rheumatic fever, viral arthritis
  f. Patient >50 y/o with chronic myalgias and arthralgias and now transient loss of

Chapter 10 Joint Pain   125

unilateral vision, think of PMR, TA, or stroke
- g. Patient with RA and new onset multiple organ changes (digital gangrene, large skin ulcers, simultaneous peripheral nerves involved as mononeuritis multiplex, mesenteric ischemia, coronary arteritis), think of systemic necrotizing vasculitis
- h. Focal weakness and severe pain on passive stretching of the muscles, think of compartment syndrome (following some trauma) or bacterial tenosynovitis
- i. Diffuse weakness and any one UMN sign (hyperreflexia, Babinski), think of spondylitic myelopathy
- j. New onset polyarticular arthritis with high BP, fever, new rash, think of vasculitis
- k. Joint pains and fever, think of septic arthritis, infective endocarditis, vasculitis, disseminated gonococcus, SLE, gout

3. Admit to the hospital or have a specialist consult as soon as appropriate if there is:
   - a. Elderly patient with new neck pain radiating into the shoulder, arm, hand, think of cervical radiculopathy due to spondylosis
   - b. Chronic inflammatory monoarticular arthritis (often the knee), think of fungal arthritis, TB arthritis, foreign body synovitis
   - c. Patient with chronic RA and new onset of eye pain and tenderness, think of scleritis, acute glaucoma
   - d. Hip pain in a patient taking long term steroids or having sickle cell anemia, think of osteonecrosis (aseptic necrosis)
   - e. Significant OA in a patient <50 y/o, think of secondary causes e.g. occupational, morbid obesity, metabolic causes (see Section E.1.a.4 for a list of causes)
   - f. Gradual onset (<1-2 days) of significant inflammatory joint pain, think of infectious causes e.g. disseminated gonococcemia, infective endocarditis
   - g. Joint disease with fever, weight loss, malaise, high ESR, think of infection, systemic vasculitis, sepsis, autoimmune disease (RA, SLE)
   - h. Shoulder pain with any motion and restricted active and passive ROM, think of "frozen shoulder"
   - i. Weakened and painful shoulder on active abduction, but much less pain on passive movement, think of rotator cuff tear
   - j. Diffuse muscle pain and tenderness, think of thyroid disease, Cushing's syndrome, poly- or dermatomyositis, medications
   - k. Shoulder pain with associated abdominal complaints, think of referred pain from gallbladder, diaphragm, liver disease

C. Make a quick diagnosis if it's obvious.
Is it an easily diagnosed condition or a medication that is responsible for the pain? In most patients you will be highly confident of a common cause of the symptom by now. If not, one or more of the following tests may exclude an organic disease and increase your confidence in your working diagnosis: CBC, ESR, RF, ANA

Recognize an easily diagnosed cause of the "joint" pain:
1. Pain is not intra-articular e.g. either bursitis, tendinitis, fibromyalgia, or myofascial pain
2. Medication side effect

---

1. Periarticular soft tissue diseases *viz* bursitis, tendinitis, tenosynovitis
   - a. Pain with active ROM is significantly worse than with passive ROM testing
   - b. Inflammatory symptoms and signs may occur but they do not signify intra-articular disease
   - c. Mostly the pain seems superficial, as contrasted with the "deep inside" feeling of arthritis, so there is exquisite focal tenderness over the involved site or with maneuvers
   - d. Common sites and causes of periarticular pain
     - (1) Shoulder
       - (a) Subacromial bursitis–occurs together with rotator cuff tendinitis with the same signs and symptoms (see below)

(b) Subcoracoid bursitis–pain over the coracoid process and medial shoulder; restricted forward arm elevation and arm adduction
(c) Rotator cuff tendinitis–pain when sleeping on the affected side; severe pain on active abduction of the affected arm, especially the arc between 60-120°; focal tenderness over the lateral aspect of the humeral head just below the acromion
(d) Bicipital tendinitis–anterior shoulder pain radiating down the biceps into the forearm; shoulder abduction and external rotation of the arm provokes the pain, as does resisting supination of the forearm with the elbow flexed at 90°; bicipital groove is very tender to palpation
(e) Adhesive capsulitis ("frozen shoulder")–pain at rest and markedly restricted ROM, both active and passive; may follow an episode of bursitis or tendinitis or be associated with RSD
(f) Rotator cuff tendon rupture–severe pain and weakness holding the arm at 90° abduction (drop arm sign)
(g) Cervical radiculopathy–C5 commonest
(h) Referred–diaphragm, gall bladder disease, subphrenic abscess, inferior MI, PE, Pancoast tumor
(2) Elbow
   (a) Olecranon bursitis–swelling and tenderness of the posterior point of the elbow
   (b) Lateral epicondylitis (tennis elbow)–associated with any activity involving repeated motions of wrist extension and supination against resistance; pain is provoked by shaking hands or turning a doorknob
   (c) Medial epicondylitis (golfer's elbow)–pain provoked by resisting wrist flexion and forearm pronation with the elbow extended
(3) Wrist and hand
   (a) Dorsum hand and wrist tenosynovitis–soft tissue swelling and localized warmth; hold the wrist in a neutral position and have him flex the digits distal to the MCP joint which causes wrist pain; think of gonococcal infection, gout, other inflammatory arthritides
   (b) deQuervain's tenosynovitis–the wrist pain is provoked by the Finkelstein test (thumb flexed across the palm, fist clenched, and wrist flexed downward provokes pain)
   (c) CTS–paresthesias 1 first 3½ digits; pain forearm to thenar eminence; increased pain at night
   (d) Cubital tunnel syndrome (at medial elbow)–ulnar nerve compression; paresthesias 4-5th digits; decreased grip strength
   (e) OA of the 1st CMC joint–pain lateral wrist, distal to the wrist crease at the base of the thumb
   (f) C_7 cervical radiculopathy–paresthesias digits 2-4; sensory symptoms provoked by neck movements
(4) Hip
   (a) Trochanteric bursitis–hip and back pain; patient supine, press bilaterally over the greater trochanters to provoke pain (point tenderness over the affected bursa)
   (b) Ischial bursitis–back, buttock, leg pain; point tenderness of the bursa overlying the ischial tuberosity; as he sits, palpate under his buttock to provoke pain at the tuberosity
   (c) Iliopsoas bursitis–groin pain over and lateral to femoral

Chapter 10 Joint Pain 127

vessels, and pain is worsened by hip hyperextension; patient tries to flex and externally rotate the hip for pain relief
- (d) Iliotibial band syndrome–painless snapping with walking; dull ache lateral hip and thigh
- (e) Entrapment lateral femoral cutaneous nerve–meralgia paresthetica; pain or dysesthesias unrelated to walking
- (f) Lumbar radiculopathy
- (g) Osteonecrosis femoral head
- (h) Referred pain–kidney stone, knee OA

(5) Knee
- (a) Patellar tendinitis–tender supra- or infrapatellar insertions; pain on climbing stairs
- (b) Prepatella (housemaid's knee)–pain provoked by kneeling
- (c) Osgood-Schlatter disease–adolescent with tenderness at tendon attachments on the tibia
- (d) Pes anserine bursitis–anteromedial tibia, 2" below the tibial tubercle; pain on climbing stairs
- (e) Iliotibial band syndrome–focal tenderness lateral femoral condyle above the lateral joint line
- (f) Chondromalacia patellae–increased pain descending stairs or squatting; crepitus and pain on knee extension
- (g) Referred from hip–positive Patrick test
- (h) L-S radiculopathy–reproduce knee pain with SLR test
- (i) Trauma–get XR, if he can't bear weight or he can't flex 90° or point tender patella
- (j) Posterior knee pain–Baker's cyst

(6) Foot and ankle
- (a) Achilles tendinitis–tendon pain on plantar flexion
- (b) Posterior calcaneal bursitis–posterior heel pain distal to Achilles tendon insertion
- (c) Plantar fasciitis–commonest heel pain; most severe early in the day; tender medial calcaneal tuberosity plantar surface
- (d) Intracalcaneal bursitis–increased pain with activity; focal pain midpoint calcaneus
- (e) Tarsal tunnel syndrome–plantar foot paresthesias, pain at the ankle and sole; nocturnal pain
- (f) Hallux rigidus–1st MTP chronic pain at the end of a step i.e. dorsiflexion
- (g) Morton's neuroma between 3-4 or 2-3 distal MTs; squeeze the MTs together and point pressure between the digits causes pain
- (h) Metatarsalgia–pain along MT heads
- (i) Stress fracture of MTs occurs with sudden increased activity; negative XR early

2. Fibromyalgia
  a. Insidious onset of pain in a patient <45-50 y/o; <u>not articular</u> and <u>no inflammation</u>; <u>no limitation of joint ROM</u>. Different from other causes, there is heightened sensitivity to pain everywhere (determine general sensitivity to pain by pressing hard over a "control" point e.g. thumbnail or midforehead, which causes pressure but <u>not</u> pain)
  b. Tender points can be elicited in a number of predictable sites, and the tenderness is <u>bilateral</u> and approximately symmetrical (neck, upper back, upper chest, buttocks)
  c. Characteristic associated symptoms in about 80% of patients are

chronic fatigue, nonrestorative sleep, morning stiffness
  d. Multiple somatic complaints occurring in > 25% of patients (suggesting systemic involvement) are LBP, neck-shoulder pain, IBS, irritable bladder, hand-wrist arthralgias; no objective signs on exam except the tender points
3. Myofascial pain with TrP
  a. Similar to fibromyalgia in that it may have chronic pain, but it also may cause new onset pain
  b. Different from fibromyalgia: there is only <u>focal tenderness</u> in a tense, taut muscle in a local or regional area, i.e. <u>unilateral</u>; also there is <u>restricted ROM</u> of the affected region
  c. Pressure over the TrP reproduces the patient's complaint (local pain and sometimes, the referred pain)
  d. Injection of the TrP brings almost immediate relief
4. PMR–differs from fibromyalgia in that onset is in a patient >50 y/o and rather rapid onset of widespread stiffness and aching especially in the proximal muscles (shoulder, pelvic girdle); also, significant limitations of ROM, high ESR, associated with TA
5. Palindromic rheumatism–onset and severity of pain like gout; negative tap; episodic attacks (last <2 d) of arthritis of the same joints as in RA but nondestructive synovitis
6. Medications causing allergic or hypersensitivity reactions and joint pain:
  a. Serum sickness includes arthralgias, fever, urticaria, lymphadenopathy occurring <2-3 weeks following drug initiation, or in 2-4 days if the drug previously has been ingested: carbamazepine, cefaclor, ciprofloxacin, fluoxetine, indomethacin, itraconazole, iron dextran, minocycline, pentoxifylline, phenytoin
  b. Drug-induced vasculitis causing arthralgias, palpable purpura, maculopapular rash, renal or liver involvement: allopurinol, azathioprine, carbamazepine, cephalosporins, cimetidine, ciprofloxacin, clarithromycin, furosemide, hydralazine, hydrochlorothiazide, L-tryptophan, mefloquine, methotrexate, naproxen, nizatidine, ofloxacin, penicillin, phenytoin, phenylbutazone, procainamide, propylthiouracil, sotalol, sulfadiazine, terbutaline, torsemide, valproate, warfarin, zidovudine
  c. Autoimmune drug reactions may induce a lupus-like syndrome after months to years of ongoing therapy: anticonvulsants, β-blockers, chlorpromazine, estrogen, hydralazine, interferon, isoniazid, methyldopa, minocycline, penicillamine, procainamide, quinidine, sulfasalazine, terbinafine, zafirlukast

D. **Identify your patient's worries and wants.** Complaint of joint pain occurs in at least 20% of people <60 y/o and in almost all people >65 y/o, yet only few of these consult. During your interview and exam, try to intuit or discover why your patient is here today, and not previously, for this problem. Don't necessarily ask directly, but try to get some ideas from your patient's responses to questions about his perception of the joint pain itself. You can't completely help your patient unless you know what worries him about the joint pain and what he wants from you. That's why he is here to see you--to satisfy his worries and wants! Here are only some of the possible worries and wants of your patient with joint pain. You must discover his specific needs
1. Common worries are:
  a. That the cause of the joint pain is a dangerous etiology e.g. septic arthritis, an inflammatory arthritis, e.g. RA or SLE
  b. That the etiology is some rare disease e.g. SLE, scleroderma, Dengue fever
  c. What other fears or anxieties might be troubling your patient? For example, he may have had joint pain for many years, and only now does he come for help.

Chapter 10 Joint Pain

What has changed? Perhaps a friend or relative, who had similar joint pain, recently has been diagnosed with SLE. There are many other possibilities–think of them

2. Your patient wants:
   a. You to perform a thorough physical exam focused on possible causes of the joint pain and he wants appropriate tests and imaging studies
   b. A plausible explanation of the cause of the joint pain
   c. Confident reassurance from you that it is not a dangerous or rare etiology. Tell him--"The good news, it's not lupus"(or whatever you believe his real worry is)

> During your exam, discover your patient's worries (e.g. "lupus,"infectious arthritis, RA) and wants (e.g. reassurance that it is benign, pain relief), so that you can respond to his specific needs as soon as possible.

   d. To know the prognosis, short term (effects on job, home life, marriage; how soon he will be back to normal) and long term (if recurrences are possible; how to prevent recurrences; if it will cause any disability)
   e. Treatment to stop the joint pain now and to prevent recurrences
   f. A specialist (rheumatologist) referral if he believes you are not confident of the diagnosis

E. Know the symptoms that differentiate the 2 common causes of joint pain.

1. The commonest cause is primary OA, which accounts for at least 80% of joint pain seen in the office
   a. Characteristics of OA
      (1) The pain is due to <u>intra-articular</u> disease, and there is <u>no synovitis</u>. The joint pain is an isolated symptom, i.e. no associated symptoms suggesting any systemic disease or secondary causes of the OA
      (2) Characteristic joints involved are:
         (a) Weight bearing joints of hips, knees and spine

> The causes of most pain due to intra-articular disease are:
> 1. OA–onset of pain in a patient >50 y/o, no sign of synovitis
> 2. RA–onset of pain usually in a patient <50 y/o, signs of synovitis, morning stiffness >30-45 min; typical inflamed joints

         (b) Small joints of hands and feet viz DIP, PIP, 1st CMC and 1st TMT
      (3) Onset of pain is insidious, mostly in patients >50 y/o, and the course is chronic with additive joint involvement; no joint pain at rest, and there is negligible morning stiffness
      (4) Secondary OA due to trauma or over-use of specific joints may result in atypical OA, which is suggested by younger age of onset of joint pain and may involve joints different from the usual for OA
         (a) Ankles and feet (ballet dancer); MCP joints (boxer); knees (roofer, football, basketball); elbow and shoulder (tennis, golf, baseball); specific joints related to work of farmers, miners, dock workers, repetitive factory work

(b) Congenital (Legg-Perthes disease, unequal lengths of lower extremities) or acquired diseases (Charcot joints due to DM; joint damage due to RA, gout, infection, or past history of hemarthroses)
(c) Endocrine or metabolic diseases
  (i) Hypothyroid–low fT4 (FTI) and appropriately elevated TSH
  (ii) Acromegaly–elevated serum IGF-1
  (iii) Hyperparathyroidism–hypercalcemia and inappropriately high serum PTH
  (iv) Diabetes mellitus–hyperglycemia
  (v) Obesity–especially BMI >40 i.e. morbid obesity
  (vi) Hemochromatosis–elevated serum ferritin and high transferrin saturation index
  (vii) Ochronosis–dark urine on standing (alkaptonuria); high urine homogentisic acid
  (viii) Hyperlipoproteinemias–inherited ones e.g. familial hypercholesterolemia, familial combined hyperlipoproteinemia
  (ix) Wilson's disease–unexplained liver disease and early onset OA
b. What suggests it might not be OA
  (1) Anytime there is a symptom or sign suggesting a dangerous cause (see above, Section B)
  (2) If there is any sign of inflammation in the involved joints
  (3) If pain and tenderness are not localized to the involved joints, i.e. the pain is not intra-articular
  (4) If ulnar wrist or MCP joints show signs of disease
  (5) If there is any constitutional symptom early in the disease process e.g. fever, weight loss, prolonged (>30-45 min) morning stiffness
  (6) If, early in the disease process, there is complaint of significant pain at rest, or the pain occurring with activity does not go away with rest e.g. pain awakens him at night
2. Common look-alike causing joint pain and how it differs from OA
a. Rheumatoid arthritis (RA)
  (1) Inflammatory symptoms and signs are due to <u>intra-articular</u> disease, and <u>synovitis</u> i.e. the whole circumference of the joint is swollen, tender, warm (not red); there is significantly decreased ROM of the affected joints
  (2) Onset is gradual in patients <50 y/o, but about 20% may have onset >60 y/o
  (3) Joint pain occurs at rest and morning stiffness lasts >30-45 min (often >2 hr)
  (4) Common joints involved are wrist, MCP, MTP, and PIP; <u>almost never DIP or spine</u> (except cervical spine); pattern of synovitis is additive
  (5) Typically it is a symmetrical polyarthritis, but at onset about 20% will have a monoarthritis with unilateral signs
  (6) Constitutional symptoms and signs (low grade fever <101°F (38.3°C), weight loss, prolonged morning stiffness) and other organs may be involved, but often not at the onset of disease
  (7) Question the diagnosis of RA if:
    (a) Predominantly involved joint early in the course either is DIP or thoracolumbar spine (LBP) or hips
    (b) Temp >101°F (38.3°C), be alert to infection, systemic or local

(c) The joint is actually red and hot, think gout or septic arthritis (joint is rarely red in RA)
(d) There is no involvement of MCP or wrist
(e) Repetitive flares (intermittent episodes of synovitis with periods of complete remission) are occurring; these are common in gout, spondylitis, IBD, psoriatic arthritis
(f) ESR is not elevated (still ESR may be normal in active RA)
(g) Synovial fluid analysis shows crystals (uric acid or calcium pyrophosphate), but RA can coexist with either gout or pseudogout
(h) Bilateral sacroiliitis is present <u>with</u> reactive bony sclerosis on XR

F. Use this summary for efficient diagnosis of a common cause.
With the information from Sections A-E in mind, here is the rapid approach to diagnosis of joint pain.

1. You already have determined:
   a. In Section A, by H&P of the involved joints, whether it is intra-articular pain, and if there is synovitis.
   b. In Section B, that there is no evidence in the H&P of any one dangerous cause of the joint pain.
   c. In Section C, that neither an easily diagnosed condition (bursitis, tendinitis, fibromyalgia, myofascial pain syndrome) nor a medication is likely responsible for the pain.
2. From the focused H&P almost always you should quickly be confident of a working diagnosis. Confident final diagnosis is made only in followup the next few weeks or months when the response to treatment or nontreatment is appropriate to your working diagnosis.
   a. If there is the slightest suspicion that it may be a septic joint, or even 1-3 septic joints, perform arthrocentesis stat.
   b. If the pain is due to intra-articular disease and there is no sign of joint inflammation (synovitis) with onset in a patient >50 y/o, diagnose primary OA and treat appropriately. If onset of the OA is <40 y/o be certain there is no treatable secondary cause of the OA.
   c. If the pain is due to intra-articular disease and there are signs of inflammation (synovitis) and other characteristics (morning stiffness >30 min, typical joints) of rheumatoid arthritis, diagnose and treat appropriately.
3. Answer your patient's worries and wants that you determined early on during the exam (Section D). Have you done everything you can to help him?
4. You now have a working diagnosis, but only with followup, sometimes long term, can you be highly confident it is correct. In return visits you are always testing by H&P that your working diagnosis is correct.

G. Abandon your working diagnosis and look for an uncommon cause only if:
1. Any <u>one</u> dangerous symptom or sign (see above, Section B.) occurs in followup of weeks, months, or years. Quickly obtain a specialist consult or send the patient to the hospital as appropriate
2. The joint pain does not respond to treatment as you expect or the natural history of your working diagnosis does not occur. OA should respond within days to treatment with acetaminophen (up to 4000 mg/d). RA requires aggressive treatment with

methotrexatae or azathioprine by your rheumatology consult

Don't spend time and money looking for one of the following etiologies until you are sure your patient doesn't have either OA or RA causing his joint pain. Nevertheless, it may be he has an uncommon or rare cause of the joint pain. These are important to recognize because each has different treatment or prophylaxis

a. Unusual forms of OA with inflammatory components
   (1) Erosive OA–episodic "flares" of synovitis, especially DIP and PIP; ulnar wrist and MCP not involved; there is much greater destruction and functional loss than usual OA
   (2) Generalized OA–episodes of "flares" with swollen, warm, tender joints; may be high ESR, negative RF
b. Inflammatory arthritis, may have positive serum RF but it's not RA:
   (1) SBE–leukocytosis and fever >38°C (100.4°F); may be cardiac murmur
   (2) Lyme disease–clinical picture indistinguishable from RA; history of summer rash in particular locales
   (3) Sarcoidosis–bilateral hilar lymphadenopathy, dry cough, DOE, high ESR
   (4) Viral infections e.g. IM, HBV, HCV
   (5) Oral contraceptives–arthralgias, morning stiffness, polyarticular synovitis
   (6) Chronic bacterial infections–TB, syphilis
   (7) Palindromic rheumatism

> If your patient's symptoms do not respond as expected to your management, he may have an uncommon or rare cause listed in Section G.2 that you can diagnose and treat. Or you may want to refer your patient to a specialist.

c. Inflammatory polyarthritis and negative serum RF
   (1) Seronegative spondyloarthropathies:
      (a) Inflamed joints are asymmetric and predominantly lower extremity
      (b) Inflammatory LBP, improves with activity
      (c) Individual diseases are:
         (i) Psoriatic arthritis is the commonest; look for any evidence of psoriasis viz scalp, ears, umbilicus, perianal, nails (onycholysis, pitting, yellowing); may be inflamed DIP joints
         (ii) Enteropathic arthritis i.e. any signs or symptoms of IBD
         (iii) Ankylosing spondylitis--20-30 y/o with unusual presentation of LBP and morning stiffness; enthesitis at Achilles tendon or manubriosternal joint ("chest pain"); bilateral sacroiliitis (Gaenslen's test), while the other spondyloarthropathies may have unilateral sacroiliitis
         (iv) Reactive arthritis–nongonococcal urethritis or cervicitis or diarrheal illness in the past 3-4 weeks; enthesitis at Achilles tendon and plantar fascia (fasciitis); painless ulcer of the glans penis, psoriaform lesions of the soles
   (2) Gout– like RA it may present with inflamed small joints of the hands, as may be the case with longstanding gout; arthrocentesis must be done to exclude septic joint
   (3) Pseudogout–rarely polyarticular; diagnosis by arthrocentesis
   (4) Relapsing polychondritis–inflamed cartilage especially external ear and nose; episodes of asymmetric arthritis that resolve spontaneously in weeks without deformity
   (5) Hypertrophic osteoarthropathy (acropachy)–clubbing of the digits, hands and feet; chief complaint may be bone pain when the legs are in a dependent position (periostitis); clue to lung malignancy or chronic lung infections
   (6) Glucocorticoid withdrawal–diffuse polyarticular hand pain
   (7) HIV–acute polyarthritis and fever in an at-risk patient
   (8) Infectious arthritis–symmetric polyarthritis may follow fever, ST, cervical lymphadenectasis due to HBV, EBV, adenovirus, echovirus, *M. pneumoniae*, rheumatic fever
   (9) Malignancy– synovial metastases causing monoarthritis; nonHodgkins lymphoma
   (10) Rheumatic fever–in adults, additive, symmetric large joint polyarthritis of lower extremities rapidly developing over a week; painful tenosynovitis; pain responds to salicylates
   (11) Hypothyroidism–joint effusions, high CPK

Chapter 10 Joint Pain   133

  (12) Calcific periarthritis–skin is red over affected joints; no joint effusion, and passive ROM less pain than active ROM
  (13) FMF–abdominal pain, large joint oligoarthritis
  (14) Hemochromatosis–bony enlargement of MCP joints but not synovitis
  (15) Sickle cell disease–oligoarthritis associated with painful crises
  (16) Hemophilic arthropathy–hemarthroses result in a proliferative synovitis
  (17) Hyperlipoproteinemia–Achilles tendinitis, tenosynovitis, oligoarticular synovitis without morning stiffness
  (18) Angioimmunoblastic lymphadenopathy–nonerosive polyarthritis, large joints, lymphadenectasis, rash, hypergammaglobulinemia
  (19) Amyloidosis–arthralgias due to amyloid deposits in synovial tissues e.g. CRF
  (20) Idiopathic hypereosinophilic syndrome–myalgias, arthralgias, pericarditis, high eosinophilia
  (21) Pigmented villonodular synovitis–chronic synovitis, often monoarthritis of the knee
  (22) Whipples' disease–rapid onset migratory arthritis in a white man >age 40, chronic diarrhea
  (23) Thyroid (acropachy)--mild synovitis with Graves disease; clubbing rare
  d. Diffuse connective tissue diseases– all may begin with systemic symptoms and mild polyarthritis of PIP and MCP i.e. just like RA–so what differentiates each one?
  (1) SLE--like RA, symmetric small joint polyarthritis of hands, wrists, feet and chief complaint may be the joints; organized synovitis causing erosion is rare but deformities are common due to inflamed tendons and joint capsule. Key to diagnosis is finding associated symptoms: Raynauds (history of digital ulcers, "can't get things from the freezer"), mucosal ulcers, skin lesions, alopecia, multi-organ involvement, photosensitivity e.g. "sick" (serositis or fevers) after being in the sun; ANA positive; 30% positive RF
  (2) Vasculitides–polyarthritis is asymmetric but joints are rarely the chief complaint; rather the dominant symptoms reflect which organs are most affected e.g. rash in hypersensitivity angiitis or neuropathy in PAN or CRF
  (3) Polymyositis/Dermatomyositis–diffuse muscle pain, tenderness, and weakness; increased serum CPK; proliferative synovitis is rare so key is to determine that it is a "non-joint" problem; 20% positive RF
  (4) Scleroderma (systemic sclerosis)--diffuse musculoskeletal pain due to skin thickening; rarely inflamed joints, so mostly a "non-joint" problem; 20% positive RF
  e. Episodic arthritis
  (1) FMF–typical ancestry, attacks lasting 1-3 d, fever, abdominal pain
  (2) Hyperimmunoglobulinemia D syndrome–similar symptoms, attacks 3-7 d, north Europeans, high serum IgD
  (3) Palindromic rheumatism–(see above, Section C.5)
  (4) Intermittent hydrarthrosis–knee, hip
  (5) Eosinophilic synovitis–synovial fluid eosinophilia

H. Use the glossary for precise thinking and accurate diagnosis.

1. **Acropachy**–(Greek *akron* meaning "extremity" and *pachys*, "thick.") It literally means thickened extremities i.e. clubbing. Acropachy is another name for hypertrophic osteoarthropathy, which may be primary or secondary, and Graves disease is one cause.
2. **Additive**–Symptoms begin in one or more joints and symptoms in these joints persist even as symptoms begin in other joints, e.g. in rheumatoid arthritis, SLE, OA.
3. **Anaphylaxis** (Greek *an* meaning "without" and *phylaxis,* "protection.") Originally it was thought that the first injection of an antigen reduced the immunity to the drug and the individual then was left without protection against a second dose. We now know it is just the opposite, too much reaction and protection.
4. **Angioedema** (Greek *angeion* meaning "vessel" or a conduit for any fluid e.g. blood vessel, and *oidema*, "swelling.")
5. **Ankylosis** (Greek *ankylos* meaning "bent or crooked.") It indicates a so fixation of joints by disease or iatrogenic causes, often in a bent configuration.
6. **Antalgic** (Greek *an* meaning "without" and *algia*, "pain.") it means he assumes a posture or gait that lessens the pain.
7. **Arthralgia** (Greek *arthron* meaning "joint" and *algia,* "pain.") It is joint pain only, without inflammation (synovitis), swelling or limitation of range of motion.
8. **Arthrocentesis** (Greek *arthron* meaning "joint" and *kentesis*, "puncture.") It is needle aspiration of joint fluid.

9. **Chondritis** (Greek *chondros* meaning "cartilage" and *itis*, "inflammation.") It is inflammation leading to destruction of cartilage.
10. **Constitutional** (symptom)--symptom suggesting whole body reaction to a localized disease (fever, fatigue, malaise, anemia, weight loss), as opposed to a symptom emanating from the diseased organ itself e.g. pulmonary disease causing hemoptysis, dyspnea, cough.
11. **Contracture** (Latin *contractus* meaning "drawn together.") It is loss of full range of movement of a joint due to a fixed resistance; it could be reversible muscle spasm or permanent periarticular fibrosis.
12. **Crepitus** (Latin *crepitus* meaning "a rattle or crackling sound.") Now it is used for the coarseness of joint movement palpated in advanced joint damage in osteoarthritis.
13. **Dactylitis** (Greek *daktylos* meaning "finger" and *itis*, "inflammation.") It literally means inflammation of a finger or toe, but it refers to a diffuse swelling of a single finger or toe, resembling a "sausage digit"; it is distinctive of spondyloarthropathies including psoriatic arthritis.
14. **Deformity**–Abnormal shape or size of a structure, for example resulting from bony hypertrophy, malaligned articulating structures, damage to periarticular supporting structures; examples in OA would be Heberden's nodes (DIP) and Bouchard's nodes (PIP).
15. **Diarthrodial** joint (Greek *diarthrosis* meaning a "movable articulation" or joint.)
16. **Dislocation** (Latin *dis* meaning "apart" and *locare*, "to place.") It is an abnormal displacement of articulating surfaces so they don't contact properly.
17. **Effusion** (Latin *effusio* meaning "a pouring out.") It is an escape of fluid into a tissue or space, either transudate or exudate.
18. **Enervating** (Latin *enervatio* meaning languor or "lack of nervous energy.")
19. **Enthesitis** (Greek *enthesis* meaning "a putting in or insertion.") Entheses are tendinous or ligamentous insertions of muscle on bone, so it is inflammation of entheses.
20. **Epicondylitis** (Greek *epi* meaning "on, upon or over" and *kondylos*, "knob or knuckle.") It is inflammation of the rounded prominence at the end of bone.
21. **Girdle**, shoulder or hip–Encircling structure or anything that encircles a joint.
22. **Gout** (Latin *gutta* meaning "a drop of fluid.") Ancient theory was that concretions in the joint were due to distillation "drop by drop" of bad humors in the body.
23. **Hemarthrosis** (Greek *haime* meaning "blood" and *arthron*, "joint.") It is extravasation of blood into a joint space.
24. **Insidious** (Latin *insidiosus* meaning "deceitful or treacherous.") A symptom coming on so subtly over a long period of time that he can't tell you exactly when it began.
25. **Migratory** –Even as one diseased joint improves or returns to normal, symptoms begin in another joint, e.g. gonococcal arthritis, rheumatic fever.
26. **Myelopathy** (Greek *myelos* meaning "marrow or inmost core" and *pathos*, "disease.") It can refer to bone marrow or the "marrow" of the CNS esp. spinal cord, so any disease of the spinal cord.
27. **Oligoarthritis** (Greek *oligo* meaning "few" and *arthron*, "joint.") It is so inflammation of 2-3 joints. Note oligo- is Greek, and *pauci-* is Latin, both meaning "few."
28. **Onycholysis** (Greek *onyx, onychos*, meaning "nail" and *lysis*, "dissolution.") It is separation of the nail plate from the nail bed beginning at the distal free margin.
29. **Osteoarthritis** (Greek *osteon* meaning "bone" and *arthron*, "joint.") It is not inflammatory clinically i.e. no evidence of synovitis.
30. **Osteophyte** (Greek *phyton* meaning "plant.") It is a bony outgrowth.
31. **Palindromic** (rheumatism)–(Greek *palin* meaning "again" and *dramein*, "to run.") In literature, a word or sentence that is the same read forward or backward. In medicine it refers to the rapid appearance and rapid disappearance of the arthritis.
32. **Paraparesis (spastic)** (Greek *para* meaning "beyond" and *paresis*, "paralysis.") Now, it means a partial paralysis of the lower extremities.
33. **Pauciarticular** (Latin *paucus* meaning "few" and *articularis*, "pertaining to a joint.") It means few, for example, 2-3 joints inflamed, in contrast to polyarticular, meaning >3 joints inflamed.
34. **Pes anserine (bursa)** (Latin *pes* meaning "foot" and *anserinus*, "like a goose foot.") The tendinous insertions resemble a goose's foot.
35. **Podagra** (Greek *pod* meaning "foot" and *agra*, "seizure.") The pain was like a seizure, as if the foot were caught in a trap.
36. **Polyarthritis** (Greek *polys* meaning "many" and *arthron*, "joint.") It indicates many (≥ 4) joints are inflamed.
37. **Radiculopathy** (Latin *radicula* meaning "radicle" or the smallest extension of a nerve or vessel, likened to "a little root.") Now it is used for compressive disease of the nerve roots causing radiating pain.

Chapter 10 Joint Pain   135

38. **Range of motion**–The arc (in degrees) of movement through which a diarthrodial joint moves in a single plane, either by active or passive movement.
39. **Rheumatism** (Greek *rheuma* meaning "flowing like a stream," i.e. any watery discharge.) Only in the 17th century was *rheumatismos,* watery effusion in joints, applied to all connective tissues. Now, "rheumatism" of joints is called arthralgia or arthritis, whereas "soft tissue rheumatic pain" refers to muscles, bursae, tendons, fibrous tissue.
40. **Rheumatoid**–Resembling rheumatism, but different in its systemic or extraarticular manifestations.
41. **Sclerosis** (Greek *skleros* meaning "hard or tough.") In osteoarthritis, focal bone thickening causes joint surfaces to be bright white on radiography.
42. **Sicca** (Latin *siccus* meaning "dry.") The Greek word for dry is *xero,* e.g. xerostoma, xerophthalmia, xerosis.
43. **Spondyloarthropathy** (Greek *spondylos* meaning "a vertebra" and *arthro,* "joint" and *pathos*, "disease.") It is arthritis, usually polyarthritis along with associated spinal inflammation. All entities are seronegative i.e. negative for rheumatoid factor.
44. **Spondylosis** (Greek *spondylos* meaning "a vertebra" and *osis*, a general term for disease or morbid process.) It is degenerative change of a vertebra due to osteoarthritis.
45. **Subluxation** (Latin *sub* meaning "under or less than" and *luxare*, "to put out of joint.") It is a partial dislocation.
46. **Synovitis** (Greek *syn* meaning "associated with or endowed with" and *oon,* "egg" and *itis*, "inflammation.") It is inflammation of the synovium. Normal synovial fluid resembles egg white and it is secreted by synovial membranes, which enclose joint spaces, bursae and tendon sheaths.
47. **Tenosynovitis** (Greek *tenon* meaning "tendon" but originally it meant "to stretch.") It is any inflammation of a tendon sheath.

136 *Werner's* Office Diagnosis

Chapter 11
Low Back Pain (LBP)

Questions on Low Back Pain

A. In a patient with complaint of "My back hurts," the most important
   1. Historical information is:
   2. First physical exam maneuver is:
B. In the office the commonest cause of LBP and its distinguishing characteristics are:
   1.
      a.
      b.
      c.
C. The other 3 common causes of LBP in the office, and their distinguishing characteristics are:
   1.
      a.
      b.
      c.
   2.
      a.
      b.
      c.
   3.
      a.
      b.
      c.
D. Of the above 4 common causes (in questions B and C), you would expect a positive SLR test in:

E. You have 4 patients, each bringing their MRI of the low back showing a lesion at a different level. For each patient, the root that likely is compressed, and the physical exam findings you would expect to find if that particular nerve root is causing your patient's pain, are the following:
   1. Protuberant disc between L_{4-5}
      a. Root:
      b. Expected findings on exam:
   2. Protuberant disc between L_5-S_1
      a. Root:
      b. Expected findings on exam:
   3. Protuberant disc between L_{3-4}
      a. Root:
      b. Expected findings on exam:
   4. Protuberant disc between L_{1-2}
      a. Root:
      b. Expected findings on exam:
F. Your patient is 70 y/o and has new onset LBP beginning "about 2 weeks ago." Neurological exam is normal except the left patellar reflex is 4/6 and the right patellar reflex, as well as other DTRs, are 1/6
   1. On history, you additionally want to know:
   2. Other than provide an analgesic, your management:

Chapter 11 Low Back Pain 137
Answers on Low Back Pain (LBP)
A. Be certain of your patients' symptom and its distinguishing characteristics
   1. "Show me exactly where you are hurting." You are looking for pain that originates centrally over the spine and between vertebrae L_4-S_1. Use the spinous process at the level of the iliac crest (L_{3-4}) to estimate the level of the pain site at the involved vertebra.
   Then, "What were you doing before the pain began?" i.e. anything unusual just before and also the previous 1-2 days. "When did the pain begin?" and "Have you ever had similar back pain before now?" You want to be certain whether it is either new onset pain, or episodic pain, or chronic, almost daily, back pain
   2. If there is complaint of pain radiating into the leg, perform a SLR test to determine if the SLR maneuver <u>exactly reproduces</u> the radiating pain, suggesting radiculopathy. Caution, radiating pain that does not go below the knee could represent referred pain from a lesion in the abdomen or pelvis
B. The commonest cause of LBP and its characteristics
   1. Lumbosacral strain syndrome (LSS)
      a. <u>New</u> LBP in a patient <50 y/o
      b. Rapid or gradual onset (<48 hr) after injury or unusual activity
      c. LBP is the dominant, isolated symptom
C. The other 3 common causes of LBP and their distinguishing characteristics
   1. Herniated disc with radiculopathy
      a. <u>New</u> LBP in a patient <50 y/o
      b. Rapid or gradual onset (after injury or unusual activity)
      c. LBP <u>and</u> radiating pain are equally dominant, and almost always unilateral
   2. Spinal stenosis
      a. <u>Episodic</u> back, buttock or leg pain in a patient >50 y/o
      b. No history of injury or unusual activity preceding the pain; it only occurs during normal walking or standing for 5-10 minutes, then rapid onset of the pain radiates into the buttocks or legs
      c. Dominant pain is in buttocks and legs, and it may be bilateral
   3. Psychological disorder e.g. MD, GAD, somatization
      a. <u>Chronic daily</u> LBP, onset at any age
      b. Insidious onset
      c. LBP is but one of a number of other chronic symptoms
D. Only one of the common causes has a positive SLR test
   Only in a patient with possible herniated disc causing radiculopathy should you perform a SLR test. Provoking only back pain upon doing the SLR e.g. in a patient with LSS, is <u>not</u> a positive test. You must perform the SLR test correctly–see the appendix in Section G.3
E. There is a false positive rate of 40% for protruding disk by MRI
   Be sure your patient's symptoms and signs are consistent with the MRI findings. The root crossing any lumbar intervertebral disc exits at the next lower vertebra, so the compressed root takes its level from the lower vertebra
   1. Lesion between L_{4-5} on the MRI
      a. L_5 root
      b. No DTR innervation by L_5; decreased sensation dorsal digits 2-4; decreased strength great toe dorsiflexion; decreased strength ankle dorsiflexion, thus difficulty walking on his heel on the involved side

2. Lesion between L_5-S_1 on MRI
   a. S_1 root
   b. Achilles reflex may be decreased or absent; decreased sensation dorsum of 5th digit; decreased plantar flexion of the ankle, thus decreased ability to walk on his toes on that leg
3. Lesion between L_{3-4} on MRI
   a. L_4 root
   b. Patellar reflex may be decreased or absent; decreased sensation dorsum of the great toe; decreased quadriceps strength, so difficulty rising from a squat position
4. Lesion between L_{1-2} on the MRI
   a. L_2 root
   b. Not a cause of LBP; neither a cause of radiating pain (radiculopathy) into the leg, nor a cause of a positive SLR test

F. Recognize a sign of danger in a patient with LBP
Nothing, because new onset LBP in a patient >50 y/o is a dangerous symptom. The finding of a sign (dangerous) of an UMN lesion i.e. hyperactive unilateral patellar reflex, tells you that the patient's LBP likely is referred pain from a spinal cord lesion. No other information is needed because you are going to get a spinal MRI at once. Remember that the spinal cord ends at about vertebra L_1, and LBP is caused almost always by a lesion between vertebrae L_4 and S_1. Thus a single lesion anywhere between vertebrae L_4-S_1 cannot cause or account for both his UMN sign (due to a lesion above L_1) and LBP (roots L_4, L_5, S_1)

Chapter 11 Low Back Pain 139

Low Back Pain (LBP)

Differential diagnosis: the 4 common causes of LBP
1. LSS–<u>new</u> LBP in a patient <50 y/o; history of recent injury or unusual exertion
2. Herniated disc with radiculopathy–<u>new</u> LBP and pain radiating down the leg; history of recent injury or strain; patient <50 y/o
3. Spinal stenosis–<u>episodic</u> LBP; patient >50 y/o; rapid onset of pain during walking or standing; no recent injury
4. Psychological disorder–chronic <u>daily</u> LBP; insidious onset; typical psychological symptoms; onset of pain in patient <50 y/o

A. **Be certain of the symptom and its distinguishing characteristics.** Your patient's problem or chief complaint is "My back aches" or "I hurt my back again"
1. First, be certain the problem is pain originating in the spinal or paraspinal area, and be certain the pain is located in the lumbar area of the back. For further orientation, identify the L_{3-4} interspace at the level of the top of the iliac crest. Ask him to "Show me where the pain is," and don't ask him to point. With the usual causes of LBP, he may voluntarily point with 1-2 fingers to the painful site. Not pointing may suggest diffuse referred pain caused by abdominal or pelvic visceral disease. Be sure the pain origin is over the vertebrae or paraspinous muscles, and not the CVA area. Determine if there is radiation of the pain–"Show me exactly where the pain goes." Finally, "When did the back pain begin?" and "Tell me how it started, and what you were doing the previous 1-2 days"
2. Almost all LBP you will see in the office had its onset the previous few days. A new onset of LBP may:
   a. Last a short time, and not happen again ever;
   b. Last a short time, then recur once or more over the next months or years, and this is "episodic LBP"; or
   c. Persist almost daily and become chronic LBP.
   Determine which of these is your patient. If your patient's back pain persists daily or occurs on most days of the month, a different approach to diagnosis is needed (see Section G.2)
3. Physical examination
   a. Back–
      (1) Percuss the spine for point tenderness and test ROM for any limitation (lateral ROM and extension, expect 30°; flexion, expect 80-90°)
      (2) Palpate for paraspinal muscle spasm and check for flattening of normal lordosis
      (3) Palpate the paraspinal muscles, posterior pelvis and gluteal areas for TrP of myofascial pain syndrome and greater trochanters for bursitis or tender points of fibromyalgia
      (4) Perform a supine SLR test if symptoms suggest radiculopathy, or do a <u>sitting</u> SLR test (see Appendix, Section G.3.a) if you suspect malingering
   b. Abdomen–

(1) Palpate and percuss for any suggestion of disease causing referred pain
(2) Palpate for tenderness or a pulsatile mass
(3) Percuss for CVA tenderness with the patient supine (use the lower ribs as control points)

Be certain:
1. Whether the pain is in the lumbosacral spine area or if it radiates down the leg
2. Whether any injury or unusual activity occurred in the previous 1-2 days
3. Whether it is either new pain or episodic pain or daily pain

(If it is chronic, persistent LBP, >3 months, see Section G.2).

---

c. Hip and sacroiliac joint disease–
   (1) Patrick test–heel to the opposite knee, press down on the ipsilateral knee; pain suggests either hip or sacroiliac disease
   (2) Laguerre's test (passive internal and external rotation of the hip joint while you hold the patient's heel) is more specific for hip disease
d. Neurological–
   (1) LBP radiculopathy indicates L_4, L_5 or S_1 root is possibly affected
   (2) Your exam really is to confirm what you already know from the history, or to find an unexpected dangerous sign
   (3) Pain radiation to the great toe suggests L_4; to the little toe S_1; to the area in between, L_5
   (4) DTRs are decreased or absent at the patella (L_4) or Achilles (S_1)
   (5) L_5 has no DTR, but it enables dorsiflexion of the great toe and ankle, so its loss would not allow normal heel walking. Loss of S_1 would not allow normal walking on his toes

By now you should be confident your patient has LBP, whether it is new, episodic or chronic, daily pain, and if it remains localized to the back or radiates down the leg. In almost all instances you now have the information you need for diagnosis of the obvious causes (Section C) and the common causes (Section E). In the rare instance that your patient appears different clinically from the usual office patient with LBP, be certain (Section B) that he does not have a symptom or sign of a dangerous disease

B. Be confident it's not a dangerous disease.
1. Send immediately to the ED by ambulance if there is:
   a. New onset UMN sign (unilateral hyperreflexia, Babinski, spasticity, lower extremity weakness) with the LBP, think of a spinal cord lesion e.g. tumor or epidural abscess
   b. Abrupt onset of severe LBP unassociated with activity and the patient is on anticoagulants, think of retroperitoneal hemorrhage
   c. New onset of back pain along with a pulsating abdominal mass, think of a rupturing abdominal aortic aneurysm
   d. Back pain with rapid onset of urinary retention, bilateral weakness or numbness, think of cauda equina syndrome
   e. Constant back pain at night, think of cauda equina syndrome, compression fracture, tumor, abscess
2. Admit at once to the ED or hospital if there is:

Chapter 11 Low Back Pain 141

   a. Abrupt onset of very severe back pain without an obvious precipitating event, think of compression fracture, referred pain (AD, ruptured viscus, ectopic pregnancy, nephrolithiasis, spinal vascular accident)
   b. Back pain with associated neurological symptoms e.g. bladder or rectal incontinence, erectile dysfunction, sensory level, lower extremity weakness, think of cord compression due to tumor, hematoma, epidural abscess
   c. Back pain with associated fever, weight loss , anemia, high ESR, malaise, think of osteomyelitis or epidural abscess; if also a murmur, think of SBE
   d. Localized area of spinal tenderness, pain at rest and high ESR, think of osteomyelitis, epidural abscess, malignancy, MM
   e. Sciatica that is gradually and progressively worsening, think of an enlarging lesion
3. Admit to the hospital or have a specialist consult as soon as appropriate if there is:

Be certain in the first minutes of your exam, that there is no evidence of any <u>one</u> dangerous symptom or sign associated with the back pain:
1. New or different back pain in a patient >50 y/o
2. New onset severe back pain without a precipitating event
3. Insidious onset, but progressively worsening back pain
4. Focal neurological signs, e.g. altered bowel or bladder dysfunction, leg weakness
5. Unexplained fever or weight loss
6. Pain worse at night or with recumbency
7. Radiculopathy with recent trauma

Any suggestion of a dangerous disease, send your patient to the ED.

---

   a. Any suggestion of referred pain causing the LBP (no precipitating event, usual changes in position do not aggravate or alleviate pain, any radiating pain into the leg that does not go below the knee, leg pain that occurs alone or precedes the LBP), think of disease of another organ and look for symptoms and signs of that organ, e.g. pancreas, stomach, gallbladder, aorta, uterus, ectopic pregnancy, endometriosis
   b. New or different back pain in a patient >50 y/o, think of tumor, infection, referred pain
   c. Back pain not relieved by recumbency or it awakens him at night, think of spinal cord tumor or infection
   d. Back pain and unexplained occult hematuria, think of referred pain from kidney infection or tumor
   e. In a patient <30-40 y/o with back pain unrelieved by rest and recumbency, pain worse at night, high ESR, think of ankylosing spondylitis, infection, tumor
   f. Back pain with history of malignancy or a new malignancy, think of metastasis to bone or spinal cord
   g. Back and leg pain that occur only after walking or running some distance and the pain is relieved after standing a couple of minutes, think of vascular claudication due to PVD; if relieved much <u>quicker</u> by sitting or leaning forward, think of spinal stenosis
   h. LBP associated with an UMN sign e.g. unilateral hyperreflexia, Babinski, spasticity, clonus, think of a spinal cord lesion
   i. LBP and bilateral radiculopathy with bilateral neurological deficits or bladder, rectal or sexual symptoms, think of a large central herniated disk
   j. LBP that radiates into the leg but not below the knee, think of referred pain from abdomen or pelvis
   k. Unexplained significant worsening of the LBP (diagnosed as LSS) with conservative therapy, think of an alternative, possibly dangerous etiology
   l. Back or rib pain precipitated by movement in a patient >40 y/o with history of injury, think of multiple myeloma

C. **Make a quick diagnosis if it's obvious.** Is it an easily diagnosed condition or a medication that is likely responsible for the LBP? In most patients you will be <u>highly</u> confident of a common

cause of the symptom by now. If not, one or more of the following tests may exclude an organic disease and increase your confidence in your working diagnosis: CBC, ESR
1. Extraspinal disease
   a. Hip joint disease–Patrick test or Laguerre's test is positive
   b. UTI, kidney tumor, nephrolithiasis–symptoms of urinary tract disease, unilateral CVA tenderness
   c. Coccydynia–painful coccyx; psychological or secondary to forgotten trauma
   d. Ischial bursitis–due to prolonged periods of sitting; very tender ischial tuberosity; pain may simulate radiculopathy i.e. back, buttock, thigh pain
   e. Trochanteric bursitis–tender ipsilateral bursa provoked by pressing on both trochanteric bursae simultaneously
   f. Iliolumbar syndrome–when testing spinal lateral ROM away from the painful side, pain is reproduced or worsened, and contralateral ROM is decreased

---

Recognize any easily diagnosed cause of the LBP:
1. Extraspinal disease e.g. UTI, pyelonephritis, hip disease, bursitis, myofascial pain
2. Pregnancy; morbid obesity
3. Medication side effect e.g. anticoagulant, glucocorticoids

---

   g. Piriformis syndrome–may be positive SLR test, but no neurological symptoms; with patient sitting and knees together, his trying to spread his knees against your resistance provokes the pain
   h. Myofascial pain syndrome–palpate for painful TrP in the paraspinal and gluteal muscles and at their insertions on the posterior pelvis
2. Pregnancy, usually third trimester; morbid obesity (BMI >40 i.e. >200 lb for 5 ft person then add 8 lb for each additional inch in height e.g. 5'6" > 250 lb; 5'9" > 275 lb; 6' >300 lb)
3. Medications
   a. Anticoagulants–associated with retroperitoneal hemorrhage
   b. Glucocorticoids–increased osteoporosis, risk of compression fractures, unusual back infections
   c. LBP can occur short term with infusion of streptokinase or anistreplase
   d. Nitrofurantoin can cause LBP associated with an acute lung reaction, high fever, dyspnea

D. **Identify your patient's worries and wants.** LBP occurs annually in up to 70% of people, and only a few consult about it. During your interview and exam, try to intuit or discover why your patient is here today, and not previously, for this problem. Don't necessarily ask directly, but try to get some ideas from your patient's responses to questions about the LBP itself. You can't completely help your patient unless you know what he really worries about and wants from you. That's why he is here to see you–to satisfy his worries and wants! Here are only some of the possible worries and wants of your patient with LBP. You must discover his specific, unique ones
1. Common worries are:
   a. That the cause is a dangerous etiology e.g. nerve or spinal cord damage, "broken back," cancer

b. That the etiology is some rare disease e.g. Lyme disease, GBS, malaria
c. What other fears or anxieties might be troubling your patient? For example, he may have had LBP for many years, and only now does he come for help. What has changed? Perhaps a friend or relative, who had similar episodic LBP, recently has been diagnosed with a tumor. There are many other possibilities–think of them
2. Your patient wants:

> During your exam, discover your patient's worries (e.g. cancer, infection, nerve damage) and wants (e.g. pain relief, reassurance if it's benign), so that you can respond to his specific needs as soon as possible.

  a. You to perform a thorough physical exam focused on possible causes of the LBP and he wants appropriate tests and imaging studies
  b. A plausible explanation of the cause of the LBP. Spend time educating him about his symptoms. Avoid terms such as "ruptured" disc or even "degenerative" disc. If appropriate to his diagnosis, emphasize the cause is "muscle or ligament strain." Even radiculopathy due to herniated disc is successfully treated conservatively in almost all instances
  c. Confident reassurance from you that it is not a dangerous or rare etiology. Tell him--"The good news, it's not nerve or spinal cord damage" (or whatever you believe his real worry is)
  d. To know the prognosis, short term (effects on job, home life, marriage; how soon he will be back to normal) and long term (if recurrences are possible; how to prevent recurrences; if it will cause any disability). Educate him regarding the excellent prognosis for either LSS or radiculopathy due to herniated disc
  e. Treatment to stop the LBP now and to prevent recurrences; provide exercises for back strengthening
  f. A specialist referral (neurologist) if he believes you are not confident of the diagnosis

E. Know the symptoms that differentiate the 4 common causes of low back pain.

1. The commonest cause is lumbosacral strain (LSS)
   a. Characteristics of LSS
      (1) New or episodic LBP (first episode <50 y/o)
      (2) The LBP is an <u>isolated</u> symptom
      (3) He can tell you exactly when the pain began and it commonly began during, or within 12-48 hours of some precipitating activity e.g. bending, lifting, gardening
      (4) Back movements (especially flexion) aggravate the pain, and motionless recumbency relieves the pain; he often is <u>least</u> comfortable sitting, even if motionless
   b. What suggests it might not be LSS
      (1) Anytime there is an associated symptom or sign suggesting a dangerous cause of the back pain (see above, Section B)
      (2) If the LBP is just one of a number of complaints, e.g. additional symptoms suggesting referred pain due to abdominal, pelvic or hip diseases
      (3) If motionless recumbency does not almost totally relieve the pain, or if sitting motionless <u>does</u> totally relieve the pain
      (4) If there are associated symptoms and signs suggesting the presence of radiculopathy or systemic disease
2. Common look-alikes and how each differs from LSS
   a. Herniated disc with radiculopathy
      (1) It is similar to LSS in all respects, except the LBP is not

isolated; that is, in addition to the LBP, there is radiating pain into the ipsilateral buttock, thigh, calf, and commonly, the foot; the radiating pain is aggravated by any Valsalva maneuver, such as cough, sneezing, BM

Common causes of most new or episodic LBP in the office patient:
1. LSS–<u>new</u> LBP in a patient <50 y/o; history of recent injury or unusual exertion
2. Herniated disc with radiculopathy–<u>new</u> LBP and pain radiating down the leg; history of recent injury or strain; patient <50 y/o
3. Spinal stenosis–<u>episodic</u> LBP; patient >50 y/o; rapid onset of pain during walking or standing; no recent injury
4. Psychological disorder–<u>daily</u> LBP; insidious onset; typical psychological symptoms; onset of pain in patient <50 y/o

---

    (2) SLR test on the affected side should <u>exactly</u> reproduce the patient's radiating pain into the leg (see Appendix, Section G.3.a)
  b. Spinal stenosis
    (1) <u>Episodic</u> LBP or numbness radiating into one or both legs only during walking or standing for some period of time
    (2) Almost always onset of LBP is in a patient >50 y/o
    (3) The pain is quickly relieved by flexing the spine e.g. sitting or bending forward while standing, but <u>not</u> quickly relieved by standing erect
    (4) SLR testing usually is negative
  c. Psychological disorder
    (1) It is <u>chronic</u> LBP, occurring almost daily
    (2) <u>Insidious onset</u>, usually he can't tell you when it began
    (3) LBP is just one of a number of symptoms, and these other symptoms are unrelated to a specific organ, which would suggest organic disease
    (4) Symptoms of a psychological disorder are present e.g. anhedonia (MD) excess worrying (GAD), multi-organ pains (somatization), alcoholism, substance abuse. It is important to treat these psychological disorders, because untreated, at a minimum they will prolong recovery from any LBP, even when LSS or radiculopathy are the cause.

F. Use this summary for efficient diagnosis of a common cause. With the information from Sections A-E in mind, here is the rapid approach to diagnosis of LBP.
1. You already have determined:
  a. In Section A, by H&P that it is LBP and whether it is either new, episodic or chronic daily pain.
  b. In Section B, that there is no evidence in the H&P of any <u>one</u> dangerous cause of the back pain.
  c. In Section C, that neither an easily diagnosed extraspinal disease or a medication is likely responsible for the LBP.
2. From the focused H&P almost always you should quickly be

Chapter 11 Low Back Pain 145

confident of a working diagnosis. Confident final diagnosis is made only in followup the next few weeks or months when the response to treatment or nontreatment is appropriate to your working diagnosis.
  a. If this is new LBP following some unusual exertional or strenuous event, and there is no radiating pain into the thigh or leg, it is likely lumbosacral strain (LSS).
  b. If the new LBP radiates into the buttock and lower extremity and it is relieved by supine position but not by sitting, and the SLR test exactly reproduces the patient's radiating pain, it is likely radiculopathy due to a herniated disc between vertebrae L_3-S_1.
  c. If the LBP or radiating pain is episodic in a patient >50 y/o, and it occurs only with standing for 5-10 minutes or walking some distance and it is quickly relieved by sitting, it is likely spinal stenosis.
  d. If the clinical picture associated with the daily LBP is unusual or bizarre, and there are associated symptoms of a psychological disorder, diagnose the psychological cause and treat it appropriately.
3. Answer your patient's worries and wants that you determined early on during the exam (Section D). Have you done everything you can to help him?
4. You now have a working diagnosis, but only with followup can you be highly confident it is correct. In return visits you are always testing by H&P that your working diagnosis is correct.

G. Abandon your working diagnosis and look for an uncommon or rare cause only if:
1. Any one dangerous symptom or sign (see above, Section B) occurs in the following days, weeks, or months. Quickly obtain a specialist consult or send the patient to the hospital as appropriate

If your patient's symptoms do not respond as expected to your management, he may have an uncommon or rare cause listed in Section G.2 that you can diagnose and treat. Or you may want to refer your patient to a specialist.

2. The course of your patient's recovery is not as you expect. If he has followed the usual prescribed conservative treatment, at least 80-90% of patients with LSS or those with herniated disk and radiculopathy are markedly improved in <4 weeks, and the other 10-20% are not worse. If in the next days or weeks, the symptoms become more intense, or if the symptoms change, examine the patient again, looking for a different, possibly dangerous, etiology.
Don't spend time and money looking for one of the following etiologies until you are sure your patient doesn't have one of the 4 common causes of episodic or new LBP above. If he doesn't have one of those causes, it may be that the correct cause was one of the uncommon causes listed below. These are important to recognize, because each has different treatment or prophylaxis
Although these etiologies usually present as chronic persistent back pain for >3 months, you may see the patient early in the course.
  a. Spondyloarthropathy–in addition to LBP there are other symptoms--morning stiffness (>30 minutes) of the spine, insidious onset of the LBP usually in a patient <30-40 y/o, other symptoms of psoriasis, IBD, Reiter's syndrome or ankylosing spondylitis; lateral flexion of the spine is <30° usually
  b. Spondylolisthesis–if severe, he also may have radiculopathy; diagnosis is by imaging studies when LBP continues unabated despite conservative therapy
  c. Very severe scoliosis or kyphosis

- d. Postural–patient is seemingly healthy, but just very bad posture; some aggravating causes are significant obesity in a young person, or increasing weight in an older person, who had bad posture all his life; also, 2% of adults have one leg shorter by at least 2 cm, so a special shoe may relieve or prevent the LBP
- e. Severe spondylosis (spine OA) in the elderly is a common cause of persistent back pain
- f. MM–patient >40 y/o, unexplained back or rib pain precipitated by movement; anemia
- g. Uncommon causes that mimic the radiating pain of sciatica; think of them if no history of injury or exertion
  - (1) Obturator neuritis–due to obturator hernia; loss of thigh adduction
  - (2) Meralgia paresthetica (dysesthesias lateral thigh surface)--due to obesity, arthritis, psoas abscess, wearing tight "hip huggers"
  - (3) Ankylosing spondylitis–as above
  - (4) Lumbosacral tumor–multiple nerve root symptoms
  - (5) Trauma–compression fracture
  - (6) Sciatic neuritis–DM, vasculitis, trauma
  - (7) Spondylolisthesis
  - (8) Paget's disease–high alkaline phosphotase
  - (9) Herpes zoster–pain may precede the dermatomal rash by 7-10 days
  - (10) Pyriform syndrome–a patient <40 y/o, pain increased by hip extension or abduction
  - (11) Peroneal nerve entrapment–dysesthesias of the anterior lower leg and dorsum foot; weak ankle dorsiflexion
  - (12) Iliolumbar syndrome–unilateral tenderness posterior iliac crest; pain worsened by lateral spine flexion away from the painful side
  - (13) Ischial bursitis–point tenderness by sitting on the affected ischial tuberosity
  - (14) Coccydynia–focal tenderness at the coccyx
- h. Referred pain causing LBP–think of it if no localized tenderness or muscle spasm in the lumbar area; low back ROM normal; if referred pain does radiate into the leg, it does not radiate below the knee e.g. during the SLR test
  - (1) Upper abdomen refers pain to the upper lumbar area–stomach, gallbladder, duodenum, pancreas
  - (2) Lower abdomen refers to the lower lumbar area–lower small intestine, retroperitoneal lesions, colon, aortic aneurysm
  - (3) Pelvic organs refer to sacral, buttock, thigh areas–uterus, prostate, ureteral stones

3. Appendix
   - a. Aspects of the SLR test for reproducing the pain of radiculopathy:
     - (1) Sensitivity of the test is best for L_5 and S_1 nerve root disease; less sensitive for L_4 and no good for roots above L_4 i.e. L_2 or L_3 nerve roots
     - (2) SLR test is performed with the patient supine (originally described with patient sitting), legs fully extended, and you lift each leg one at a time, at the heel
     - (3) A positive test is reproduction of your patient's pain and paresthesias when the leg is lifted to between 30-70%; just increased pain localized to the low back is not positive, and only hamstring tightness is a negative test. If the test seems equivocal, ankle dorsiflexion at 70° may provoke the pain of sciatica and be a positive test. Also to get more confidence a test is positive, bring the leg down to say 60°, i.e. just to where the pain disappears and then dorsiflex the foot; if the sciatica again is elicited, you can have more confidence the test is positive. Occasionally, simultaneous Valsalva or "cough" at 70° may provoke the radiating pain, again a positive test. If not positive, suspect a psychogenic cause except in the elderly, where a false negative SLR test may occur. If you are confident of your patient's pain, a negative SLR test suggests another cause of the "sciatica" e.g. bursitis, referred pain, nerve entrapment (see above, Section G.2.g)
     - (4) A positive test suggests lower lumbar disc herniation as the cause of the patient's pain (sciatica) radiating down the buttock, leg, and foot
     - (5) A positive "crossed" SLR (symptoms also elicited upon lifting the contralateral leg) suggests a large disc herniation with an extruded fragment
     - (6) Confirm a positive SLR by testing for the "flip sign," i.e. do the SLR with the patient sitting; test is positive if he falls back to maintain his back straight
     - (7) The older the patient with complaints consistent with sciatica, the more likely there is a negative SLR; probably because it's due to non-mechanical causes, so search carefully for serious disease e.g. referred pain in these elderly patients
     - (8) If radicular (sciatica) pain is elicited by SLR at much <30°, suspect a psychogenic etiology, because the nerve root and surrounding dura do not move in the foramen until about 30°

Chapter 11 Low Back Pain 147

- b. Almost all (90-95%) lumbar disc herniations occur at nerve root L_5 (herniation at the L_4-$_5$ space) or root S_1 (herniation at the L_5-S_1 space), so focus your thinking on these areas when doing your exam:
  - (1) L_5 root--pain and numbness radiating from low back to posterior thigh, anterolateral leg, median and dorsum of foot and great toe; may be weakness dorsiflexion foot and great toe; difficult to heel walk; DTRs unaffected usually
  - (2) S_1 root--pain and numbness of buttock, posterior thigh and leg, posterolateral foot and lateral toes; weakness of plantar flexion foot and toes (usually late); Achilles reflex may be decreased or absent
  - (3) L_4 root--much less common; pain radiation anterior leg with weakness of knee extension (quadriceps); sensory loss anteromedial surface of the thigh down to medial foot; patellar reflex decreased or absent
- c. Clues to a nonorganic etiology of LBP (Spine 5, 117, 1980)
  - (1) History
    - (a) Overreaction during the H&P--collapsing, tremor, bizarre facial expression, exaggerated verbalization, inappropriate gait
    - (b) Pain is constant 24 hours or "always there"
    - (c) "Whole leg gives way"
    - (d) Pain and numbness are not in a physiologic distribution (e.g. involves the whole leg)
    - (e) Pain is localized only to the coccyx or rectum
    - (f) "Intolerance" to many treatment modalities
    - (g) Frequent prior visits ER without a diagnosis
    - (h) Multiple other somatic complaints of equal severity to the LBP (suggesting somatization)
  - (2) Physical exam–suspect a psychologic disorder if any of the following occurs:
    - (a) Patient standing, you put axial pressure or loading on his head and he says it increases the LBP (axial loading may increase cervical or thoracic pain, but cannot increase lumbar pain)
    - (b) SLR is positive, say at 60°, but then the pain is not relieved by your flexing his knee at that angle (pain should be relieved if radiculopathy)
    - (c) SLR is positive when he is tested supine, but then the flip test is negative (that is, a negative SLR test in the sitting position, and he doesn't "fall back" to maintain a straight back as you lift and extend his knee)
    - (d) Toe flexion test–patient prone, knees flexed and heels face the ceiling and you flex or extend his toes; if either movement worsens LBP or provokes sciatica
    - (e) Simulated rotation reproduces LBP i.e. patient standing, feet together and arms fixed firmly to his lateral body; you then passively rotate his torso and LBP occurs or is worsened or sciatica occurs

H. Use the glossary for precise thinking and accurate diagnosis.

1. **Ankylosing spondylitis** (Greek *ankylos* meaning "bent or crooked" and *spondylos*, "vertebra.") It denotes fusion of vertebrae due to inflammation.
2. **Arthrodesis** (Greek *arthro* meaning "joint" and *desis*, "binding.") It is surgical fusion of joint surfaces
3. **Cauda equina** (Latin meaning literally "horse's tail.") The nerve roots below L_1 descending down the vertebral canal resemble a horses' tail.
4. **Causalgia** (Greek *kausos* meaning "heat" and *algia*, "pain.") It is any burning pain.
5. **Claudication** (Latin *claudicatio* meaning "limping or lameness.") The word was first used for an exercising horse that came up lame, but soon recovered with rest. Vascular claudication is due to ischemia of exercising muscle so there also is pain, but claudication itself is not pain. Formerly there was also "pseudoclaudication," which resembled vascular claudication, but there was no vascular disease on angiography. We now call this neurogenic claudication or spinal stenosis.
6. **Discitis** (septic) (Greek *diskos*, later Latin *discus*, meaning "a circular or round flat plate.") Now it is inflammation of an intervertebral disk.
7. **Extraspinal** (Latin *extra* meaning "outside of" or "unrelated to" and *spinalis*, "spinal or vertebral column.")
8. **Formication** (Latin *formica* meaning "ant.") It is a tactile hallucination of insects crawling over the skin.
9. **Herniation** (Greek *hernos* meaning "a sprout" like the bud of a plant.) Now it is any protrusion through an abnormal opening.
10. **Kyphosis** (Greek *kyphos* meaning "bent or bowed.") The present restricted use is to bowing of the dorsal spine.
11. **Lordosis** (Greek *lordos* meaning "bent backward.") It is an exaggerated anterior convexity of the lumbar spine.
12. **Malinger** (French *malingre* meaning "sickly.") Now it is willful faking or

exaggeration of symptoms of illness for some desired end or gain.
13. **Meralgia paresthetica** (Greek *meros* meaning "thigh" and *algia*, "pain" and *paresthesia*, "abnormal perception.") It indicates abnormal sensations (burning, tingling, formication) along the lateral thigh.
14. **Osteomalacia** (Greek *osteon* meaning "bone" and *malakia*, "softness.") Now it is soft, weakened bone due to demineralization, especially calcium loss due to vitamin D deficiency.
15. **Osteomyelitis** (Greek *osteon* meaning "bone" and *myelos*, "marrow" and *itis*, "inflammation.") It is infection and inflammation of any part of bone.
16. **Osteophytes** (Greek *osteon* meaning "bone" and *phyton*, "plant.") It is any bony outgrowth resembling a plant.
17. **Osteoporosis** (Greek *osteon* meaning "bone" and *poros*, "passage.") It suggests passages or pores due to loss of bone mass.
18. **Osteosclerosis** (Greek *osteon* meaning "bone" and *sklerosis*, "hardening.") It is abnormal increased density of bone e.g. due to Paget's disease.
19. **Paraplegia** (Greek *para* meaning "resembling" and *plege*, "stroke.") It is paralysis of both legs and lower body; if paraparesis, then it is weakness of the legs and lower body.
20. **Radiculopathy** (Greek *radicula* meaning "smallest branch of a nerve or vessel" and *pathos*, "disease.") Literally, it is nerve root disease.
21. **Sciatica** (Greek *ischiadikos* meaning "subject to trouble in the hips.") The original *nervus ischiadicus* is now our sciatic nerve, and sciatica refers to pain anywhere along its course.
22. **Scoliosis** (Greek *skoliosis* meaning any "bending or curvature.") Now the restricted meaning is lateral curvature of the spine.
23. **Spondyloarthropathy** (Greek *spondylos* meaning "vertebra" and *arthron*, "joint" and *pathos*, "disease.") It is disease of the intervertebral joints.
24. **Spondylolisthesis** (Greek *spondylos* meaning "vertebra" and *oliothanein*, "to slip.") It is a forward slipping or displacement of one vertebra over another one
25. **Spondylolysis** (Greek *spondylos* meaning "vertebra" and *lysis*, "dissolution.") It indicates dissolution or breakdown of a vertebrae
26. **Spondylosis** (Greek *spondylos* meaning "vertebra" and *osis*, "disease or morbid process.") It is a general term for degenerative changes of vertebral osteoarthritis.
27. **Stenosis** (spinal) (Greek *stenosis* meaning "narrowing of a duct or canal.") It is a narrowed spinal canal usually due to spondylosis.

Chapter 12 Presyncope

Questions on Presyncope

A. In your patient with complaint of "dizziness," the most important
  1. Historical information is:
  2. First physical exam maneuvers are:
B. In the office, the commonest cause of presyncope, and its 4 major distinguishing characteristics, are:
  1.
     a.
     b.
     c.
     d.
C. The other 2 common causes of presyncope in the office, and how you can differentiate them from the commonest cause and from each other are:
  1.
     a.
     b.
     c.
     d.
  2.
     a.
     b.
     c.
     d.
D. Your patient is a 19 y/o sophomore at West Texas A&M University. She has "never been sick." While running wind sprints yesterday, she "almost passed out." Otherwise she always has been perfectly well and your exam is normal. Will you reassure her "not to worry"? Or?

E. Your patient is a 75 y/o woman with "dizziness when I stand up." You immediately do a "tilt test" and find she has neither orthostatic hypotension (by measurements supine and standing) nor orthostatic symptoms even during 10 minutes standing. Her neurological exam is unremarkable. Her likely diagnosis is:

Answers on Presyncope
A. Be certain that the symptom is presyncope
  1. Determine quickly if the "dizziness" (a very general nonspecific term your patient almost always uses) is either vertigo or presyncope or disequilibrium. Vertigo suggests vestibular (peripheral or central) disease, and it is a spinning or illusion of movement. Disequilibrium suggests disease of posterior column or peripheral neuropathy, and it is a feeling of imbalance or difficulty only while walking or standing. Presyncope suggests cardiac disease or decreased brain nutrition (either of perfusion, oxygen or glucose), and it is a feeling of about to pass out or lose consciousness. Also determine whether it is new onset or episodic or chronic, almost daily "dizziness"
  2. On physical exam, quickly do <u>provocative</u> tests to help confirm which of the above 3 types of "dizziness" is most likely present in your patient:
     a. Vertigo– do the Dix-Hallpike maneuver to provoke vertigo, if present, and to interpret any nystagmus
     b. Disequilibrium–determine if the "dizziness" is reproduced by the Romberg test
     c. Presyncope–test for orthostatic hypotension to see if it provokes your patient's symptoms
     d. You may have certain patients:
        (1) Hyperventilate–deep sighing respirations 15-20 per minute for 3 minutes, trying to provoke her specific symptoms of dizziness
        (2) Walk up and down the hall–observe her gait for abnormalities e.g. syndrome of multiple sensory deficits in the elderly; psychogenic gait
B. Commonest cause of presyncope and its distinguishing characteristics
  1. Prodrome of simple faint, previously called vasovagal syncope, now neurocardiogenic syncope
     a. <u>New onset</u> (or a previous similar episode)
     b. Onset in a patient <40 y/o
     c. Rapid onset (over 5-10 minutes) with an increasingly worsening feeling of about to pass out; associated symptoms of nausea, sweating, hot flush
     d. Symptoms occur during standing for some length of time, but they are <u>not</u> reproduced by testing for orthostatic BP changes
C. The other 2 common causes of presyncope and distinguishing characteristics of each
  1. Orthostatic "dizziness" (including orthostatic hypotension, POTS, MOI)
     a. <u>Episodic</u> dizziness
     b. Onset at any age
     c. Rapid (seconds-minutes) onset of dizziness or "lightheadedness"
     d. Dizziness <u>only</u> on moving from the supine or sitting position to standing; dizziness is reproducible by correctly testing for orthostatic BP changes, even though BP may not decrease
  2. Panic attack
     a. <u>Episodic</u> dizziness
     b. Onset <40 y/o
     c. Rapid onset (seconds to minutes) of dizziness and other symptoms of panic e.g. chest pain
     d. Onset of dizziness is not related to position or changes in position
D. Recognize a dangerous sign of presyncope

Chapter 12 Presyncope   151

<u>You</u> should be very worried. Anybody who has presyncope or syncope during or after vigorous exercise has a cardiac etiology until proven otherwise. You may not hear the murmur of hypertrophic cardiomyopathy (HCM) unless you auscultate her heart for a systolic murmur, which increases in intensity <u>after</u> you have her squat, then rise to a standing position

E. Multiple sensory deficits are a common cause of "dizziness" in the elderly

Revisit the history. "What exactly do you mean when you said you only get dizzy after you stand up?" She tells you–"Oh, I meant, when I stand up and start walking." Observe her gait as she walks in the hall. Note that she gradually weaves from one object to the next, touching the wall or chair for sensory guidance. She likely has "multiple sensory deficits" of afferent input for balance. Get her eyeglasses changed, hearing aid if needed, physical therapy and exercise prescription. Test her hearing aid by cupping your hand over it. A functioning battery will make a "beep" noise; a dead battery will make no noise that you can hear

Presyncope

Differential diagnosis: the 3 common causes of presyncope
1. Faint prodrome–<40 y/o patient; symptoms only during standing >15-20 min
2. Orthostatic intolerance–any age; symptoms begin seconds or minutes after rising from sitting or supine position
3. Panic attack–<40 y/o patient; symptoms unrelated to position; typical associated hyperarousal symptoms e.g. chest pain, SOB, paresthesias, palpitations

A. **Be certain of the symptom and its distinguishing characteristics.** Your patient's problem or chief complaint is "I felt dizzy and I think I blacked out." Dizziness is a term patients often use to describe feelings of a spectrum of disorders, from the benign (anxiety, fatigue) to the dangerous (TIA, neuromuscular weakness). The patient knows no other way to describe the feeling, so you must discover and interpret precisely what she felt before and during the "dizziness." Think of dizziness as composed of 3 subtypes, and the subtype can suggest the organ involved
   1. Most dizziness is not presyncope, so first, you must be confident it is not one of the other two types of dizziness
      a. Vertigo is an illusion that either she or things around her are spinning or rotating or tilting; she may feel pulled to one side or even toward the ground, but there is no feeling of possibly losing consciousness; vertigo suggests disease of the vestibular system
      b. Disequilibrium is an imbalance or feeling that she might fall, but the sensation that she might pass out is absent; thus, it occurs only while she is walking or standing or turning, and it suggests posterior column disease or peripheral neuropathy
      c. Presyncope is a feeling that she is about to pass out or about to "faint," and no symptoms suggesting vertigo or disequilibrium; these are the same symptoms a patient with syncope has in the moments before losing consciousness; presyncope suggests cardiac or neurological disease, the same causes as for syncope
   2. To help determine the subtype of dizziness, ask "Tell me about a typical episode (or the episode if only one)." "Start with what you were doing earlier in the day, up to when the dizziness started," then "Tell me exactly what you were feeling before and during the episode–and don't use the word dizzy or vertigo." "How did you feel afterwards–what did you think was happening?" If it did not frighten her, think possibly it is a psychological disorder, especially if it is chronic almost daily dizziness
   3. Next, is the "dizziness" new or episodic? "When is the last time you had a similar episode of "dizziness" anything like this episode?" and "When before the last time?" Positive answers to both questions suggest either episodic or chronic, almost daily dizziness. Recurrences over a number of years without progressively worsening symptoms <u>may</u> be reassuring, whereas, recent onset with

Chapter 12 Presyncope 153

or without recurrence, especially in an elderly patient, suggests a dangerous cause. In some patients you might ask "How many different kinds of dizziness do you get?" "Now tell me about this one dizziness"

Be certain:
1. The symptom is presyncope (feeling of about to pass out) and not vertigo (illusion of motion, spinning) or disequilibrium (imbalance when walking or standing)
2. Whether the symptom is either new onset or episodic dizziness
3. What the patient was doing (e.g. position or change in position) just before the dizziness started
4. What other symptoms occurred just before or during the dizziness

---

4. Physical examination–From the questions above you should recognize presyncope; still, always do the dizziness simulation tests to be more confident it is presyncope. Both Dix-Hallpike and Romberg tests should be negative if she has presyncope alone. Sometimes, however, especially in the elderly, the cause of the dizziness is multifactorial, so more questions may need to be answered in some elderly patients, to be confident presyncope is at least one factor. For example, a patient may have asymptomatic carotid insufficiency, then she gets dehydrated or a new antihypertensive medication is started, and then presyncope occurs
    a. Dix-Hallpike maneuver–with her sitting, extend her head back 20-30°, eyes straight ahead. Then slowly rotate her head back and forth alternating 30° right, then 30° left, every few seconds, 5-10 times. Reproduction of the "dizziness" suggests vertigo. If still in doubt it might be vertigo, and not presyncope, spin her repeatedly in a swivel chair, have her stand, and if it exactly reproduces her "dizziness," it is vertigo
    b. Romberg test–have her stand, feet together, arms outstretched in front. If, on closing her eyes, marked imbalance occurs (e.g. she has to move one foot to maintain balance), it is a positive test and suggests she has disequilibrium. Then watch her gait as she walks up and down the hall. If this, or pivoting, reproduces the complained of dizziness, it suggests disequilibrium, and not presyncope
    c. Test for orthostatic intolerance–have her resting supine at least 10 minutes, then measure BP and pulse. Again measure BP and pulse immediately after she stands, and (if necessary) repeat the BP and pulse readings every 30-45 seconds while she remains standing still, for up to 5-10 minutes. At each measurement, ask "How does that make you feel?" or "Does that make you feel better," but don't ask "Does that make you dizzy?" What you really are looking for is her volunteering "That's it, now I'm dizzy" or "That's the feeling I get."
    Calculate the mean arterial pressure: (MAP) = [DBP + 0.4 (SBP - DBP)] for the supine reading and any significantly changed standing reading. The difference in MAP from supine to standing in a

normal patient does not decrease more than 1-2 mmHg, so any significant decrease in the MAP with concomitant reproduction of the patient's "dizzy" symptom suggests that orthostatic hypotension is causing her dizziness. In control patients without hypotension, heart rate increases 6-18 bpm on standing so the rate should increase higher with orthostatic hypotension

By now you should be confident your patient has presyncope, whether it is new or episodic presyncope, what she was doing just before the presyncope occurred, and if there were any concomitant symptoms. In almost all instances you now have the information you need for diagnosis of the obvious causes (Section C) and the common causes (Section E). In the rare instance that your patient appears different clinically from the usual office patient with presyncope, be certain (Section B) that she does not have a symptom or sign of a dangerous disease

B. Be confident it's not a dangerous disease.

1. Send immediately to the ED by ambulance if there is:
   a. New onset of presyncope accompanied by any one of the following:
      (1) Abrupt onset of a very severe headache, think of SAH
      (2) Palpitations or chest pain, think of myocardial ischemia, AD, PE
      (3) Abdominal pain, think of ruptured aortic aneurysm, ruptured ectopic pregnancy
      (4) Narrow pulse pressure, think of severe aortic stenosis
   b. Presyncope in a pacemaker-dependent patient, think of pacemaker failure
   c. Evidence of dyspnea, hypotension, arrhythmias, EKG ischemic changes, think of silent MI in a diabetic or elderly patient
   d. New presyncope in a patient with past history of severe carotid disease causing stroke, think of a new TIA or stroke due to obstruction of the other carotid
   e. Presyncope with abrupt onset of either dyspnea or tachypnea or pleuritic chest pain, think of PE
   f. Presyncope and neurological symptoms (diplopia, dysphagia, dysesthesias,

---

Be certain in the first minutes of your exam that there is no evidence of any <u>one</u> dangerous symptom or sign associated with the presyncope:

1. New onset presyncope in a patient >50 y/o
2. During or following vigorous exercise
3. Chest pain or palpitations
4. Abrupt onset of dyspnea
5. Unexplained marked tachycardia
6. Mental status change or abnormal neurological sign or symptom e.g. diplopia, dysarthria, dysphagia

Any suggestion of a dangerous disease, send your patient to the ED.

---

dysarthria, ataxia) suggesting brain stem ischemia, think of vertebrobasilar TIA

2. Admit at once to the ED or hospital if there is:
   a. Presyncope during or following exertion, think of aortic stenosis, HCM, pulmonic stenosis
   b. Presyncope in a patient with T2DM on a sulfonylurea, think of prolonged hypoglycemia
   c. Marked orthostatic hypotension, think of severe hypovolemia (blood loss, dehydration), Addison's disease
   d. Presyncope in a patient at high risk of sudden death (PMH of ventricular tachycardia, MI, valvular heart disease, CHF)
   e. Presyncope in an elderly patient while supine or sitting or who previously had an

Chapter 12 Presyncope 155

episode of syncope, think of cardiac or CNS disease
3. Admit to the hospital or have a specialist consult as soon as appropriate if there is:
   a. Unexplained new onset presyncope in a patient >50 y/o
   b. New presyncope in a patient on medications associated with dangerous arrhythmias e.g. digitalis, quinidine, procainamide, TCA, phenothiazines
   c. Presyncope associated with change in body position e.g. turning on one side in bed, think of left atrial myxoma
   d. Presyncope with head movements (twisting the neck, head upward looking) or a tight collar, think of carotid sinus hyperactivity
   e. Presyncope following performance of a Valsalva maneuver (defecation, sneeze, cough) in an elderly patient, think of chronic pulmonary hypertension
   f. Unexplained presyncope in a patient with a systolic murmur, think of severe aortic stenosis, HCM, pulmonic stenosis; if a diastolic murmur, think of atrial myxoma; if a loud S2, think of pulmonary hypertension
   g. Presyncope and orthostatic hypotension on exam, think of Addison's disease, pheochromocytoma, hypoaldosteronism, severe hypokalemia

C. **Make a quick diagnosis if it's obvious.** Is it an easily diagnosed condition or a medication that is responsible for the presyncope? In most patients you will be highly confident of a common cause of the symptom by now. If not, one or more of the following tests may exclude an organic disease and increase your confidence in your working diagnosis: EKG, glucose, electrolytes, Ca

---

Recognize any easily diagnosed cause of presyncope:
1. Metabolic causes, e.g. hypoglycemia or hypoxia
2. Spot diagnoses
3. Medication side effect

---

1. Metabolic causes–hypoglycemia, hypoxia, hypocapnia, hypokalemia, hypocalcemia will be found by laboratory test if suggested by H&P
2. Spot diagnosis of conditions known to provoke presyncope in susceptible individuals; explanation and reassurance is needed
   a. Extremely common in patients <40 y/o is mild dizziness ("lightheaded") almost immediately on standing from supine. Precise research BP measurements in the first 30 seconds detect a 20-30 mmHg momentary decrease in normals, and younger patients often sense this drop in BP that occurs before we can obtain measurements
   b. Valsalva-related, *viz* cough, micturition, defecation, swallowing, retching; isometric athletics e.g. weight lifting, diving, stretching
   c. Severe pain, for example, neuralgias *viz* glossopharyngeal, trigeminal
   d. Carotid sinus hypersensitivity–symptoms only with her head turning; men while shaving, tight collar
   e. Iatrogenic causes e.g. venipuncture, procedures associated with suffocating feelings (dental, bronchoscopy, esophagoscopy)
   f. Late pregnancy; gestational HTN and a side-effect of methyldopa
   g. Mobilization after prolonged bed rest
   h. Postcibum (postprandial) hypotension may occur commonly in the elderly patient soon after a large meal, especially breakfast. If she is diabetic, everyone assumes it is hypoglycemia, instead it is hypotension
   i. Multiple sensory deficit in the elderly presents as disequilibrium, but she may have presyncope also. Uncertain gait, she touches the

wall or furniture for reassurance while walking. There may be peripheral neuropathy (DM, B12 deficiency) or just poor vision or hearing or physical condition; blunted physiological reflexes of aging; then addition of a multidrug regimen and presyncope occurs. Treat all the deficiencies–glasses, hearing aid, physical therapy

3. Medications–any <u>one</u> medication may be responsible for new dizziness (90% of oral meds listed in the PDR list dizziness as a side effect); so look for a temporal relationship between any new presyncope and the time the new medication was started. The following medications may cause or aggravate orthostatic intolerance:
   a. Any antihypertensive agent but especially peripheral vasodilators e.g. ACEI, α-receptor blockers (prazosin), hydralazine, guanethidine, methyldopa, CCBs
   b. Sometimes β-blockers (note that these drugs are effective treatment in neurocardiogenic syncope), anticonvulsants, antidepressives
   c. Ototoxic–loop diuretics, salicylates, aminoglycoside, quinine, quinidine
   d. Miscellaneous: TCAs, diuretics, nitrates, antipsychotics, sedatives, hypnotics, bromocriptine, opiates, ethanol, sildenafil

D. **Identify your patient's worries and wants.** Up to 20% of young healthy adults have experienced at least one episode of syncope, and very few sought medical attention. During your interview and exam try to intuit or discover why your patient is here today, and not previously, for this problem. Don't necessarily ask directly, but try to get some ideas about her particular worries from her responses to questions about the dizziness itself. You can't completely help your patient unless you know what she really worries about and wants from you. That's why she is here to see you--to satisfy her worries and wants! Here are only some of the possible worries and wants of your patient with presyncope. You must discover her specific, unique ones

1. Common worries are:
   a. That the cause of the dizziness is a dangerous etiology e.g. heart disease, stroke, TIA, brain tumor
   b. That the etiology is some rare disease e.g. WNV encephalitis, Lyme disease, MS
   c. What other fears or anxieties might be troubling your patient? For example, she may have had dizziness for many years, and only now does she come for help. What has changed? Perhaps a friend or relative, who had a similar dizziness, recently has been diagnosed with MS. There are many other possibilities–think of them

---

During your exam, discover your patient's worries (e.g. stroke, brain tumor, heart problem) and wants (e.g. tests, treatment), so that you can respond to her specific needs as soon as possible.

---

2. Your patient wants:
   a. You to perform a thorough physical exam focused on possible causes of the dizziness and she wants appropriate tests and imaging studies
   b. A plausible explanation of the cause of the dizziness
   c. Confident reassurance from you that it is not a dangerous or rare etiology. Tell her–"The good news, it's not a stroke" (or whatever you believe her real worry is)
   d. To know the prognosis, short term (effects on job, home life, marriage; how soon she will be back to normal) and long term (if recurrences of dizziness are possible; how to prevent recurrences; if it will cause any disability)
   e. Treatment to prevent recurrences of presyncope, especially education
   f. A specialist referral (cardiologist, neurologist) if she believes you are not confident of the diagnosis

Chapter 12 Presyncope 157

E. Know the symptoms that differentiate the 3 common causes of presyncope.
1. The commonest cause is the prodrome of simple faint (neurocardiogenic or vasovagal syncope)

Common causes of most presyncope in the office patient:
1. Faint prodrome–<40 y/o patient; symptoms only during standing >15-20 min
2. Orthostatic intolerance–any age; symptoms begin seconds or minutes after rising from sitting or supine position
3. Panic attack–<40 y/o patient; symptoms unrelated to position; typical associated hyperarousal symptoms e.g. chest pain, SOB, paresthesias, palpitations

---

   a. Characteristics of simple faint prodrome
      (1) The presyncope is an isolated symptom in a patient <40 y/o; she is well except during the episode, and no symptoms suggesting disease of other organs occur before or during the presyncope
      (2) The presyncope occurs almost always while she is standing, rarely while sitting, never while supine. Often there is associated emotional distress, mental or physical, e.g. pain or fear, or the distress may not be obvious, e.g. in a crowd, standing in line, in hot or uncomfortable (physical or emotional) surroundings
      (3) The presyncopal sensations have a gradual onset over a few minutes usually, and include autonomic nervous symptoms of nausea (not vomiting) or a queasy feeling, flushing sensation, sweating, palpitations, tightness in the throat, increased salivation, paresthesias. These symptoms gradually worsen over a few minutes ending in black spots, blurred vision, visual field constriction and a feeling of about to pass out. Lying down quickly relieves the "dizziness" but some of the other symptoms may last 1-2 minutes
   b. What suggests it might not be prodrome of simple faint
      (1) Anytime there is an associated symptom or sign suggesting a dangerous cause (see above, Section B)
      (2) If the dizziness feeling has an abrupt onset or there are no associated prodromal symptoms or if it occurs while she is supine
2. Common look-alikes and how each differs from faint prodrome
   a. Orthostatic intolerance is of 4 kinds, and each may be identified during an orthostatic test lasting 5-10 minutes as needed to reproduce the patient's dizziness:
      (1) Orthostatic hypotension–significantly decreased MAP occurs almost immediately on standing up from the supine, and it is accompanied by appropriate increased pulse rate (usually >20 bpm); it may be secondary to:
         (a) Hypovolemia–dehydration, severe diarrhea or emesis, decreased thirst mechanism in the elderly
         (b) Venous pooling–fever, sepsis, vigorous exercise, hot shower,

alcohol
- (c) Heart pump failure–MI, severe aortic stenosis, arrhythmia, Addison's disease
- (d) Neurological causes–neuropathy (DM, alcoholism, amyloidosis)
- (2) Delayed orthostatic hypotension and appropriate increased pulse occurs within 5-10 minutes of standing from the supine; criteria of hypotension are met and concomitant orthostatic symptoms occur
- (3) Postural tachycardia syndrome (POTS) does not have inducible hypotension on rising and standing for up to 10 minutes; its hallmark is a pulse increase ≥ 30 bpm and absolute heart rate ≥ 120/min and concomitant orthostatic symptoms
- (4) Mild orthostatic intolerance (MOI) also has no orthostatic hypotension during the 10 minute tilt test, but the standing pulse rate increases by ≥ 30 bpm compared to supine resting rate and there are typical orthostatic symptoms

Orthostatic symptoms common to all 4 types of orthostatic intolerance are: dizziness, tiredness or fatigue, blurred vision and symptoms of sympathetic activation *viz* nausea, palpitations, tremulousness, SOB. Also, these patients commonly complain of many daily symptoms including dizziness, chronic fatigue, palpitations, tremulousness, sweating, inability to concentrate

b. Panic attack
- (1) Onset <40 y/o patient and dizziness is unrelated to position
- (2) Prior to dizziness there may be abrupt onset of intense anxiety that an unspecified event might occur; search for this anticipatory anxiety in your history
- (3) Over the next 5-10 minutes multiple hyperarousal symptoms including "dizziness" (palpitations, sweating, trembling, SOB, chest or abdominal pain, headache, paresthesias) along with feeling of loss of control, feeling of unreality or fear of dying
- (4) Panic attacks occur in >40% of patients with each of the following chronic psychological disorders:
  - (a) GAD–she is the "worry wart" of the family, she worries most of the day and can't go to sleep at night because of worrying; she worries about catastrophes that conceivably could happen, but are extremely unlikely
  - (b) MD should always be detectable by some evidence of anhedonia, i.e. she no longer is doing one or more of the enjoyable things she used to do
  - (c) In somatization syndrome, though characterized primarily by pain symptoms in a number of organ systems, presyncope occasionally may be a dominant symptom along with pains

F. **Use this summary for efficient diagnosis of a common cause.** With the information from Sections A-E in mind, here is the rapid approach to diagnosis of presyncope.
1. You already have determined:
   a. In Section A, by H&P, that it is presyncope and not vertigo (spinning) or disequilibrium (imbalance)
   b. From Section B, that there is no evidence in the H&P of a dangerous cause of the dizziness
   c. In Section C, that there is neither an easily diagnosed cause nor a

medication that is likely responsible for the presyncope
2. From the focused H&P almost always you should quickly be confident of a working diagnosis. Confident final diagnosis is made only in followup the next days, weeks, or months when the response to treatment or nontreatment is appropriate to your working diagnosis
   a. If your patient is <40 y/o, and the clinical picture is consistent with the prodrome of simple faint, and the tilt test is normal in the office, make the diagnosis and treat appropriately
   b. If MAP significantly decreases, heart rate appropriately increases and "dizziness" occurs together either almost immediately upon standing or within 5-10 minutes of standing, diagnose orthostatic hypotension and treat appropriately.
   c. If your patient has no change in MAP, but she has a heart rate increment ≥ 30 bpm sometime during 5-10 minutes of standing and heart rate exceeds 120 bpm and orthostatic symptoms occur, diagnose POTS and treat appropriately.
   d. If she has no change in MAP, but she has a heart rate increment ≥ 30 bpm sometime during 5-10 of standing, and orthostatic symptoms occur, diagnose MOI and treat appropriately.
   e. If she has abrupt onset of severe apprehension about some future possible event, and dizziness (among other symptoms) follows in minutes, diagnose panic attack.
   f. If your patient with dizziness meets criteria for either GAD, panic disorder, or MD, diagnose and treat the psychological disorder appropriately.
3. Answer your patient's worries and wants that you determined early on during the exam (Section D). Have you done everything you can to help her?
4. You now have a working diagnosis, but only with followup can you be highly confident it is correct. In return visits you are always testing by H&P that your working diagnosis is correct.

G. Abandon your working diagnosis and look for an uncommon or rare cause only if:

1. Any one dangerous symptom or sign (see above, Section B) occurs in followup of days, weeks, or months. Quickly obtain a specialist consult or send the patient to the hospital as appropriate

> If your patient's symptoms do not respond as expected to your management, he may have an uncommon or rare cause listed in Section G.2 that you can diagnose and treat. Or you may want to refer your patient to a specialist.

2. The cause of the dizziness does not respond to treatment as you expect or the natural history of your working diagnosis does not occur. The common causes should all respond to treatment. If new dizziness occurs after adequate treatment for the presyncope, be sure there is not a new kind of dizziness e.g. vertigo or disequilibrium, and proceed as appropriate
   Don't spend time and money looking for one of the following etiologies until you are sure your patient doesn't have one of the 4 common causes of presyncope above. If she doesn't have one of those common causes, it may be that the correct cause is one of the uncommon etiologies listed below. These are important to recognize, because each has different treatment or prophylaxis

a. Causes of orthostatic hypotension with characteristic orthostatic symptoms (i.e. like immediate or delayed orthostatic hypotension):
   (1) Pure autonomic failure (PAF)–isolated hypotension, impotence, bladder dysfunction, i.e. no CNS symptoms
   (2) Multiple system atrophy (Shy-Drager syndrome)–starts as PAF, then CNS symptoms (tremor, rigidity, eye movement paresis)
   (3) Autonomic neuropathy (alcohol, porphyria, amyloidosis)
   (4) Severe diabetic autonomic neuropathy–gastroparesis, hypotension, loss of reactive symptoms of hypoglycemia
   (5) Olivopontocerebellar atrophy–ataxia and symptoms of parkinsonism; may lack rest tremor
   (6) Parkinson's disease or parkinsonism–rest tremor, rigidity, bradykinesia
b. Causes of orthostatic symptoms without concomitant orthostatic hypotension i.e. like POTS (Mayo Clin Proc 70, 617, 1995)
   (1) Milder autonomic neuropathy
   (2) Nonspecific dysautonomia i.e. idiopathic autonomic deficits
   (3) Mild diabetic autonomic neuropathy
   (4) Olivopontocerebellar atrophy
   (5) Hypothyroidism
   (6) Parkinson's disease

H. Use the glossary for precise thinking and accurate diagnosis.

1. **Aphasia** (Greek *a* meaning "negative" and *phasis,* "speech.") It indicates the patient's inability to comprehend another person's speech or writing, or inability to express herself in speech or writing. It is due to injury or disease of brain centers of comprehension or speech, *viz* Broca's.
2. **Diaphoresis** (Greek word for "profuse sweating.")
3. **Diplopia** (Greek *diplo* meaning "double or twice" and *opsis,* "sight or vision.") The patient sees 2 images of a single object.
4. **Disequilibrium** (Latin *dis* meaning "deprived of" and *equilibrium*, "balance.") It is imbalance.
5. **Dizzy** (Anglo-Saxon *dysig* meaning "foolish.") Now it's a lay term for broad range of feelings.
6. **Dysarthria** (Greek *dys* meaning "difficult or disturbed" and *arthroun*, "to utter distinctly" and *ia,* "state or condition.") It is disturbed articulation of words due to neuromuscular disease, usually CNS or peripheral nerve disease.
7. **Neurocardiogenic** syncope (Greek *neuron* meaning "nerve" and *kardia*, "heart," and *genesis,* "bringing into being.") It emphasizes the combination of neural and cardiac changes resulting in syncope. The former designation was "vasovagal" for similar pathogenesis.
8. **Orthostatic** (Greek *orthos* meaning "straight or erect" and *statikos,* "causing to stand.") It strictly refers to symptoms occurring when she stands up. "Postural" is a more general term referring to symptoms occurring with any change in position.
9. **Postcibum** (Latin *post* meaning "after" and *cibum,* "meal.") It refers to anything occurring soon after any meal. "Postprandial" is used similarly, but strictly speaking, know that *prandium* means "breakfast."
10. **Prodrome** (Greek *pro* meaning "in front of" and *dromos*, "a running.") It refers to symptoms preceding the dominant symptom. A syndrome (*syn* meaning "together") may include prodromal symptoms "together" with the dominant symptoms.
11. **Syncope** (Greek *syngkope* meaning "a cutting to pieces" or "a fainting spell.") Literally, it refers to a cutting off of consciousness. Today's use of the term syncope is the same, that is, loss of consciousness and concomitant falling. Syncope occurs because "nutrition" to both cerebral hemispheres is decreased to some critical level. Thus, sufficiently decreased blood flow or glucose or oxygen will cause syncope. Presyncope represents the symptoms that occur as the diminished functioning of the brain approaches, but does not reach, the critical level to cause loss of consciousness and falling.
12. **Vasovagal** (Latin *vas* meaning "vessel" for carrying fluid e.g. blood, and *vagus*, "wandering" nerve i.e. tenth cranial nerve.) Presyncope due to causes tending to decrease blood pressure–vasodilation (decreased peripheral resistance) and bradycardia (vagal stimulation). Sometimes "vasodepressor" syncope is used and it emphasizes the vasodilation aspect of causation over the vagal induced bradycardia..
13. **Vertigo** (Latin *vertere* meaning "to turn" and *igo,* "a condition.") It represents the spinning or hallucination of movement, either of self or of surrounding objects.

CHAPTER 13 RASH
Questions on Rash

A. To identify the cause of any rash, first observe a typical lesion using the ophthalmoscope (10-40x); the names of each of the following lesions are:

1. Flat <1cm diameter: > 1 cm diameter:
2. Elevated with watery fluid <1cm: > 1 cm:
3. Elevated with pus <1cm: > 1 cm:
4. Elevated ad solid <1cm: > 1 cm:
   > 1 cm but originating deep in the skin:

B. The commonest rash seen in the office patient is a maculopapular, generalized, bilaterally symmetrical red rash. The 2 common causes and how you differentiate each from the other are:
   1. Common cause:
      a. Characteristic:
   2. Common cause:
      a. Characteristic:

C. The commonest cause of red rash and its distinguishing characteristics are:
   1.
      a.
      b.
      c.
      d.

D. The commonest cause of eczema and its distinguishing characteristics are:
   1.
      a.
      b.
      c.
      d.

E. Three other common causes of red rash and their distinguishing characteristics are:
   1.
      a.
      b.
      c.
      d.
   2.
      a.
      b.
      c.
      d.
   3.
      a.
      b.
      c.
      d.

F. If it is a papulosquamous rash (papules with scaling), but it is not pityriasis rosea or psoriasis, always do the following tests:
   1.
   2.

G. You know about tinea corpus and tinea pedis–what is tinea incognito?

H. Your favorite topical steroid for each of the following body areas is:
   1. Face, axilla, genitals, groin
   2. Chest, arms, legs

Answers on Rash
A. Describe the individual lesions of a rash
  1. Macule; patch
  2. Vesicle; bulla
  3. Pustule; abscess
  4. Papule; plaque; nodule
B. Quickly identify the 2 very common generalized maculopapular rashes
  1. Viral infection (exanthem)–look for associated symptoms of the infection e.g. rhinorrhea, cough, myalgias, arthralgias, headache, low grade fever
  2. Medication side effect–no symptoms of infection; rash onset is usually 7-14 days after starting a new medication
C. The commonest cause of red rash and its distinguishing characteristics
  1. Eczema (of various causes) has signs of epithelial disruption (10-40X)
     a. Lesion is moist or weeping
     b. Some evidence of crusting (dried serum proteins)
     c. Excoriations (scratch marks) causing erosions (removal of pieces of epidermis)
     d. Minimal epithelial disruption may show only yellowish scales and thin red lines (fissures)
D. The commonest cause of eczema and its distinguishing characteristics
  1. Atopic eczema
     a. Intense pruritus and uncontrollable scratching, especially at night
     b. Isolated lesions may be papules with little scaling; signs of epithelial disruption e.g. weeping, crusting
     c. Rash location is flexor surface of neck, elbows, wrist, knees, dorsum of hands and feet, chest, groin
     d. Rarely facial lesions
E. Three other common red rashes and their distinguishing characteristics
  1. Seborrheic dermatitis
     a. Mild pruritus
     b. Isolated lesions are plaques with much scaling, like "dandruff"
     c. Rash locations are hairy areas (scalp, eyebrows) with itchy scalp, and glabrous skin or sternum
     d. Commonly <u>facial</u> involvement (nasolabial folds, ear canals, glabella)
  2. Psoriasis
     a. Mild pruritus
     b. Isolated lesions are red plaques with silver scales
     c. Rash locations are scalp, knees, elbows, umbilicus, gluteal folds
     d. Rarely facial lesions
  3. Pityriasis rosea
     a. Mild pruritus
     b. Isolated lesions are papules
     c. Rash location is truncal, and the rash is symmetrical in an evergreen tree pattern
     d. Rarely facial lesions
F. Don't miss 2 common treatable causes of a papulosquamous rash
  Two masqueraders–tinea and secondary syphilis, so always (if in

doubt) do KOH preparation of the lesion for tinea and some test for syphilis e.g. VDRL or RPR
G. Expect "tinea incognito" in your new, but previously treated patient with rash
If the inflammation (erythema) of acute tinea has been treated with topical corticosteroids without treating the infection, the resulting "chronic rash" may have neither the erythema nor the scaling. Thus, the rash may be impossible to identify, i.e. "incognito." A similar masking process can occur with scabies treated only with topical steroids
H. Know thoroughly one topical steroid for the various sensitivities of skin areas
  1. Hydrocortisone 1-2.5%
  2. Triamcinolone 0.1%
  Apply topical steroids no more than bid

Rash

Differential diagnosis: the 4 common causes of rash
1. Eczemas–intense pruritus; most have onset <50 y/o (types–atopic eczema, pompholyx eczema, lichen simplex chronicus); same therapy initially for each
2. Seborrheic dermatitis–"dandruff" of scalp, eyebrows, glabrous skin; "itchy" scalp; only common rash involving the <u>face</u>
3. Psoriasis–red plaques and silvery scale; scalp, elbows, knees
4. Pityriasis rosea–<30 y/o; "herald lesion"; Christmas tree pattern on the trunk

Note that all of the above rashes may need treatment with topical steroids.

A. **Be certain of the symptom and its distinguishing characteristics.** Your patient's problem or chief complaint is "I have a rash." A rash (eruption) is merely the presence of many skin lesions, often grouped together in a characteristic distribution. Have her show you everywhere the "rash" is located. If there are no lesions it may be that she had a "flushing" episode (see below, Section G.2.a). If there are lesions, ask her:
1. "Exactly when did the rash begin and where did it start and what did it look like at the beginning?" You may need to show her pictures of vesicles, bullae, or pustules to help her identify her early lesions for you, as this can be extremely important
2. "What has the rash done since it began?" Change in distribution? Is it getting better or worse? "What have you treated it with?" Examine a typical lesion, expecting solid, red lesions. You already are familiar with non-red rashes, vesicular rashes (*H. simplex, H. zoster*), bullae rashes (poison ivy, oak), pustular rashes (acne, folliculitis)
3. "If you didn't have this rash, would you feel perfectly well?" If not, "Exactly what else has changed?" You want to know if there are associated symptoms with the rash, local or systemically. Most importantly, determine the intensity of itching, and especially nocturnal itching–"What time of day is the itching worse."
4. Physical examination in dermatology usually is more important than history for correct diagnosis:
   a. Look for any sign of systemic disease. Fever is extremely important to identify, first being certain no antipyretic has been taken in the past 4-6 hours. Rectal temperature should be obtained in every patient with a rash who is ill-appearing, as some dangerous diseases present with fever and rash
   b. Find a typical lesion and examine it carefully, in good light and with a 5-10X lens, or better yet, the ophthalmoscope at 10-40X
      (1) Is the typical lesion flat (<1cm, macule; >1 cm, patch) or elevated?
      (2) If elevated, does it contain watery fluid (<1cm, vesicle; >1 cm,

Chapter 13 Rash

bulla) or pus (<1cm, pustule; >1 cm, abscess)?
(3) If elevated and solid, is it <1 cm (papule) or >1 cm (plaque)? A nodule also is >1 cm and solid, but it originates deeper in the skin; you can feel its deeper base

---

Be certain:
1. That your patient has a rash
2. Whether it is new or episodic or chronic rash
3. Where the rash started and what the first lesions looked like
4. Where the rash is located now, especially if the face is involved
5. If there is epithelial disruption (an eczema)
6. If there are associated symptoms, e.g. intense pruritus

---

(4) Search for signs of epithelial disruption indicating an eczema. Excoriations (scratch marks on the skin surface due to pruritus) cause erosions (tiny ulcer-like lesions due to loss of only the epidermal layer). Deeper loss of some or all the dermis defines an ulcer. A fissure also penetrates into the dermis, but you see it as a linear lesion or only a red line at 10-20X. Lesions with epithelial disruption are moist or show weeping with resultant crusting, i.e. dried serum proteins due to a disrupted, leaking epidermis. Dermatitis has inflammation (erythema) but not epithelial disruption
(5) Scales <u>must</u> be found if present (only red rashes have scales), so scrape the lesion if necessary and look at 10-40X. Lichenification is thickened epidermis secondary to itchy lesions being chronically rubbed, instead of scratched; it becomes obvious at 10-40X and resembles the bark of a tree
  c. Equally important, examine the whole <u>exposed</u> body and determine the areas affected by the rash, its distribution, and equally important, which areas are spared e.g. face, palms, soles

By now you should be confident it is a red rash, whether it is new, episodic or chronic rash, if it is an eczema, the intensity of pruritus, and the body areas affected. In almost all instances you now have the information you need for diagnosis of the obvious causes (Section C) and the common causes (Section E). In the rare instance that your patient appears different clinically from the usual office patient with rash, be certain (Section B) that she does not have a symptom or sign of a dangerous disease

B. **Be confident it's not a dangerous disease.**
1. Send immediately to the ED by ambulance if there is:
   a. Rash, hoarseness, dysphonia, dysphagia, think of anaphylaxis
   b. New rash and dyspnea, think of anaphylaxis, allergic reactions, urticaria
   c. Inspiratory stridor, think of laryngeal edema due to anaphylaxis, allergic reaction, hereditary angioedema
   d. Rash, high fever, hypotension, think of toxic shock syndrome, acute meningococcemia, purpura fulminans, disseminated *Vibrio.vulnificus*
   e. Hypotension or angioedema i.e. facial swelling (lips, lids) with or without urticaria, think of anaphylaxis, hereditary angioedema
   f. Systemic symptoms (vomiting, dyspnea, hypotension) accompanying urticaria, think of anaphylaxis, hereditary angioedema, hypocomplementemic vasculitis
   g. A very ill patient (fever, toxic) with large bullae or erosions of both skin and mucosal membranes (eyes, mouth, genitals), think of Stevens-Johnson syndrome

h. Trunk lesions of large bullae or erosions, sloughing epidermis, think of toxic epidermal necrolysis

---

Be certain in the first minutes of your exam that there is no evidence of any <u>one</u> dangerous symptom or sign associated with the rash:
1. Severely ill patient
2. Fever >101°F (38.3°C)
3. Dyspnea, inspiratory stridor, hoarseness
4. Severe blistering or facial swelling
5. Systemic hypotension
6. Meningismus
7. Severe urticaria

Any suggestion of a dangerous disease, send your patient to the ED.

---

i. Patient on coumadin or heparin and new tender purple plaques, think of anticoagulant-induced necrosis
2. Admit at once to the ED or hospital if there is:
   a. Severe headache, rash and meningismus, think of meningitis
   b. Rash, fever, very severe headache, abdominal pain, vomiting, think of RMSF, acute meningitis
   c. Fever, rash, and cardiac murmur, think of infective endocarditis
   d. Rapid onset of a large red plaque with associated pain and tenderness, think of cellulitis
   e. Hypesthesia or blisters overlying an area of cellulitis, think of necrotizing fasciitis
   f. Cellulitis of the central face, think of it progressing to cavernous sinus thrombosis
   g. Acutely severe urticaria, think of it progressing to anaphylaxis
   h. Ill patient with fever and rash and immunocompromised conditions (HIV, asplenia, chronic steroid therapy, transplant patient--acute graft-versus-host disease), think of unusual infections
   i. Palpable purpura and petechiae with fever, think of meningococcemia, purpura fulminans
   j. Ill patient with generalized skin redness and scaling, often fever and lymphadenopathy, think of exfoliative erythroderma
   k. Urticaria during or following significant activity, think of exercise-induced urticaria
   l. Painful urticaria lasting >24 hours, think of urticarial vasculitis
3. Admit to the hospital or have a specialist consult as soon as appropriate if there is:
   a. Oral blisters or erosions that are much larger than herpes or canker sores, or upper trunk large erosions that heal unusually slowly, think of pemphigus vulgaris
   b. Erythema multiforme (target lesions on trunk, palms, soles) and oral mucosal lesions, think it may progress to Stevens-Johnson syndrome
   c. More than 50% of skin surface with eczematous lesions, think of exfoliative erythrodermatitis
   d. Rash and fever and:
      (1) Pharyngitis, think of IM, HIV primary infection, arcanobacterial pharyngitis, rheumatic fever, enteroviral infection (echovirus, coxsackie), Kawasaki's disease
      (2) Gastroenteritis symptoms, think of leptospirosis, ehrlichiosis (leukopenia), RMSF, typhoid fever, WNV, babesiosis
      (3) Arthritis, think of Still's disease, disseminated gonococcemia, Parvo B19, meningococcemia, Lyme disease
      (4) Headaches, myalgias, think of murine typhus, ehrlichiosis, leptospirosis (conjunctivitis), Lyme disease, relapsing fever (Borrelia), secondary syphilis, RMSF, WNV, babesiosis
      (5) Thrombocytopenia, think of meningococcemia, any septicemia, RMSF, typhus, IM, infective endocarditis, HPS, ehrlichiosis, babesiosis, dengue fever, malaria, CMV, *M. pneumoniae*
      (6) Scarlatiniform rash (diffuse erythema), think of scarlet fever, toxic shock syndrome (thrombocytopenia), Kawasaki's disease (thrombocytosis)

Chapter 13 Rash 167

- e. Erythroderma (most of the body is erythematous) unexplained by chronic skin disease (psoriasis, eczema) or drugs, think of malignancy, especially cutaneous T cell lymphoma (Sezary syndrome)
- f. Any papulosquamous or eczematous lesions (psoriasis, eczema) not responding to appropriate topical therapy, think of tinea, secondary syphilis, cutaneous T cell lymphoma (CTCL), allergic contact dermatitis due to the topical agent itself
- g. Atopic dermatitis localized to exposed surfaces (face, neck, dorsum, hands), think of airborne contact dermatitis, photosensitive eruption
- h. Unusually severe seborrheic dermatitis, think of HIV

C. **Make a quick diagnosis if it's obvious.** Is it an easily diagnosed cause or a medication that is responsible for the rash? In most patients you will be <u>highly</u> confident of a common cause of the symptom by now. If not, one or more of the following tests may exclude an organic disease and increase your confidence in your working diagnosis: CBC, ESR, HIV

Recognize any easily diagnosed rash or a medication side effect:
1. Non-red rashes–herpes, acne
2. Contact dermatitis
3. Exanthem–symptoms of a viral infection
4. Medication side effect

---

1. Non-red rashes–If there is significant pruritus with a non-red rash, scratching can convert it into eczema. In such a case, critical to a correct diagnosis is to find evidence that the non-red rash preceded the red rash–either by your finding an intact lesion, or by your patient describing precisely what the rash looked like at the beginning
    a. Vesicular lesions
       (1) *H. simplex*–occurs either perioral or genital area; often all vesicles are broken, and only a round red erosion with remnants of the original lesion's roof is seen at 10-40X
       (2) *H. zoster*–plaques of clustered vesicles in a line along the affected dermatome (scalp, face, trunk); the rash doesn't cross midline, and pain may precede the rash by more than a week
       (3) Dyshidrosis–very tiny vesicles along the sides of digits (you may see them only at 20X); with scratching, the lesions often are converted into dyshidrotic eczema; or due to exposure to harsh soaps or detergents, it becomes irritant contact dermatitis (dry and chapped)
    b. Bullae *viz* poison ivy, poison oak, poison sumac
    c. Pustules *viz* acne, rosacea, folliculitis, candidiasis
    d. Colored lesions e.g. actinic keratosis (skin color), pityriasis versicolor (lesions are white on dark skin, or tan on white skin)
2. Red rash, but it is a vascular reaction that does not blanch, *viz* petechiae and ecchymoses; use diascopy technique (press a glass slide on the lesions) to determine absence of blanching
3. Contact dermatitis–often it is obvious by history and location of the rash; see Section G.3
4. Viral exanthems–e.g. rubeola, rubella, EBV, echovirus, coxsackie virus, adenovirus; rash is similar to the maculopapular rash of drugs, but the viral rash may be less erythematous and less pruritic. Look

especially for the accompanying symptoms of the viral illness (prostration, myalgias, arthralgias, headache, lack of eosinophilia, and no new medication) to differentiate from a drug reaction. Caution: Follow the course of any maculopapular rash because it may be the initial rash in a dangerous disease (RMSF, meningococcus, secondary syphilis, HIV, typhoid fever)
5. Medications–almost any drug can cause a rash in any individual patient; drug reactions are very common, but drug rashes should rarely be confused with the 4 common causes of red rash e.g. no scaling, no epithelial disruption, no plaques. Most drug eruptions are either:
   a. Exanthems that account for 75% of drug eruptions (morbilliform, like measles)
      (1) Maculopapular, red rash; smaller than 5 mm lesions may become confluent as patches; low-grade fever and mild pruritus commonly occur, and lesions blanch on diascopy
      (2) Lesions begin head and neck or upper trunk and spread symmetrically outward to the limbs
      (3) Onset occurs during the first 2-3 weeks of drug ingestion, except with semisynthetic penicillins the rash often begins later
      (4) Stopping the drug results in fading and desquamation, but it may take > 2 weeks to disappear
   b. Urticaria or hives that represent about 20% of drug eruptions
      (1) Pruritic, red welts (wheals) due to localized edema, and they blanch with diascopy
      (2) Usually generalized, but mostly in covered areas–chest, trunk, buttocks
      (3) Lesions begin 1-2 days after starting the drug, and individual lesions usually last less than 1 day
      (4) Urticaria may be associated with symptoms of:
         (a) Serum sickness–starts as an exanthem (morbilliform) or urticaria, but also fever, arthralgias, myalgias
         (b) Angioedema–central face involvement, especially swelling and edema of tongue and lips
         (c) Anaphylaxis–urticaria and rapid onset of laryngeal edema, vomiting, possibly hypotension
   c. Hypersensitivity syndromes due to anticonvulsants, allopurinol, sulfonamides
      (1) Starts as a morbilliform eruption, then it worsens to eczema or exfoliation
      (2) Often also fever, lymphadenectasis, hepatitis, eosinophilia
   d. Vasculitis has palpable purpura (not blanching), often starting on the legs
   e. Fixed dry eruption has round red plaques, especially genitalia, face, hands, mucous membranes; causative drugs are barbiturates, tetracycline, sulfonamides, phenolphthalein
   f. Photosensitivity is an exaggerated sunburn-like reaction in exposed areas; fluoroquinolones, tetracyclines, thiazides are causative

D. **Identify your patient's worries and wants.** Rashes occur very commonly and few people with rash consult about it. During your interview and exam try to intuit or discover why your patient is here today, and not previously, for this problem. Don't necessarily ask directly, but try to get some ideas from your patient's responses to questions about her perception of the rash. You can't completely help your patient unless you know what she really worries about and

Chapter 13 Rash 169

wants from you. That's why she is here to see you–to satisfy her worries and wants! Here are only some of the possible worries and wants of your patient with rash. You must discover her specific, unique ones

> During your exam, discover your patient's worries (e.g. infection, SLE, HIV) and wants (e.g. antimicrobial, antipruritic), so that you can respond to her specific needs as soon as possible.

1. Common worries:
   a. That the cause of the rash is a dangerous etiology e.g. anaphylaxis, malignancy, dangerous infection, SLE
   b. That the etiology is some rare disease e.g. toxic shock syndrome, RMSF, monkeypox
   c. What other fears or anxieties might be troubling your patient? For example, she may have had rash at other times, and only with this one does she come for help. What has changed? Perhaps a friend or relative, who had similar rash, recently has been diagnosed with skin cancer or "lupus." There are many other possibilities–think of them
2. Your patient wants:
   a. You to perform a thorough physical exam focused on possible causes of the rash and she wants any other appropriate tests
   b. A plausible explanation of the cause of the rash
   c. Confident reassurance from you that it is not a dangerous or rare etiology. Tell her, "The good news, it's not lupus" (or whatever you believe her real worry is)
   d. To know the prognosis, short term (effects on job, home life, marriage; how soon she will be back to normal) and long term (if recurrences are possible; how to prevent recurrences; if it will cause any disability)
   e. Treatment to stop the rash now and to prevent recurrences
   f. A dermatology referral if she believes you are not confident of the diagnosis

E. **Know the symptoms that differentiate the 4 common causes of rash.**
   1. The commonest cause of red rash is eczema (a dermatitis or almost any skin disease may become an eczema)
      a. Dermatitis has only inflammation and mild pruritus. For any dermatitis to become an eczema, epithelial disruption must occur (lesion surface is moist or weeping; crust occurs on some lesions; erosions and excoriations; and superficial blistering; minimal epithelial disruption may show only yellowish scale and thin red fissures seen at 20X)
         (1) Eczemas with onset in a patient <45-50 y/o; usually there is intense pruritus; each is treated similarly (see Section G.4)
            (a) Atopic eczema– uncontrollable nocturnal scratching also occurs with scabies or dermatitis herpetiformis; if it is neither of these, diagnosis likely is atopic eczema; flexor surfaces of elbows, knees, wrist, neck, ankles
            (b) Pompholyx eczema (dyshidrotic dermatitis)–hands only or hands and feet; may see darkened vesicles on palms or soles
            (c) Lichen simplex chronicus (neurodermatitis)–as with atopic dermatitis, the scratching precedes the inflammation; differs in that additional areas are affected–sides of the neck, back, lateral leg, upper thighs and anogenital areas; inflammation becomes lichenified chronically
            (d) Any skin disease can become a secondary eczema in a patient prone to scratching
         (2) Dermatidides usually with onset in a patient >45-50 y/o; there is mild pruritus, but scratching commonly converts it to an eczema

> Common causes of most red rashes in adults:
> 1. Eczemas–intense pruritus; most have onset <50 y/o (types–atopic eczema, pompholyx eczema, lichen simplex chronicus); same therapy initially for each
> 2. Seborrheic dermatitis–"dandruff" of scalp, eyebrows, glabrous skin; "itchy" scalp; only common rash involving the <u>face</u>
> 3. Psoriasis–red plaques and silvery scale; scalp, elbows, knees
> 4. Pityriasis rosea–<30 y/o; "herald lesion"; Christmas tree pattern on the trunk
>
> Note that all of the above rashes may need treatment with topical steroids.

(see Section G.4 for treatment)
      (a) Asteatotic (xerotic) dermatitis–severe dry skin especially anterior legs and backs of the hands
      (b) Stasis dermatitis–venous insufficiency of the legs precedes eczema
  b. What suggests it might not be an eczema
    (1) It is a red rash, but you also find a few other intact lesions e.g. vesicles, bullae, pustules, or your patient describes one of these other lesions that occurred early on
    (2) If it is a red, scaling rash, but you can find no evidence of epithelial disruption (see above) to any of the lesions, assume the rash is a papulosquamous disease e.g. pityriasis rosea, secondary syphilis, tinea, and look for its characteristics; always get KOH prep and test for syphilis (VDRL) if in doubt about the cause of any red rash
2. Common look-alikes causing red rash and how each differs from eczema
  a. Seborrheic dermatitis is very common (5% of the adult population and >20% of HIV patients)
    (1) It begins after puberty and it is a chronic disease with exacerbations and remissions like atopic dermatitis, but much less or no pruritus. The scalp almost always itches
    (2) Lesions are red plaques in any hairy areas but especially the scalp and eyebrows; nonhairy areas (glabrous skin) affected are behind and at the entrance of ear canals, nasal folds, glabella and midsternum
    (3) On the scalp the lesions are <u>poorly marginated</u> (10-40X), which may help to differentiate them from tinea capitis or psoriasis, both of which have sharp margins. Of these 3 diseases tinea alone has broken hair and focal hair loss
    (4) Lesions of seborrheic dermatitis on glabrous skin may be indistinguishable from psoriasis, unless you can find some lesions that are not sharply demarcated, unlike the sharply marginated lesions of psoriasis. Diagnostic difficulty is common even with dermatologists who call it "seboriasis" and give a treatment trial of frequent vigorous shampooing of the scalp,

even when there are only lesions of glabrous skin
  b. Psoriasis
    (1) New lesions are 1-3 mm papules. Later coalesced lesions are sharply marginated (10-40X) the whole circumference of the red plaques, which are covered by much white or silver scale. Scraping off the scale reveals bleeding points (Auspitz's sign)
    (2) Distribution of the lesions–especially scalp, elbows, knees, gluteal fold, periumbilicus, nails, and less often, extensor surfaces of arms and legs; usually spares palms, soles, face
    (3) Extracutaneous manifestations may help to confirm the diagnosis
      (a) Nails–pitting, onycholysis, discolored nails, subungal hyperkeratosis
      (b) Joints–10% of patients have joint complaints *viz* spondyloarthropathy with sacroiliitis, symmetric polyarthritis like RA, asymmetric oligoarthritis of hand joints
  c. Pityriasis rosea
    (1) Rarely occurs in patients >30 y/o; early on papular lesions predominate on the trunk and proximal extremities (neck, inner arms, inner thighs), and spare the face
    (2) Ask about a 2-10 cm "herald" lesion, but it occurs only in 50% of patients, and it often precedes the start of other lesions by 7-14 days. The "herald" lesion has scaling, and may be round (annular), suggesting tinea corporis ("ring worm"), which should be excluded by KOH exam
    (3) Following the "herald" lesion, 30-100 isolated plaques 1-2 cm in diameter erupt, and at least some are oval, shaped like a football with the long axis oriented along skin lines on the trunk
    (4) If no "herald" lesion occurred and there are very few or no oval lesions, consider tinea, secondary syphilis or guttate psoriasis. If in question, get a serologic test for syphilis and KOH preparation

F. **Use this summary for efficient diagnosis of a common cause.** With the information from Sections A-E in mind, here is the rapid approach to diagnosis of a red rash.
  1. You have already determined:
    a. In Section A, by H&P that it is a rash, its distribution, and characteristics of a typical lesion.
    b. In Section B, that there is no evidence in the H&P of any one dangerous cause of the rash.
    c. In Section C, that it is neither an easily diagnosed non-red rash nor a red rash due to contact dermatitis, viral infection, or a medication side effect.
  2. From the focused H&P almost always you should quickly be confident of a working diagnosis. Confident final diagnosis is made only in followup the next few weeks or months when the response to treatment or nontreatment is appropriate to your working diagnosis.
    a. If she is <45-50 y/o, there is intense pruritus, and signs of epithelial disruption, it is either a primary eczema (atopic eczema, pompholyx eczema, lichen simplex chronicus) or a secondary eczema (see Section G.4 for management).
    b. If your patient has minimal pruritus with the dermatitis, it likely is

either asteatotic (xerotic) dermatitis or stasis dermatitis. Use moisturizers and topical corticosteroids.
- c. If the rash begins after puberty, there is "itchy scalp" and characteristic facial distribution, diagnose and treat seborrheic dermatitis
- d. If it is a papulosquamous disease having sharply marginated, red, scaling lesions, and no signs of epithelial disruption, diagnose and treat:
  (1) Psoriasis–characteristic lesions and distribution
  (2) Pityriasis rosea–"herald" patch followed by oval lesions on the trunk.
- e. See Section G.4 for treatment of any eczema, which includes all of the above entities if scratching converts it to an eczema.
3. Answer your patient's worries and wants that you determined early on during the exam (Section D). Have you done everything you can to help her?
4. You now have a working diagnosis, but only with followup can you be highly confident it is correct. In return visits you are always testing by H&P that your working diagnosis is correct.

G. Abandon your working diagnosis and look for an uncommon cause only if:

1. Any one dangerous symptom or sign (see above, Section B) occurs in followup of days, weeks, or months. Quickly obtain a dermatology or infectious disease consult or send the patient to the hospital as appropriate.

If your patient's symptoms do not respond as expected to your management, he may have an uncommon or rare cause listed in Section G.2 that you can diagnose and treat. Or you may want to refer your patient to a specialist.

2. Your patient's response to therapy is not as you expect or if the natural history of your working diagnosis does not occur
Don't spend time and money looking for one of the following etiologies until you are sure your patient doesn't have one of the 4 common causes of her rash. Nevertheless, it may be she has an uncommon or rare cause of the red rash
   a. Transient red flushing of the face and upper chest by history only
      (1) Carcinoid syndrome, mastocytosis, pheochromocytoma (commonly pallor, very rarely flushing), MTC
      (2) Drugs especially nicotinic acid, monosodium glutamate, alcohol, nitrites, sulfites
   b. Glucagonoma syndrome–migratory necrolytic erythema; intertriginous and dependent areas; early phase resembles persistent subacute eczema
   c. Dermatomyositis–heliotrope erythema of eyelids and dark red plaques on knuckles; suspect internal malignancies
   d. Atopic dermatitis picture occurs with inherited immunodeficiencies having increased susceptibility to infections
      (1) Wiskott-Aldrich syndrome–thrombocytopenia and recurrent severe infections e.g. disseminated HSV
      (2) Ataxia telangiectasia–oculocutaneous telangiectasia
      (3) Chronic granulomatous disease and Job's syndrome–eosinophilia
   e. Similar rash to atopic dermatitis
      (1) Any of the allergic contact dermatidides
      (2) Mineral deficiency e.g. zinc
      (3) Gluten-sensitive enteropathy–desquamative dermatitis with much scaling, may resemble seborrheic dermatitis also

Chapter 13 Rash   173

      (4) Hyperimmunoglobulin E syndrome–recurrent respiratory tract infections, soft tissue abscesses, markedly increased IgE levels
- f. Pagets disease of breast and extramammary sites–eczematous lesions of one breast or vulva, scrotum, axilla; may be adenocarcinoma
- g. Diseases resembling psoriasis
  - (1) Parapsoriasis– very stable plaques, not changing constantly like psoriasis
  - (2) Mycosis fungoides–later stage of parapsoriasis
  - (3) Sezary syndrome– lymphadenopathy
  - (4) Pityriasis rubra pilaris–large plaques on the entire trunk
  - (5) Reiter's syndrome–palm and sole psoriasis and arthritis
  - (6) Bowen's disease (squamous cell carcinoma in situ)--resembles psoriasis or chronic eczema; plaque grows very slowly by lateral extension
  - (7) Bazek's syndrome–psoriaform lesions at the tips of fingers and toes; suggests GI or lung malignancy
  - (8) SLE
  - (9) Sarcoidosis
- h. Pruritus causing scratching can cause unusual rashes that do not respond to usual therapies–think of cutaneous T-cell lymphoma, Hodgkin disease, polycythemia vera, malignancies of the GI tract, lung, CNS
- i. Celiac sprue–associated with dermatitis herpetiformis; nocturnal scratching like atopic eczema; papulovasicular rash on extensor surfaces, back, intergluteal folds; concomitant diarrhea and weight loss

3. Contact dermatitis may occur at any age with variable pruritus, and it is of three major types:
   - a. Strong irritants, mostly to hands, are usually identified easily by history; mild pruritus but marked inflammation, pain and epithelial disruption
   - b. Weak irritants do one of two things:
     - (1) Dry the skin (xerosis) by solvent action e.g. soap, detergent and hot water remove skin lipids; hands are usually equally affected
     - (2) Too much moisture (maceration) e.g. sweat or water on hands, feet, intertriginous areas; mild maceration resulting in mild inflammation (chafing) is called intertrigo, whereas severe inflammation with epithelial disruption becomes irritant contact dermatitis
   - c. Allergic etiology of contact dermatitis
     - (1) Lesions are different from the above two irritant contact dermatidides, that is, more prominent redness, edema and pruritus; in acute cases there is weeping and crusting (eczema), and in chronic cases, scaling and fissuring
     - (2) First identify the allergen; often location and shape of the lesion is all that you need for diagnosis
     - (3) Clues that an environmental allergen is causative are an asymmetrical or unilateral distribution of skin lesions, and lesions that are not round, but linear or angular shaped

4. Treatment of severe rash or eczema sometimes depends less on specific diagnosis of disease causation, and more on what you observe:
   - a. Pruritus first must be alleviated to stop any itch-scratch cycle; after scratching stops, characteristic lesions can be diagnosed
     - (1) Systemic H2 antihistamines
       - (a) Sedating e.g. hydroxyzine, diphenhydramine
       - (b) Nonsedating e.g. loratadine, cetirizine, doxepin
     - (2) Topical anesthetic e.g. pramoxine, doxepin (Zonalon)
     - (3) Mentholated lotion e.g. Sarna, calamine lotion
     - (4) Cool tub bath with colloidal oatmeal (Aveeno)
   - b. Cold, wet dressings with tap water or Burow's solution for 10-20 minutes tid, for acute inflammation
   - c. Topical corticosteroid appropriate type and concentration for the skin area inflamed
   - d. Topical antibacterial ointment for secondary infection
   - e. Systemic glucocorticoids as needed (single dose IM Kenalog, 1 mg/kg; oral prednisone 1 mg/kg, tapered over 2-3 weeks)
   - f. Dry skin (xerosis) needs treatment with a moisturizer
     - (1) Daily bathing, then ointment-based emollient applied bid e.g. Moisturel, DML Forte, Curel, Eucerin
     - (2) Humectant e.g. Lac-Hydrin 12% lotion, OTC alpha-hydroxy preparation
   - g. Severe atopic eczema that is unresponsive to topical steroids, may try pimecrolimus

H. Use the glossary for precise thinking and accurate

diagnosis.

1. **Abscess** (Greek *apostema* meaning "a drawing off" referring to "bad humors" removed systemically to a specific site.) Now it is a >1 cm elevated pustular lesion.
2. **Atopy** (Greek *atopos* meaning "out of place" or affecting only a minority of the population.) It is hereditary predisposition to develop some sort of allergic disease e.g. allergic dermatitis, atopic dermatitis, allergic rhinitis, asthma.
3. **Comedo** (Latin *comedere* meaning "to eat up.") A comedo refers to a filled ("blackhead") sebaceous gland in skin; when squeezed a wormlike fragment is expressed and ancients thought this was the remains of a worm that burrowed into skin to devour flesh.
4. **Diascopy** (Greek *dia* meaning "through" and *skopein*, "to examine.") Pressing a glass slide against skin, empties dermal blood vessels, and allows observation of changes in the underlying skin. Hemorrhage or extravasated RBCs (petechiae, ecchymosis) do not blanch.
5. **Dyshidrosis** (Greek *dys* meaning "disordered, abnormal" and *hidrosis*, "a sweating.") It originally was thought to represent a skin disease due to retention of sweat.
6. **Eczema** (Greek *ek* meaning "out" and *zeein*, "to boil" so anything thrown out by heating.) To the ancients, such a rash or eruption was boiling over of body humors onto skin. Now it indicates more than simply dermatitis (inflammation of skin). In addition to redness, there also is epithelial disruption (oozing, crusting, superficial blisters, excoriation, erosions).
7. **Emollient** (Latin *emollire* meaning "to soften or make mild.") It is a cream or ointment that softens or soothes damaged skin or irritant lesions.
8. **Erythema** (Greek word for "redness in the skin, or a blush.") Erythema is now used to describe redness of any external or internal surface.
9. **Erythroderma** (Greek *erythro* meaning "red" and *derma*, "skin.") It indicates widespread red skin, and it suggests exfoliative dermatitis, which can be an emergency.
10. **Enanthem** (Greek *en* meaning "in" and *anthema*, "a blossoming.") It is an eruption localized to mucous membranes, e.g. due to a virus.
11. **Exanthem** (Greek *exanthema* meaning "a breaking out," such as blooming of flowers, e.g. *anthos* means "flower bloom or blossom.") Now we recognize two kinds of exanthem–either a red maculopapular (morbilliform) or a diffuse erythema (scarlatiniform), and they are generalized rashes (compared to enanthems).
12. **Excoriation** (Latin *excoriare* meaning "to flay" or tear away strips of skin.) Now it means a scratching of skin that causes erosions, that is, tearing away of pieces of the epidermal layer.
13. **Excrescence** (Latin *excrescere* meaning to "grow out or rise up.") It is any lesion growing out above normal surface.
14. **Glabella** (Latin *glaber* meaning "hairless, smooth.") It refers to the smooth area on the frontal bone between the superciliary arches, and the smooth hairless area between the eyebrows.
15. **Glabrous** (Latin *glaber* meaning "hairless or bald.") It is skin typically devoid of hair.
16. **Guttate** (psoriasis) (Latin *gutta* meaning "a drop.") Young adult may suddenly develop >50 small, nonconfluent papules (as opposed to the usual plaque of psoriasis) over the trunk and proximal extremities.
17. **Herpes zoster** (Greek *herpes* meaning "to creep" and *zoster*, "belt or girdle."); Unlike a girdle, H. zoster lesions do not cross the midline.
18. **Humectant** (Latin *humectare* meaning "to be moist.") It refers to any moisturizer.
19. **Intertrigo** (Latin *inter* meaning "between" and *terere*, "to rub.") It now refers to a mild dermatitis occurring where apposed surfaces of skin come together, e.g. creases of the neck, folds of the groin, armpits, under breasts. These areas, therefore, are called intertiginous areas. Intertrigo is caused by moisture retention (maceration), warmth, friction.
20. **Lichenification.** Due to chronic rubbing of an itchy lesion, the epidermis becomes obviously thickened. The normal skin markings or striae stand out, and their criss-cross pattern encloses shiny smooth quadrilateral facets best seen at 10-40X.
21. **Maceration** (Latin *maceratio* meaning "softening of a solid by soaking.")
22. **Morbilliform** (Latin *morbilli* meaning "measles" and *forma*, "shape.") It is a rash resembling measles (rubeola) i.e. maculopapular, red, nonpruritic.
23. **Ointment** (Latin *ungere* meaning "to anoint or apply oil.") The Old French *oignement* was an "annointing" or the substance itself.
24. **Onycolysis** (Greek *onyx* meaning "nail" and *lysis*, "dissolution.") It is separation of the nail plate from the nail bed, beginning at the free margin and moving proximally.

Chapter 13 Rash   175

25. **Papulosquamous** (Latin *papula* meaning "small elevation" of skin and *squamosos*, "scaly.") It indicates a group of skin diseases with scaly, papular lesions e.g. psoriasis, pityriasis rosea.
26. **Paronychia** (Greek *para* meaning "alongside of" and *onyx*, "nail.") It is inflammation at the margins of the nail bed of a finger or toe.
27. **Petechia and ecchymosis** (Latin words for pinpoint and larger, respectively, intradermal extravasations of RBCs or hemorrhage.) Because of their color, they are both "purpura" i.e. the Latin word for "purple."
28. **Pilosebaceous** (unit) (Latin *pilus* meaning "hair" and *sebum,* "grease.") It is the hair and oil-producing gland in skin. The hair originates in deep dermis, and the sebaceous gland resides in superficial dermis.
29. **Pityriasis.** Hippocrates used the word to describe a scruffy excrescence on the skin, because the scruff or dandruff resembled a husk of cereal grain called a *pityron.*
30. **Pompholyx** (Greek word meaning "bubble.") It describes a vesicular eruption.
31. **Pox** (Norman French *poquet* meaning "a little pocket" in the skin.) Previously "pox" was the generic term for a variety of pustular eruptions; the "great pox" was syphilis, more feared than the "small" pox.
32. **Pruritus** (Latin *pruire* meaning "to itch.") Note that it is not spelled *puritus* or *pruritis*.
33. **Psoriasis** (Greek word denoting any "itchy or scaling condition" in Hippocrates time.) The word *psora* was a specific disease "the itch or mange," which included under the larger category, psoriasis. Now it is only one of the papulosquamous diseases *viz* red scaling lesions that may itch mildly, but no epithelial disruption is present.
34. **Rash** (Latin *rasi* meaning "to scrape or scratch.") Originally it implied redness resulting from scraping skin away; now rash implies only multiple skin lesions. Don't say "skin rash"–it's redundant.
35. **Scabies** (Latin word for "the itch" and it is related to *scabere*, "to scratch.") To the Romans, scabies was a larger category of any itchy, mangy skin disease. The Anglo-Saxon word *scab* for "crust on a sore" probably derived from scratching scabies lesions.
36. **Seborrhea** (Latin *sebum* meaning "tallow, suet, grease" and Greek *rhoia,* "a flowing.") It is excessive elaboration of oil by skin glands.
37. **Shingles** (Latin *cingulum* meaning "a girdle.")
38. **Tachyphylaxis** (Greek *tachy* meaning "rapid or fast" and *phylaxis*, "a guarding or protection.") It is a decreased response to a drug after daily dosing. For example, topical steroids in cream tid for 4 days rapidly lose effect, which is regained 3-4 days after stopping the steroid, so apply topical steroids by interrupted dosing.
39. **Telangiectasia** (Greek *telos* meaning "end," and *angi*, "vessel" and *ectasia*, "dilatation.") The end branches of terminal arterioles and capillaries are permanently dilated causing focal red lesions in the dermis, and they blanch by diascopy.
40. **Trunk or truncal** (Latin *truncus* meaning "stem" like a trunk of a tree.) It represents the main part of the body to which the head and limbs are attached (back, buttocks, chest, abdomen, pelvis).
41. **Urticaria** (Latin *urtica* for the plant called stinging nettle.) When the plant is touched it produces a stinging sensation and inflammation of the skin. *Urticaria* is what touching the nettle did to the Roman's skin, causing a red, pruritic plaque (now called a wheal). Hives is a lay term for urticaria. Angioedema (soft tissue swelling lips, lids) may occur with wheals and progress to anaphylaxis, or it may occur with no wheals in hereditary angioedema.
42. **Xerosis.** (Greek word meaning "abnormal dryness," e.g. of the eyes, mouth, skin.) If severe it results in asteatotic dermatitis.

Chapter 14
Shortness of Breath (SOB)

Questions on Shortness of Breath

A. In your patient with complaint "I can't get my breath," the most important
   1. Historical information is:
   2. Physical exam is:
B. In the office, the 2 common causes of SOB and their distinguishing characteristics are:
   1.
     a.
     b.
     c.
   2.
     a.
     b.
     c.
C. All patients with dyspnea have SOB, but not all patients with SOB have dyspnea. The 4 characteristics of dyspnea are:
   1.
   2.
   3.
   4.
D. If your patient has dyspnea, you immediately consider that the cause might be disease of one of 2 organs:

E. You think your patient might have a PE, if he has any one of the three following respiratory symptoms:
   1.
   2.
   3.
F. Your patient is 25 y/o and abruptly awakens at 0200 hr with severe SOB and frantically gets out of bed. You immediately consider 2 likely diagnoses:
   1.
   2.
   The same symptoms in a 70 y/o patient make you consider 2 other dangerous causes:
   3.
   4.

Answers on Shortness of Breath (SOB)
A. Be certain of your patient's symptom and its distinguishing characteristics
   1. You want to identify immediately if your patient has dyspnea, that is, a very uncomfortable awareness of working to breathe. Dyspnea suggests organic disease of either the heart or lungs. Patients with dyspnea always have SOB. Most patients who come to the office with SOB, however, do not have dyspnea. They don't have the uncomfortable and labored breathing of dyspnea, instead they feel they can't get enough air into their lungs, and they may feel as if they are suffocating. If he has to "work" to breathe, that is dyspnea. Except with severe, clinically obvious heart or lung disease, dyspnea only occurs chronically with some increased exertion or exercise; new onset dyspnea occurs at rest with PE, pneumonia, pneumothorax
   2. Search for any sign of heart or lung disease, the commonest causes of dyspnea. Auscultate the lungs for any evidence of adventitious sounds, that is, either crackles or wheezes, and the heart for abnormalities of rhythm or valve murmur. Examine for extra-cardiopulmonary signs *viz* JVD, hepatojugular reflux, pretibial edema
B. The 2 common causes of SOB in the office and their distinguishing characteristics
   Neither of the following common causes has any symptom or sign on exam of cardiac or lung disease. They differ in the following characteristics:
   1. Psychological causes
      a. Patient <40-50 y/o with episodic SOB
      b. It is not dyspnea
      c. SOB almost always occurs at rest, and when it occurs with activity, SOB is inappropriately worse than the degree of exertion
   2. Lifestyle causes (cigarette smoker, obesity, "couch potato")
      a. Patient >45-50 y/o with daily SOB and gradually worsening as he gets older
      b. It is dyspnea
      c. SOB is episodic, only during exertion, and the dyspnea is appropriate for the degree of exertion
C. Characteristics of dyspnea
   1. A very uncomfortable sensation in the chest, often called "chest pain" by the patient
   2. Awareness of labored or difficult breathing; he really is working to breathe
   3. Over months or years, it progressively worsens; at the start, it is only on exertion (DOE), then later it occurs even at rest
   4. It prevents the patient from doing certain physical activities
   (In non-dyspneic SOB, the patient is not working to breathe, he just "can't get enough air in," there is not progressive worsening over time, and it does not prevent physical activities)
D. The implications of your patient having dyspnea
   It is heart or lung disease until proven otherwise
E. Symptoms that make you think of PE
   1. Abrupt onset of unexplained dyspnea or
   2. Abrupt onset of unexplained tachypnea or

3. New onset of unexplained pleuritic chest pain
   So the presence of any <u>one</u> of these symptoms should make you think of a possible PE. Still, only about 20% of these patients have PE. Concomitant presence of any <u>one</u> risk factor (morbid obesity, recent immobilization, recent pelvic or hip surgery) increases the likelihood of PE in your patient
F. Recognize of the importance of age (geriatrics) in disease prevalence:
   1. Acute asthma
   2. Panic attack
   3. CHF i.e. paroxysmal nocturnal dyspnea (pulmonary edema)
   4. PE

Shortness of Breath (SOB)

> **Differential diagnosis: the 2 common causes of SOB**
> 1. Psychological entities–<u>episodic</u> SOB (but <u>not dyspnea</u>) at rest; onset <40 y/o; unpredictable onset; symptoms of MD, GAD, panic attack
> 2. Lifestyle–<u>daily</u> dyspnea; onset >40 y/o; predictably occurs with exertion (DOE)

A. **Be certain of the symptom and its distinguishing characteristics.** Your patient's problem or chief complaint is "Sometimes I can't get my breath." First, be certain whether his SOB is dyspnea or not. Dyspnea is a subset of SOB, that is, all patients with dyspnea (an uncomfortable <u>working to breathe</u>) have SOB, but many patients with "SOB" do not have dyspnea. Dyspnea is <u>not</u> tachypnea (rapid respiratory rate), nor is it hyperpnea (excessively deep respirations), nor is it hyperventilation (tachypnea and hyperpnea together). Hyperventilation is overbreathing relative to the need for bodily metabolism, and it almost always occurs at rest or with minimal activity. Dyspnea, in contrast, almost always occurs during some period of increased exercise. It is the feeling of having to work to breathe fast enough to compensate for the increased metabolic needs due to exertion

1. Have him describe precisely what is new about his SOB and don't

> Be certain:
> 1. That the symptom is SOB and if it is dyspnea (<u>working</u> to breathe)
> 2. Whether it is either new onset SOB or episodic SOB or chronic, daily SOB
> 3. Whether the onset of SOB was abrupt, gradual or insidious
> 4. If the SOB occurs only with exertion

let him use the phrase "short of breath" in the description. "Tell me exactly what you feel during a typical episode." Let him tell you at length all he can volunteer about his SOB, especially the very first time he noticed it, what brings it on, time of day when it occurs, what relieves it. Ask him, "What exactly does your SOB prevent you from doing?" Dyspnea will prevent him from doing certain physical activities. Aim to identify dyspnea as soon as possible, because it strongly suggests pulmonary or cardiac disease. Is the SOB of new onset, episodic attacks, or chronic, persistent SOB?

2. Ask him, "In a typical episode, what happens just before you get SOB, that is, what do you find brings it on?" Episodic or chronic SOB that is <u>never</u> provoked by or aggravated by physical exercise

or exertion is not likely dyspnea, and SOB that occurs as an isolated symptom is almost certainly not dyspnea. Continue to ask "What do you mean by that?" until you have clearly in your mind, exactly what change has occurred in his breathing from when it was normal; pulmonary diseases, as well as many cardiac diseases, almost always have dyspnea on exertion as an early symptom, and as the pulmonary or cardiac disease progressively worsens over months, dyspnea at rest occurs

3. Physical examination
   a. Examine for obvious causes of restrictive hypoventilation– kyphoscoliosis, thyromegaly, ascites, skin disease, chest wall tenderness; and signs of CHF (JVD, bilateral pretibial edema)
   b. Auscultate the chest for wheezes, crackles, murmurs
   c. Determine if hyperventilation (20-30 short inspirations and prolonged expirations) reproduces your patient's symptoms e.g. paresthesias, lightheadedness, chest pain, palpitations

By now you should be confident if it is dyspnea, whether it is new or chronic SOB, if onset was abrupt or insidious, and if there are activities he can not do. In almost all instances you now have the information you need for diagnosis of the obvious causes (Section C) and the common causes (Section E). In the rare instance that your patient appears different clinically from the usual office patient with SOB, be certain (Section B) that he does not have a symptom or sign of a dangerous disease

B. **Be confident it's not a dangerous disease.**
1. Send immediately to the ED by ambulance if there is:

Be certain in the first minutes of your exam that there is no evidence of any one dangerous symptom or sign associated with the SOB:
1. Abrupt onset of unexplained dyspnea or tachypnea or pleuritic chest pain
2. Any new onset of severe or worsening dyspnea
3. Severely ill appearing patient
4. Unstable vital signs e.g. hypotension, tachycardia, tachypnea
5. Inspiratory stridor
6. Loss of consciousness (syncope)
7. ST without pharyngeal erythema

Any suggestion of a dangerous disease, send the patient to the ED.

   a. Abrupt onset of new SOB (dyspnea) at rest, think of PE, pneumothorax
   b. Rapid onset of unexplained new dyspnea, think of PE, MI, pneumothorax, foreign body aspiration, pneumonia
   c. Dyspnea and severely ill appearance, think of any catastrophic cause e.g. silent MI, PE, shock
   d. Dyspnea and inspiratory stridor or hoarseness, think of obstructed upper airway due to foreign body, angioedema, thyromegaly, laryngospasm
   e. Dyspnea and JVD while sitting up, think of pericardial tamponade, severe CHF
   f. New dyspnea and ST with minimal pharyngeal erythema, think of epiglottitis
   g. Recent history of severe weakness (lower extremity or generalized) and new onset of prominent dyspnea at rest, think of GBS, myasthenic crisis
   h. New dyspnea and hypotension or syncope, think of anaphylaxis (wasp sting, food allergy)

Chapter 14 SOB   181

2. Admit at once to the ED or hospital if there is:
   a. Abrupt onset of unexplained dyspnea or tachypnea in a young patient (including pregnancy), think of noncardiogenic pulmonary edema (PE, narcotic overdose, bilateral RAS, eclampsia)
   b. Prominent dyspnea and pulsus paradoxus, think of pericardial tamponade, severe acute asthma
   c. New onset of prominent unexplained dyspnea, think of asthma, MI, PE, pneumothorax
   d. New onset or worsening orthopnea, think of CHF, COPD, asthma
   e. Recent symptoms suggesting URI or acute bronchitis, but now dyspnea, think of pneumonia
   f. Dyspnea and unilateral wheezes, think of PE, bronchial obstruction, lung cancer
   g. Dyspnea and basilar crackles, think of CHF, pneumonia
   h. Dyspnea, fever, focal crackles not clearing with cough, think of pneumonia
   i. Dyspnea and relative bradycardia (high fever and inappropriately low pulse rate), think of Legionella
   j. Dyspnea and relative tachycardia (no or low fever, high pulse rate), think of thyroid storm
   k. Tachypnea (but not dyspnea) or hyperventilation, think of any metabolic acidosis (DKA, salicylates, methanol, ethylene glycol, or lactic acidosis from sepsis)
   l. Severe dyspnea and diffuse bilateral wheezes, think of bronchial asthma, pulmonary edema
   m. New onset SOB and pleuritic chest pain, think of PE, pneumothorax, pneumonia, pleurisy
   n. New or episodic dyspnea associated with palpitations, think of cardiac arrhythmia
   o. New dyspnea and urticaria, think of angioedema
   p. Episodic dyspnea and severe headache, especially wintertime, think of carbon monoxide poisoning
   q. New dyspnea and thrombocytopenia, think of HPS
   r. New dyspnea, urticaria, pruritus, facial edema, think of anaphylaxis
   s. New onset of dyspnea a few days after lung injury (toxic inhalation, aspiration of gastric contents or near drowning, hemorrhagic pancreatitis, severe pneumonia, radiation pneumonitis, sepsis syndrome), think of noncardiogenic pulmonary edema i.e. ARDS
3. Admit to the hospital or obtain a consult as soon as appropriate if there is:
   a. Episodic dyspnea and exertional pain located <u>anywhere</u> between the ear lobes and umbilicus, think of angina pectoris
   b. Chronic dyspnea and crackles on exam, think of cardiomyopathy, interstitial lung disease
   c. Chronic, unexplained dyspnea, think of cardiopulmonary causes, anemia
   d. New dyspnea and signs of unexplained systemic disease (anorexia, weight loss, malaise), think of lung malignancy, atrial myxoma, SBE
   e. Dyspnea only on exertion, think of cardiopulmonary causes, severe anemia
   f. Nocturnal SOB, think of bronchial asthma, CHF, panic attack, chronic bronchitis
   g. Platypnea or trepopnea, think of cardiopulmonary causes
   h. Prominent dyspnea and shifted trachea, think of pneumothorax, pleural effusion
   i. DOE and systolic murmur, think of aortic stenosis, HCM; if there is a diastolic murmur, think of mitral stenosis, atrial myxoma, SBE
   j. Unexplained dyspnea and dry cough, think of *P. carinii* pneumonia in an HIV patient
   k. Dyspnea in a patient with recurrent lung infections, chronic purulent sputum, think of bronchiectasis
   l. New dyspnea with severe pharyngitis, think of Group A streptococcal pneumonia

C. **Make a quick diagnosis if it's obvious.** Is it an easily diagnosed condition or a medication that is responsible for the SOB? In most patients you will be <u>highly</u> confident of a common cause of the symptom by now. If not, one or more of the following tests may exclude an organic disease and increase your confidence in your working diagnosis: CBC, Chem 7, CXR, EKG, albumin, creatinine, UA, TSH
1. Systemic disease may be undiagnosed, so obtain appropriate diagnostic studies as determined by your H&P *viz* spirometry with bronchoprovocation, echocardiography
   a. Heart–cardiomyopathy, CAD, CHF, valve disease

b. Lung–bronchial asthma, COPD, interstitial lung disease, bronchiectasis, pulmonary hypertension
2. Obvious causes of SOB due to restricted lung expansion are pregnancy, ascites, severe kyphoscoliosis, pectus excavatum, *H. zoster*, costochondritis, chest trauma, any cause of pleuritic chest pain

---

Recognize any easily diagnosed cause of SOB:
1. Heart or lung disease–either undiagnosed disease or symptoms of disease exacerbation in a patient with known cardiopulmonary disease, e.g. asthma, COPD, CHF
2. Obvious restrictive causes of hypoventilation–pregnancy, ascites, pleural effusion, kyphoscoliosis, *H. zoster*, chest wall pain, pleuritic chest pain
3. Medications–onset of SOB temporally related to starting the medication

---

3. Medications associated with dyspnea
   a. Nitrofurantoin, ACEI, neuroleptics, NSAIDs
   b. Those causing interstitial lung disease: cytotoxic agents (bleomycin, methotrexate, cyclophosphamide); gold salts; penicillamine; cardiac (amiodarone, β-blockers)
   c. Noncardiogenic pulmonary edema–heroin, methadone, propoxyphene
   d. Airway obstruction–β-blockers, NSAIDs, penicillins, cephalosporins, cholinergic drugs, tartrazine (yellow dye additives)

D. **Identify your patient's worries and wants.** About 25% of people in various studies of symptom prevalence complained of SOB, yet only a few consult about it. During your interview and exam try to intuit or discover why your patient is here today, and not previously, for this problem. Don't necessarily ask directly, but try to get some ideas from your patient's responses to questions about his perception of the SOB itself. You can't completely help your patient unless you know what he really worries about and wants from you. That's why he is here to see you--to satisfy his worries and wants! Here are only some of the possible worries and wants of your patient with SOB. You must discover his specific, unique ones

---

During your exam, discover your patient's worries (lung cancer, heart disease, infection) and wants ("x-ray," antibiotics), so that you can respond to his specific needs as soon as possible.

---

1. Common worries are:
   a. That the cause of the SOB is a dangerous etiology e.g. lung cancer, heart disease, emphysema, TB, HIV
   b. That the etiology is some rare disease e.g. HPS, WNV, inhalation anthrax
   c. What other fears or anxieties might be troubling your patient? For example, he may have had SOB at other times, and only now does he come for help. What has changed? Perhaps a friend or relative, who had similar SOB, recently has been diagnosed with "heart failure"? There are many other possibilities–think of them
2. Your patient wants:

Chapter 14 SOB

   a. You to perform a thorough physical exam focused on possible causes of the SOB and he wants appropriate tests and imaging studies
   b. A plausible explanation of the cause of the SOB
   c. Confident reassurance from you that it is not a dangerous or rare etiology. Tell him--"The good news, it's not lung cancer" (or whatever you believe his real worry is)
   d. To know the prognosis, short term (effects on job, home life, marriage; how soon he will be back to normal) and long term (if recurrences are possible; how to prevent recurrences; if it will cause any disability)
   e. Treatment to stop the SOB now and to prevent recurrences
   f. A specialist referral if he believes you are not confident of the diagnosis

E. Know the symptoms that differentiate the 2 common causes of SOB.

Common causes of SOB seen in the office:
  1. The commonest cause is SOB due to psychological causes

> Common causes of most SOB in office patients:
>   1. Psychological entities–<u>episodic</u> SOB (but <u>not dyspnea</u>) at rest; onset <40 y/o; unpredictable onset
>   2. Lifestyle–<u>daily</u> dyspnea; onset >40 y/o; predictably occurs with exertion (DOE)

   a. Characteristics of psychological SOB
      (1) Onset of SOB in a patient <40 y/o
      (2) SOB is a solitary symptom i.e. no associated symptoms of any cardiopulmonary disease
      (3) The SOB is <u>episodic</u>; it fluctuates in severity unpredictably, frequently occurs at rest, or is much worse than the degree of any concomitant exertion
      (4) It is not dyspnea; in his description of the SOB there is no evidence of an awareness that he has to work to breathe, it is just "I can't get enough air in." Inspiration usually is much more difficult than expiration. Auscultation during an attack may confirm this, that is short inspiration and prolonged expiration (sighing), and no adventitious sounds during either phase; between attacks, auscultation reveals equal length of inspiratory and expiratory phases
      (5) Symptoms of hyperventilation (lightheadedness, paresthesias of fingers and perioral area, chest discomfort) may occur during an attack, and these symptoms often can be reproduced by having him take 20-30 short inspiratory breaths with long expirations. Hyperventilation syndrome is not a diagnosis in itself; think of it as the common resultant of a number of causes, many of which are psychological, but the cause occasionally may be organic (Thorax 52, 530, 1997)
      (6) Common psychological etiologies with SOB, <u>not</u> dyspnea
         (a) MD—anhedonia, depressed mood, early morning insomnia, worries (guilt) about past actions
         (b) GAD–"worry wart" of the family, worries constantly about future but improbable catastrophes, can't fall asleep at night for worrying
         (c) Panic attack—rapid onset of SOB with other characteristic hyperarousal symptoms; fear of dying during the episode and

he may frantically try to flee from the situation; panic attacks are common with other psychological disorders
  b. What suggests it's not psychological SOB
    (1) Anytime there is an associated symptom or sign suggesting a dangerous cause (see above, Section B) or if dyspnea is the symptom
    (2) If the severity of SOB is proportional to the amount of exertion, or the SOB never occurs at rest, that is, the SOB occurs only on exertion, and the greater the exercise, the greater the SOB
    (3) Any one concomitant symptom or sign suggesting cardiac or lung disease (cough, hemoptysis, chest pain, pretibial edema, crackles, wheezes)
2. Common look-alike causing SOB and how it differs from psychological causes of SOB
  a. Lifestyle
    (1) SOB is a solitary symptom
    (2) It is chronic, daily SOB
    (3) It is dyspnea, he really works to breathe when he walks or climbs stairs, i.e. DOE
    (4) Onset of dyspnea is usually in a patient >45-50 y/o, but the exact onset is determined by his unique combination of lifestyle factors contributing to lung dysfunction
      (a) Obesity–Calculate BMI in $kg/m^2 = [lb/(inches)^2]$ x 703. BMI $\geq$ 30 may have SOB on moderate exertion, BMI $\geq$ 40 ("morbid obesity") may have SOB on lesser exertion and BMI >50-60 may have SOB at rest
      (b) Tobacco abuse–increasing pack years of smoking
      (c) Deconditioning–lack of any regular exercise, almost total sedentary life
      (d) Decreasing lung function with normal ageing

F. **Use this summary for efficient diagnosis of a common cause.** With the information from Sections A-E in mind, here is the rapid approach to diagnosis of SOB in the office patient.
  1. You already have determined:
    a. In Section A, by H&P, that your patient has SOB, and if the SOB is dyspnea (working to breathe).
    b. In Section B, that there is no evidence in the H&P of a dangerous cause of the SOB.
    c. In Section C, that there is neither an easily diagnosed cardiopulmonary disease or localized cause of hypoventilation; nor a medication that is likely responsible for the SOB.
  2. From the focused H&P almost always you should quickly be confident of a working diagnosis. You will admit to the hospital any patient with new, unexplained significant dyspnea and patients with dyspnea due to exacerbations of cardiopulmonary disease. Other episodic or chronic SOB complaints usually can be diagnosed in the office by exam and appropriate tests. Confident final diagnosis is made only in followup the next weeks or months when the response to treatment is appropriate to your working diagnosis.
    a. If your patient is <40 y/o and has new onset SOB or episodic SOB, and it definitely is not dyspnea, look for symptoms

suggesting associated psychological disease e.g. panic attack or GAD, diagnose and treat it appropriately.
   b. If your >40-50 y/o patient has chronic dyspnea of insidious onset, and he has some combination of marked obesity, smoking, lack of exercise, diagnose deconditioning syndrome and help him change his lifestyle
   c. If your patient does not respond to treatment or if there is any suggestion of the presence of heart or lung disease causing the SOB, obtain appropriate tests *viz* CXR, EKG, spirometry with bronchoprovocation (for hyperreactive airway diseases) and echocardiography.
3. Answer your patient's worries and wants that you determined early on during the exam (Section D). Have you done everything you can to help him?
4. You now have a working diagnosis, but only with followup can you be highly confident it is correct. In return visits you are always testing by H&P that your working diagnosis is correct.

G. Abandon your working diagnosis and look for an uncommon cause only if:
1. Any one dangerous symptom or sign (see above, Section B) occurs in the following weeks, months or years. Quickly obtain a consult or send your patient to the hospital as appropriate.

If your patient's symptoms do not respond as expected to your management, he may have an uncommon or rare cause listed in Section G.2 that you can diagnose and treat. Or you may want to refer your patient to a specialist.

2. The SOB does not respond to treatment as you expect or the natural history of your working diagnosis does not occur. The SOB due to panic attack or other psychological causes should disappear with treatment of the psychological disorder. Dyspnea caused by lifestyle factors will resolve only to the degree he can institute lifestyle changes e.g. adequate weight loss (Arch Int Med 160, 1797, 2000), exercise program
Don't spend time and money looking for one of the following etiologies until you are sure your patient doesn't have one of the 2 common causes of SOB above. Nevertheless, it may be he has an uncommon cause of the SOB. These are important to recognize, because each has different treatment or prophylaxis
   a. GERD may be obvious from a history of burning chest pain and regurgitation of acid or it may be occult; confident diagnosis only by curing the dyspnea with aggressive PPI therapy
   b. PNDS–history of throat clearing and sensation of postnasal drip; treat as detailed in Chapter 5 Cough
   c. Occult asthma is a common cause of "undiagnosed dyspnea" after extensive workup, including CXR and spirometry; diagnosis is only by showing bronchial hyperresponsiveness to pharmacological challenge testing using methacholine (Chest 100, 1293, 1991). Occult asthma is common in the elderly, and in many of these patients, onset of dyspnea, cough, occasional wheezing, is >60 y/o (Chest 116 603, 1999)
   d. Difficult to control systemic HTN; episodic SOB, as one of the symptoms of hyperventilation, occurs in 16% of men and 45% of women (Arch Int Med. 157, 945, 1997) in a referral practice
   e. Platypnea–orthodeoxia syndrome–dyspnea and hypoxemia induced by upright posture and due to right to left intracardiac shunting
   f. Mitochondrial myopathy–dyspnea with mild exercise, weakness, muscle pain after exercise

g. Systemic diseases–SOB and lung disease may complicate various chronic diseases
   (1) Endocrine–hyperthyroidism, acromegaly, DM, carcinoid, hypoparathyroidism
   (2) Connective tissue disease–RA, scleroderma, SLE, amyloidosis, ankylosing spondylitis, Behcet's syndrome
   (3) Renal–dialysis, CRF, any cause of metabolic acidosis
   (4) Neuromuscular–MS, MG, parkinsonism, post polio syndrome, ALS
   (5) Nutritional–malnutrition, high carbohydrate diet

H. Use the glossary for precise thinking and accurate diagnosis.

1. **Adipose** (Latin *adeps* meaning "fat, particularly lard.") It refers specifically to tissue laden with fat composed of fatty acids and triglycerides.
2. **Adventitious** (Latin *ad* meaning "to or toward" and *venire*, "to come.") It now refers to abnormal lung sounds *viz* wheezes and crackles.
3. **Angioedema** (Greek *angeion* meaning "vessel" and *oidema*, "swelling.") It refers to an allergic reaction with dilatation and increased permeability of dermal capillaries causing giant wheals.
4. **Anxiety** (Latin *anxietas* meaning "worry.") It refers to excessive worry about something that is not likely to happen.
5. **Apnea** (Greek *a* meaning "not" and *pnoia*, "breathing.") It may be voluntary or involuntary e.g. during sleep or coma, and it is now defined as cessation of airflow for ≥ 10 sec in determining criteria for obstructive sleep apnea
6. **Asthma** (Greek for "gasping or panting.") The Romans used the word for "sonorous wheezing"
7. **Dyspnea** (Greek *dys* meaning "difficult or labored" and *pnoia*, "breathing.") The normal resting patient is unaware of his breathing. Dyspnea is a very uncomfortable constant awareness of having to work just to breathe.
8. **Hypercapnea** (Greek *hyper* meaning "over or excessive" and *kapnos*, "smoke.") Now it refers to excess levels of carbon dioxide in the blood.
9. **Hypercarbia**–same meaning as hypercapnea
10. **Hyperventilation** (Greek *hyper* meaning "excessive" and Latin *ventilatio*, "fresh air.") It is a breathing rate and volume in excess of metabolic needs.
11. **Hypopnea** (Greek *hypo* meaning "under" and *pnoia*, "breathing.") It is decreased rate and depth of breathing.
12. **Interstitial** lung disease (Latin *inter* meaning "between" and *sistere*, "to set.") It is disease in the lung parenchyma including alveoli, alveolar epithelium, capillary endothelium, and spaces between these structures.
13. **Myxoma** (Greek *myxa* meaning "mucus" and *oma*, "tumor.") It is a tumor composed of primitive connective tissue cells and stroma.
14. **Obesity** (Latin *obesus* meaning "whatever has eaten itself fat.") It is eating food in excess of the amount needed to support energy needs, thus filling adipose storage sites.
15. **Orthopnea** (Greek *ortho* meaning "erect" and *pnoia*, "breathing.") Best breathing is in the erect or sitting up position, and labored breathing (dyspnea) occurs while supine. Orthopnea occurs very soon after assuming recumbency, different from paroxysmal nocturnal dyspnea, which occurs a few hours after falling asleep.
16. **Oximetry** (Greek *oxy* referring to "oxygen" and *metron*, "a measure.") It is a measurement of oxygen saturation of arterial blood. Note that values for pH and carbon dioxide are not provided as in a blood gas measurement.
17. **Paroxysmal nocturnal dyspnea** (PND) (Greek *paroxysmos* meaning "sudden recurrence of symptoms.") PND or "cardiac asthma" awakens the patient a few hours after he has been asleep. The symptoms are a frightening suffocating feeling and wheezing.
18. **Pickwickian (syndrome)**–(coined in 1956) allusion to the sleepy, extremely obese boy in Dickens' "Pickwick Papers." The marked obesity, flushed facies and decreased vital capacity are due to hypoventilation. It also is called "obesity-hypoventilation syndrome."
19. **Platypnea** (Greek *platys* meaning "flat" and *pnoia*, "breathing.") Best breathing is in the flat or supine position, and difficult breathing is in the upright position, just the opposite of orthopnea.
20. **Pneumonia** (Original Greek word meant "disease of the lungs," a generic usage.) Now pneumonia specifically refers to infectious disease especially affecting alveoli and causing dyspnea.
21. **Pneumonitis** (Greek *pneumon* meaning "lung," and *itis*, any "inflammation.") It is a more general term of any disease of lungs due to inflammation e.g. hypersensitivity pneumonitis (chronic allergic alveolitis).

22. **Pneumothorax** (Greek *pneuma* meaning "air" and *thorax,* "chest cavity.") It refers to air accumulating inside the chest cavity, but outside the lungs.
23. **Rales** (French word for "death rattle" or the sound of mucus accumulating in the throat of a dying patient.) Laennec applied the term to similar sounds he heard over lungs with his new stethoscope. The politically correct term today is crackles.
24. **Retrognathia** (Latin *retro* meaning "backward" and *gnathos*, "jaw.") It is a backward malposition of the mandible that predisposes to obstructive sleep apnea.
25. **Spirometry** (Latin *spirare* meaning "to breathe" and Greek *metron*, a "measure.") It refers to measurement of breathing capacity of the lungs and other lung function tests.
26. **Stethoscope** (Greek *stethos* meaning "chest" and *skopein*, "to view or examine.") It is an instrument to auscultate the chest.
27. **Tamponade** (French *tamponner* meaning "to plug up.") It is constrictive pressure on the heart by rapid accumulation of a pericardial effusion, which does not allow adequate ejection of blood so the heart appears "plugged up."
28. **Telemetry** (Greek *tele* meaning "at a distance" and *metron,* "measure.") It refers to making measurements on the patient at a distance from the patient.
29. **Trepopnea** (Greek *trepein* meaning "to turn" and *pnoia,* "breathing.") Best breathing is in the recumbent (but not supine) position e.g. best on one side but it may be worse on the other side or supine.
30. **Wheeze**–musical, continuous (>250 msec) whistling sound occurring during inspiration or expiration

Chapter 15 Sore Throat (ST)
Questions on Sore Throat (ST)
A. In a patient with complaint of "sore throat," the most important
   1. Historical information is:
   2. Physical exam is:
B. In the office, the commonest cause of <u>new</u> ST and its distinguishing characteristics are:
   1.
      a.
      b.
C. There are 3 other common causes of <u>new</u> ST, each of which has marked oropharyngeal, tonsillar erythema and exudate. You can differentiate each from the others by:
   1.
      a.
      b.
   2.
      a.
      b.
   3.
      a.
      b.
D. Your next patient is a 22 year old mildly obese (BMI= 31) man who comes for an annual exam. On ROS he notes an occasional mild ST for the last 3-4 months. He has no symptoms suggesting GERD. There is no pharyngeal erythema and no exudate. He does not smoke, and he denies taking any medications. His chronic ST likely is caused by:

E. Your patient is a 23 y/o man who has had "strep throat, many times" in the past, and "penicillin always cures it." He now has dominant nasopharyngeal symptoms, mild pharyngeal erythema, no exudates and no enlarged or tender lymph nodes. You are certain it is a viral pharyngitis, but the rapid strep antigen test is positive. Your next step is:

F. Your 30 y/o patient appears ill and has a very severe ST. She has minimal pharyngotonsillar erythema and no exudate on exam. Thyroid gland is not tender to palpation, but when you ask her to swallow, she has great difficulty swallowing and the odynophagia is severe. Which antibiotic will you choose?

Chapter 15 ST

Answers on Sore Throat (ST)
A. Be certain of the symptom and its distinguishing characteristics
 1. Determine if it is a <u>new</u> sore throat; then if the associated dominant symptoms are either:
    a. Nasopharyngeal–rhinorrhea, nasal congestion, sneezing, lacrimation; <u>or</u>
    b. Oropharyngeal–ST, dysphagia, odynophagia; <u>or</u>
    c. Tracheobronchial–cough, fever; <u>or</u>
    d. Systemic–high fever, cough, myalgia, headache, malaise
 2. Immediately look at the oropharynx
    a. If there is no erythema, think of referred pain such as subacute thyroiditis or otitis media (or local causes–epiglottitis, lingual tonsillitis)
    b. If marked erythema bilaterally (and tonsillar hypertrophy or exudates), think of oropharyngeal causes
    c. If mild erythema, think of viral causes (nasopharyngeal, tracheobronchial, or systemic infections) of ST
B. The commonest cause of new ST
 1. Viral URI e.g. common cold
    a. Nasopharyngeal symptoms dominate
    b. Mild oropharyngeal erythema and no exudates or enlarged nodes
C. The 3 common causes of new onset ST having marked pharyngotonsillar erythema and exudate
 1. GABHS (strep throat)
    a. Enlarged and tender anterior cervical lymph nodes
    b. Minimal systemic symptoms, but there may be high fever, minimal cough
 2. Infectious mononucleosis (IM)
    a. Enlarged and tender lymph nodes–anterior <u>and</u> posterior cervical; also may be axillary and inguinal nodes
    b. Minimal systemic symptoms, except significant malaise, which may precede the sore throat
 3. Adenovirus
    a. No enlarged, tender nodes, but there may be conjunctivitis
    b. Systemic symptoms dominate *viz* myalgias, headache, high fever, cough
D. A common cause of episodic or chronic ST in a nonsmoker
 Laryngopharyngeal reflux, that is, he has GERD without the symptoms of esophagitis (heart burn, chest pain). In a patient of this age you could treat with a PPI, as for GERD. If he were an older patient, say 55 y/o, or he had any <u>one</u> dangerous symptom, you should refer to ENT for laryngoscopy
E. Obtain a rapid strep test only if you are uncertain of the cause of the new onset ST
 Because your clinical suspicion of GABHS was very low, you should not have done the rapid strep antigen test. What you have done is confirm that he is a strep carrier
F. Recognize the dangerous disease, epiglottitis
 None, she has epiglottitis until proven otherwise. Get her to the ED quickly, even possibly by ambulance as determined by your judgment

Sore Throat (ST)

Differential diagnosis: the 5 common causes of <u>new</u> sore throat
1. Viral URI–dominant <u>nasopharyngeal</u> symptoms e.g. sneezing, rhinorrhea, nasal congestion
2. GABHS–severe <u>oropharyngeal</u> symptoms; tender, enlarged anterior cervical nodes
3. IM–severe <u>oropharyngeal</u> symptoms; tender, enlarged posterior cervical nodes and generalized nodes; dominant malaise
4. Influenza–mild ST, dominant <u>systemic</u> symptoms
5. Adenovirus–oropharyngeal symptoms <u>and</u> systemic symptoms; conjunctivitis

A. **Be certain of the symptom and its distinguishing characteristics.** Your patient's problem or chief complaint is "I've got a ST." First, be certain the problem is oropharyngeal pain, and not mouth pain (lesions of tongue, gingiva, oral mucosa) or neck pain or dysphagia or hoarseness or dysphonia; and whether the ST is the dominant symptom
1. Ask him–"Exactly when did the pain begin?" You want to know whether it is a new pain, or an episodic pain or a chronic, persistent ST. "Show me where the pain is most severe" and "Now swallow–does that make the pain better or worse?" Swallowing will aggravate the pain (odynophagia) in almost all causes of ST, including referred pain
2. It is very important to determine whether the symptoms and signs associated with the ST are predominantly either nasopharyngeal <u>or</u> oropharyngeal <u>or</u> lower respiratory tract <u>or</u> systemic

Be certain:
1. It is pharyngitis; i.e. erythema
2. Whether it is either new pain present <2 weeks, or episodic pain, or chronic, persistent pain
3. Whether dominant associated findings either are nasopharyngeal, oropharyngeal, lower respiratory tract or systemic
4. If there are enlarged tender lymph nodes either anterior or posterior cervical, or generalized

3. Physical examination
   a. "Show me where it hurts the most." Usually he will point inside the mouth or grasp his throat; inspect the oropharynx and tonsils for expected erythema (in all causes of pharyngitis) and possible exudate (GABHS, IM, adenovirus) of the pharynx or tonsils. If

he points to the external, anterior neck (hyoid or thyroid cartilage) and there is minimal erythema of the pharynx, think of subacute thyroiditis or lingual tonsillitis, but especially worry it might be epiglottitis. Note the degree of tonsillar hypertrophy; be certain there are no danger signs e.g. unilateral disease, trismus, or uvular deviation

b. Palpate for enlarged and possibly tender neck (anterior and posterior cervical) and systemic (axillary, inguinal) lymph nodes, hepatosplenomegaly, and for a tender thyroid gland; inspect the ear canals for possible disease causing referred pain

c. Auscultate over the larynx for stridor and the lungs for adventitious sounds (wheezing or crackles)

By now you should be confident whether or not it is pharyngitis, if it is new, episodic or chronic ST, and whether the dominant associated findings are nasopharyngeal, oropharyngal, lower respiratory tract, or systemic. In almost all instances you now have the information you need for diagnosis of the obvious causes (Section C) and the common causes (Section E). In the rare instance that your patient appears different clinically from the usual office patient with ST, be certain (Section B) that he does not have a symptom or sign of a dangerous disease

B. **Be confident it's not a dangerous disease.**

1. Send immediately to the ED by ambulance if there is:
   a. Abrupt onset of severe, persistent throat pain without pharyngeal erythema, think of referred pain due to MI, AD, esophageal rupture, mediastinitis or pneumomediastinum
   b. Respiratory distress, drooling, stridor, trismus, think of epiglottitis, deep space cellulitis (Ludwig's angina), abscess
   c. Toxic appearance i.e. prostration, tachycardia, think of "complicated" ST due to cellulitis, abscess, metastatic infection (Lemierre syndrome)
   d. Minimal pharyngeal erythema, but severe dysphagia and dysphonia (muffled or changed voice, "hot potato" voice), think of epiglottitis, lingual tonsillitis
   e. Severe abdominal pain in a patient with IM and splenomegaly, think of splenic rupture

---

Be certain in the first minutes of your exam that there is no evidence of any <u>one</u> dangerous symptom or sign associated with the sore throat:

1. Toxic appearance or altered mental status
2. Respiratory distress or stridor
3. Severe dysphagia
4. Trismus
5. Abdominal pain

Any suggestion of a dangerous disease, send your patient to the ED.

---

2. Admit at once to the ED or hospital if there is:
   a. Dizziness or orthostasis, think of dehydration due to inability to drink liquids (dysphagia), caused by retropharyngeal abscess, tonsillar hypertrophy with IM
   b. Toxic appearance or confusion, think of neck deep space cellulitis, abscess, pneumonia (especially in an elderly patient)
   c. Rapid onset of hoarseness and concomitant dyspnea suggesting progression of respiratory distress, think of acute epiglottitis
   d. Progressively worsening unilateral throat pain, think of peritonsillar or

paraphryngeal abscess
- e. Progressively worsening dysphagia, think of peritonsillar abscess (quinsy)
- f. Pharyngeal ulcers or bleeding gums occurring with the ST, odynophagia, fever, think of agranulocytosis (neutropenia) or acute leukemia (neutrophilia)
- g. ST and odynophagia with minimal pharyngotonsillar erythema, think of epiglottitis, lingual tonsillitis
- h. Anytime symptoms (tachypnea, tachycardia, odynophagia) exceed the physical findings of pharyngitis, think of epiglottitis
- i. Presentation suggesting "strep throat" (pharyngotonsillar exudates, high fever) in a military recruit, but there also is cough, myalgias, hoarseness, chest pain, think of adenovirus which may be lethal
- j. Worker in a plague-endemic area (Santa Fe) with new ST, fever, cervical lymphadenitis, think of primary plague pharyngitis

3. Admit to the hospital or have a specialist consult as soon as possible if there is:
   - a. Episodic throat pain associated with exercise, anger, intercourse, think of angina pectoris
   - b. Odynophagia due to oral or esophageal candidiasis, but usual immunosuppressed states (HIV, DM, glucocorticoid therapy) are absent, think of occult malignancy
   - c. Odynophagia without pharyngeal erythema, think of infectious esophagitis *C. albicans*, HSV, CMV), pill-induced esophagitis, foreign body
   - d. Esophageal dysphagia (occurs after swallowing), think of esophageal malignancy, scleroderma
   - e. Foul breath odor and purulent exudate, think of Vincent's angina, an anaerobic pharyngitis that may worsen to peritonsillar abscess or Lemierre's syndrome (septic thrombophlebitis of internal jugular vein)
   - f. Exudative pharyngitis and cervical adenopathy associated with GI symptoms of abdominal pain or diarrhea, think of *Y. enterocolitis*
   - g. If the infectious pharyngitis is not getting better, or even is worsening after 5-7 days, think of bacterial complications of sinuses or lungs
   - h. Chronic persistent ST with anorexia, weight loss, referred otalgia, think of malignancy

C. **Make a quick diagnosis if it's obvious.** Is it an easily diagnosed noninfectious cause or a medication that is responsible for the ST? In most patients you will be highly confident of a common cause of the symptom by now. If not, one or more of the following tests may exclude an organic disease and increase your confidence in your working diagnosis: CBC

Diagnose and treat a noninfectious cause of an episodic or chronic ST:
1. Laryngopharyngeal reflux due to GERD
2. Chronic pharyngeal irritants
3. Subacute thyroiditis
4. Medication side effect

---

1. Noninfectious causes have either episodic ST or chronic, persistent ST with minimal or no erythema of the pharyngotonsillar area, and no lymphadenectasis
   - a. GERD is very common and includes patients previously diagnosed as "globus hystericus." Typical symptoms of GERD may occur as well as symptoms of a foreign body sensation in the throat causing throat clearing. Morning throat pain may occur more often after dietary or alcohol indiscretion the previous night. Treatment is PPI therapy
   - b. Laryngopharyngeal reflux has the same pathogenesis as GERD but it may lack the characteristic esophageal symptoms of GERD.

Have a high suspicion of the diagnosis (ST, hoarseness, cough) and refer to ENT for laryngoscopy if your patient is >45 y/o; otherwise, treat it with PPI
   c. PNDS e.g. allergic rhinitis has itchy eyes and palate, sneezing and watery nasal discharge; the "drip" causes the irritant ST, as well as the chronic cough
   d. Irritative environmental agents e.g. smoking tobacco or marijuana, occupational, dry air and mouth breather
   e. Subacute thyroiditis may cause "ST" but there is no pharyngeal erythema present on exam. Thyroid gland is very tender to palpation and there is high ESR. Hyperthyroidism may occur initially, and it may require treatment with propranolol (not PTU)
2. Medications
   a. Pill-induced esophagitis may cause referred "ST," i.e. no pharyngeal erythema on exam
   b. Inhalant medications for asthma or allergic rhinitis commonly cause mild erythema and ST

D. Identify your patient's worries and wants.
ST occurs almost universally (e.g. common cold may occur in adults 2-4 times yearly), and fewer than 15% of people with symptoms of a new respiratory illness consult about it. During your interview and exam try to intuit or discover why your patient is here today, and not previously, for this problem. Don't necessarily ask directly, but try to get some ideas from your patient's responses to questions about his perception of the ST itself. You can't completely help your patient unless you know what he really worries about and wants from you. That's why he is here to see you--to satisfy his worries and wants! Here are only some of the possible worries and wants of your patient with ST. You must discover his specific, unique ones
1. Common worries are:

During your exam, discover your patient's worries ("strep" throat, heart disease) and wants (antibiotic), so that you can respond to his specific needs as soon as possible.

   a. That the cause of the ST is a dangerous etiology especially "strep throat," cancer, HIV, STD
   b. That the etiology is some rare disease e.g. SARS, inhalation anthrax
   c. What other fears or anxieties might be troubling your patient? For example, he may have had ST at other times, and only with this one does he come for help. What has changed? Perhaps a friend or relative, who had similar ST, recently has been diagnosed with HIV. There are many other possibilities–think of them
2. Your patient wants:
   a. You to perform a thorough physical exam focused on possible causes of the ST, and he wants appropriate tests and imaging studies
   b. A plausible explanation of the cause of the ST
   c. Confident reassurance from you that it is not a dangerous or rare etiology. Tell him, "The good news, it's not strep throat" (or whatever you believe his real worry is)
   d. To know the prognosis, short term (effects on job, home life, marriage; how soon he will be back to normal) and long term (if recurrences are possible; how to prevent recurrences; if it will cause any disability)
   e. Treatment to relieve the pain now and to prevent recurrences
   f. A specialist referral if he believes you are not confident of the diagnosis

E. Know the symptoms that differentiate the 5 common causes of new onset ST.
1. The commonest cause is viral URI (common cold)

a. Characteristics of common cold
   (1) It is due to coryza ("head cold") in which nasopharyngeal and eye symptoms are dominant *viz* rhinorrhea, nasal congestion, sneezing, excess lacrimation
   (2) Oropharyngeal findings are minimal *viz* ST is mild, with no exudates and minimal erythema with concomitant minimal odynophagia, and systemic symptoms of headache, fever, malaise, myalgias are mild or not prominent

---

The common causes of most new sore throat:
1. Viral URI–dominant nasopharyngeal symptoms e.g. sneezing, rhinorrhea, nasal congestion
2. GABHS–severe oropharyngeal symptoms; tender, enlarged anterior cervical nodes
3. IM–severe oropharyngeal symptoms; tender, enlarged posterior cervical nodes and generalized nodes; dominant malaise
4. Influenza–mild ST, dominant systemic symptoms
5. Adenovirus–oropharyngeal symptoms and systemic symptoms; conjunctivitis

---

   b. What suggests it might not be a viral URI
      (1) Anytime there is an associated symptom or sign suggesting a dangerous cause (see above, Section B)
      (2) If there is any one of the following present: the patient has recently had close contact with a patient diagnosed with "strep throat" or he has a fever >101° (38.3°C) or tonsillar or pharyngeal purulent exudates or tender anterior cervical lymph nodes
2. Common look-alikes causing ST and how each differs from viral URI
   a. Strep throat (GABHS)
      (1) Nasopharyngeal symptoms (coryza) are minimal
      (2) Oropharyngeal signs dominate the presentation with severe throat pain, and prominent pharyngotonsillar erythema and purulent exudate; severe odynophagia accurately reflects the degree of erythema and exudates
      (3) Anterior cervical nodes may be enlarged and tender, and significant cough is absent
   b. Infectious mononucleosis (IM)
      (1) The patient almost always is <35 y/o
      (2) Myalgias and significant malaise often precede the ST and dominate the clinical picture; pharyngotonsillitis may be severe and usually is exudative, just like GABHS
      (3) Different from strep throat, there is generalized lymphadenectasis (anterior cervical, postauricular, axillary or inguinal nodes) and enlarged, tender posterior cervical nodes are distinctive for IM; splenomegaly may be present and prohibits contact sports
      (4) Absolute lymphocytosis (>4000/mm^3), relative lymphocytosis

(>50 % of WBCs) and also atypical lymphocytosis (>10%), and thrombocytopenia may occur, but sometimes only after one week of symptoms
(5) Almost all young adults with IM will have mildly elevated LFTs, which also help differentiate from "strep" throat; when the patient with IM is >35-40 y/o, the ST may be mild, enlarged lymph nodes may be absent, but liver abnormalities and prolonged fever may dominate (JAMA 281, 454, 1999)
c. Influenza
(1) Rapid onset of systemic (nonrespiratory) symptoms *viz* high fever, chills, myalgias, headache, malaise, arthralgias, anorexia, and dry cough dominate the clinical picture
(2) Although both nasopharyngeal and oropharyngeal symptoms may occur, they are not dominant; there may be mild to severe pharyngitis, but without exudate or tender nodes
d. Adenovirus
(1) The presentation mimics a combination of GABHS and influenza, i.e. severe ST with exudates (like GABHS), but also prominent systemic symptoms of high fever, chills, myalgias, malaise (like influenza)
(2) One-half of patients also have follicular conjunctivitis, a syndrome called "pharyngoconjunctival fever"; epidemics occur in summer in civilians and in winter in military recruits (may be lethal in recruits)
(3) Recognition of the clinical picture and a negative rapid strep test indicates symptomatic treatment

F. **Use this summary for efficient diagnosis of a common cause.** With the above information from Sections A-E in mind, here is the rapid approach to diagnosis of ST
1. You already have determined:
   a. In Section A, by H&P, that it is ST i.e. throat pain, and not referred pain.
   b. In Section B, that there is no evidence in the H&P of a dangerous cause of the ST.
   c. In Section C, that there is neither an easily diagnosed noninfectious cause, nor a medication that is likely responsible for the ST.
2. From the focused H&P almost always you should quickly be confident of a working diagnosis. Confident final diagnosis is made only in followup the next few days or weeks when the response to treatment or nontreatment is appropriate to your working diagnosis. The focus in your patient with new ST is whether or not he has strep throat. The younger the adult, the more likely he may have strep throat and the more susceptible he is to acute rheumatic fever or glomerulonephritis. Still even in young adults a new ST is low probability (<5-10%) of being GABHS.
   a. If your patient has dominant nasopharyngeal symptoms (rhinorrhea, sneezing, stuffy nose), mild pharyngeal erythema and no exudate, it likely is viral URI, so treat symptomatically.
   b. If oropharyngeal findings dominate (prominent pharyngotonsillar erythema and exudate; tender, enlarged anterior cervical nodes), think of strep throat; if there also is generalized lymphadenectasis

(posterior cervical, axillary, inguinal nodes), think of IM.
  c. If systemic symptoms of rapid onset (myalgias, headache, cough, high fever) dominate the clinical picture with associated oropharyngeal findings (pharyngeal erythema but no exudates or tender nodes), diagnose influenza and manage accordingly; if there are similar systemic symptoms, but also pharyngotonsillar exudates and conjunctivitis, diagnose adenovirus infection.
3. Answer your patient's worries and wants that you determined early on during the exam (Section D). Have you done everything you can to help him?
4. You now have a working diagnosis, but only with followup can you be highly confident it is correct. In return visits you are always testing by H&P that your working diagnosis is correct.

G. Abandon your working diagnosis and look for an uncommon cause only if:

1. Any one dangerous symptom or sign (see above, Section B) occurs in followup of days, weeks, or months. Quickly obtain a consult or send your patient to the hospital as appropriate

If your patient's symptoms do not respond as expected to your management, he may have an uncommon or rare cause listed in Section G.2 that you can diagnose and treat. Or, you may want to refer your patient to a specialist.

2. The ST does not respond to treatment as you expect or the natural history of your working diagnosis does not occur. The natural history of each of these 5 common causes is a self-limited course in which symptoms are gone or markedly less in a week, except possibly a lingering cough. If symptoms are worsening at 5-10 days, re-evaluate for complications.
Don't spend time and money looking for one of the following etiologies until you are sure your patient doesn't have a common cause of his ST. Nevertheless, it may be he has an uncommon or rare cause of the ST. These are important to identify, because each has a different treatment or prophylaxis
   a. New ST
      (1) Viral pharyngitides–all of these may have prominent pharyngitis
         (a) HSV in young adults, exudative pharyngitis; later look for vesicles and shallow ulcers on the palate and mouth
         (b) HIV primary infection
            (i) It occurs about a month after the initial infection and the pharyngitis may be severe with oropharyngeal ulcers, but there is no exudate
            (ii) Also different from GABHS, systemic symptoms are prominent *viz* fever, myalgias, malaise, arthralgias, lymphadenectasis, maculopapular rash
         (c) Measles (rubeola)
      (2) Bacterial pharyngitides–these may have high fever, but not usually purulent exudate.
         (a) *M. pneumoniae* or *C. pneumoniae*–dominant symptoms reflect a lower respiratory infection *viz* cough, dyspnea, crackles; some studies show these organisms as important causes (10%-20%) of ST in the adult
         (b) *B. pertussis*–same early catarrh, but later paroxysmal severe cough and sometimes vomiting dominate
         (c) *A. hemolyticum*–may have associated diffuse scarlet fever-type rash with exudative pharyngitis in a young adult
         (d) *H. influenza*, type B--cough, ear pain due to otitis media
         (e) *S. aureus*–think of it as a cause of ST in an immunocompromised patient
         (f) *N. gonorrheae*–most are asymptomatic, but if there is history of fellatio, may be minimal to severe pharyngitis with prominent exudate

    - (g) *C. diphtheriae*–mild pharyngitis but gray "pseudomembrane" on the tonsillar and pharyngeal mucosa
    - (h) Secondary syphilis–ST, lymphadenectasis, maculopapular or papulosquamous rash
  - b. Chronic ST
    - (1) Persistent pharyngitis--may be resistant organisms or chronic colonization or patient noncompliance with antibiotics or fungal infection e.g. candida, histoplasmosis, blastomycosis
    - (2) Neuralgias e.g. glossopharyngeal or internal laryngeal nerve--severe lancinating pain in the posterior or lateral pharynx that lasts seconds
    - (3) OSA–look for other symptoms *viz* snoring, daytime somnolence, chronic fatigue; be alert to symptoms suggesting a secondary treatable cause of OSA e.g. hypothyroidism, acromegaly
    - (4) Thyroid disorders may cause recurrent referred pain to the throat with no erythema; subacute thyroiditis, invasive fibrous thyroiditis (Riedel's struma), hemorrhage into a thyroid cyst, thyroid cancer
    - (5) Styalgia (Eagle's syndrome)–pain along the stylohyoid ligament
    - (6) STAR complex (Southern Med J 86, 521, 1994)--ST, temperature elevation, arthritis, rash; viral or autoimmune etiologies
    - (7) Globus pharyngeus (psychogenic pharyngitis)–commonly misdiagnosed in the past; many of these patients are now correctly diagnosed with laryngopharyngeal reflux or GERD

H. Use the glossary for precise thinking and accurate diagnosis.

1. **Abscess** (Greek *apostema* meaning "a drawing off" such as removing "bad humors" and accumulating them at a focal site.) Now, it is any focal collection of pus.
2. **Angina** (Latin word for "sore throat" e.g. Ludwig's angina, Vincent's angina.)
3. **Angina pectoris** (Latin *angere* meaning "to strangle or choke," and *pectus*, "chest,") The original descriptions of episodic cardiac ischemia emphasized the "choking" or sensation of taking his breath away.
4. **Aphthous stomatitis** (Greek *aphta* meaning "small ulcer" and *stoma*, "mouth.") It is the same as a canker sore, which is a small ulcer of the mouth and lips.
5. **Catarrh** (Greek *katarrhein* meaning "to flow down.") It is infection causing inflammation of mucous membranes with discharge, and for Hippocrates, it was normal humor formed in excess in the head and discharged through the nose.
6. **Cellulitis** (Latin *cellula* meaning "a small cell.") Now it indicates infection and diffuse inflammation of the deep subcutaneous tissues.
7. **Cervical** (Latin *cervix* meaning "neck.")
8. **Coryza** (ancient Greek word *koryza* for "a cold in the head.") It meant at that time to a runny nose indicating an effluent of a nasty "cold" humor responsible for the symptoms. Today it refers to an acute catarrhal response of nasal mucosa, or profuse nasal discharge.
9. **Croup** (Danish *kropja* for a particular type of cough, i.e. barking.) It is due to acute laryngotracheobronchitis in children, often with associated hoarseness and stridor.
10. **Defervescence** (Latin *defervescere* meaning "to cease boiling.") It is the period during infection when fever is diminishing.
11. **Diphtheria** (Greek *diphthera* meaning "a prepared hide or leather.") It refers to the parchment-like membrane in the throat.
12. **Dysphagia** (Greek for *dys* meaning "difficult or requiring effort" and *phagein*, "eating.") It is difficulty swallowing or significant effort needed to swallow anything.
13. **Dysphonia** (Greek *dys* meaning "difficult or with great effort," and *phone*, "voice.") It is difficulty in mechanics of speaking.
14. **Exudate** (Latin *exsudare* meaning "to sweat out" i.e. *sudor* means "sweat.") Any inflammation allows escape of protein and cellular debris from blood vessels to deposit in tissues or on their surfaces.
15. **Fever** (Latin *fervere* meaning "to seethe or to steam.")
16. **Follicular** conjunctivitis (Latin *follis* meaning a "leather bag") It refers to smooth, shiny swellings 1-2 mm in diameter, especially seen on palpebral conjunctiva.
17. **Globus** pharyngeus or hystericus (Latin word for "ball.") It is the sensation of a lump in the throat, but no difficulty swallowing; formerly it was interpreted as a sign of psychogenic dysphagia, but now it suggests GERD.
18. **Gonorrhea** (and gonococcus) (Greek *gone* meaning "seed" and *rheos,* "a flowing.") The ancients interpreted the characteristic urethral discharge as an abnormal leakage

of semen, thus the erroneous name, which we continue to use.
19. **Heterophilic** (antibodies) (Greek *heteros* meaning "other" and *philein,* 'to love.") It means affinity for antigens other than the ones that generated the antibodies.
20. **Inflammation** (Latin *inflammare* meaning "to set afire.") The features of rubor, calor, dolor, tumor suggested a smoldering fire.
21. **Lymphadenectasis** (Latin *lympha* meaning "water" and Greek *aden*, "gland" and *ektasis*, "distended.") Enlarged lymph nodes.
22. **Lymphadenitis**–A pathology term, indicating lymph node inflammation, which might be suggested clinically by tenderness of the nodes.
23. **Lymphadenopathy**–Another pathology term, but it indicates actual lymph node disease i.e. from Greek *pathos* meaning "disease."
24. **Meatus** (nasal) (Latin *meare* meaning "to go or to pass," in the sense of a channel.)
25. **Odynophagia** (Greek *odyne* meaning "pain" and *phagein,* "to eat.") It is painful swallowing.
26. **Phagophobia** (Greek *phagein* meaning "to eat," and *phobein,* "to be frightened.") It is a morbid fear of eating e.g. due to the pain that he anticipates will occur if he eats.
27. **Ptyalism** (Greek *ptyalon* meaning "spittle.") It is excessive secretion of saliva.
28. **Pyrexia** (Greek *pyrexis* meaning "feverish.") It is the Greek word for fever, which came from the Greek word *pyr* meaning "fire."
29. **Pyrosis** (Greek word meaning "burning.") It refers to retrosternal burning pain of GERD; now, heartburn is the lay term for the burning pain.
30. **Quinsy** (Greek *kyangche* meaning "a severe sore throat.") It is another term for peritonsillar abscess.
31. **Retrognathia** (Latin *retro* meaning "backward" and Greek *gnathos,* "jaw.") It is the mandible displaced backward, and it is associated with obstruction sleep apnea.
32. **Rhinorrhea** (Greek *rhinos* meaning "nose" and *rhoia,* "a flowing.") It is any runny nose. Rhinitis is a different term, and indicates actual inflammation of the mucous membranes of the nose, which often causes rhinorrhea.
33. **Struma** (Latin word for goiter)
34. **Trismus** (Greek *trismos* meaning "a squeaking.") Now it is an inability to open the jaw or mouth because of severe muscle spasm of the jaw.
35. **Xerostoma** (Greek *xero* meaning "dry" and *stoma*, "mouth.") It means dry mouth.

Chapter 16 Spells
Questions on Spells
A. The most important information suggesting your patient likely is having a spell is
1. In the history :
2. From the physical exam:

B. In the office, the 2 very common causes of "spells" and their distinguishing characteristics are:
1.
   a.
   b.
   c.
2.
   a.
   b.
   c.

C. Your next patient is a 45 y/o woman who has uncontrolled systemic hypertension. She recently began her third antihypertensive medication. The likely cause of her "resistant hypertension" if there are associated
1. Episodes of flushing without sweating i.e. "dry flushes":
2. Episodes of headache, palpitations, dizziness, paresthesias:
3. Episodes of sweating, headache, palpitations, pallor:

Answers on Spells
A. Be certain your patient is having a "spell"
 1. In a patient <45 y/o who has episodes of abrupt or rapid onset of frightening symptoms, and the symptoms are predominantly of the cardiopulmonary or neurological systems, think it might be a spell
 2. The physical exam shows not one sign consistent with the symptoms that suggest cardiopulmonary or neurological disease
B. Two common causes of spells and their distinguishing characteristics
 1. Panic attack
    a. Onset of most panic attacks is in a man or woman <35 y/o, but a second lesser peak occurs at 45-54 y/o; almost never is onset in a patient >60 y/o
    b. Rapid onset (<10 minutes) of a group of symptoms suggesting cardiopulmonary or neurological disease
    c. Episodes of symptoms, may occur weekly or monthly, or less often
 2. Perimenopause
    a. Onset in a woman between 35-50 y/o
    b. Abrupt onset of a hot flash, followed in minutes by sweating and tachycardia
    c. Episodes may occur daily or many times a day
C. Causes of spells in a patient with uncontrolled systemic HTN
 1. Any cause of "dry" flush *viz* alcohol, medication side effect such as antihypertensive vasodilators or clonidine. Alcohol intake itself can cause resistant hypertension
 2. "Anxiety-induced hyperventilation" (Arch Int Med 157, 945, 1997) does not have flushing, but paresthesias are common
 3. Pheochromocytoma almost never presents with flushing, rather pallor occurs in pheochromocytoma "spells"

Chapter 16 Spells 201

Spells

Differential diagnosis: the 3 common causes of spells
1. Panic attack–onset <40 y/o man or woman; anticipatory anxiety; rapid onset of sympathetic hyperarousal symptoms
2. Perimenopause–woman 35-50 y/o; abrupt onset hot flash, then facial flushing, sweating and tachycardia occur; if there are cyclic menses, flushing may occur before or during the period
3. Spells associated with an underlying chronic psychological disorder (GAD, MD, somatization)

A. **Be certain of the symptom and its distinguishing characteristics.** Your patient's problem or chief complaint is "I get butterflies inside. Sometimes my chest hurts, my heart pounds and I can't breathe." Be certain she is having "spells," that is, there are discrete episodes of a few symptoms occurring together. The symptoms are perplexing, that is, they do not suggest disease of any one organ, and she is well in between episodes. The complex of symptoms is more or less stereotypic in your patient, but they always include some of the following: either cutaneous flushing or "hyperadrenergic" symptoms e.g. palpitations, tachycardia, sweating, tremulousness, hot or feverish, sensation of choking, chest or abdominal distress, nausea, headache, weak all over, SOB, lightheadedness, blurred vision, paresthesias. Be certain there is no loss of consciousness; even though she may say "blackouts," almost always "blackouts" are momentary and not truly loss of consciousness
  1. Ask her–"When is the last time you had such an attack?" and "When did you have one before that one?"–positive answers to both questions tells you they are episodic. "How old were you when you had your first attack that was anything at all like these?" If the onset of symptoms definitely occurs in a patient >40-50 y/o, never diagnose a syndrome e.g. panic attack, until you are very confident by lab tests that a cardiac or neurological disease is not responsible for the symptoms
  2. "Tell me about a typical episode, what happens just before and what happens afterwards?" "What are you thinking about and feeling just before and during an episode?" "How does it begin, which symptoms occur, and is there any sequence to the symptoms e.g. one always following another?" If there is complaint of "flushing," be certain there was redness, and if so, was there a significant degree of sweating? "What do you think might be causing these symptoms? What is new in your life now?"
  3. Physical examination
     a. Look for objective evidence of systemic disease, especially fever (rectal temperature), weight loss (change in belt or pants size), orthostatic hypotension or postural dizziness (measure BP and P first, after she is supine for 10 minutes, and then standing; ask "How do you feel now?" on standing–<u>don't</u> ask "Are you dizzy?")

Be certain:
1. That your patient has self-limited spells and what symptoms characteristically occur
2. Of the interval between spells
3. Whether onset to peak severity of the symptoms is abrupt or rapid (< 5-10 minutes)
4. Of the age at onset of the spells
5. What events immediately precede the spells

   b. Physical exam is directed by the sometimes numerous symptoms, so carefully examine specific sites of pain. Very importantly, because the common causes all are syndromes, finding any one sign on physical exam must direct you toward identifying an organic disease. Pulse rate and rhythm are important–teach your patient to take her pulse rate and rhythm during the spells at home–keep a diary

   By now you should be confident that they are self-limited spells, what the age of onset was, if onset of the spell to peak severity is rapid, and what immediately precedes the spell. In almost all instances you now have the information you need for diagnosis of the obvious causes (Section C) and the common causes (Section E). In the rare instance that your patient appears different clinically from the usual office patient with spells, be certain (Section B) that she does not have a symptom or sign of a dangerous disease

B. **Be confident it's not a dangerous disease.**
   1. Send immediately to the ED by ambulance if there is:

Be certain in the first minutes of the exam that there is no evidence of any one dangerous symptom or sign associated with the spells:
1. Ongoing ischemic chest pain
2. Very ill appearing patient
3. Changed mental status
4. Significant acute respiratory difficulty
5. Severe headache with diaphoresis
6. Acute unilateral loss of vision

Any suggestion of a dangerous disease, send your patient to the ED.

   a. Ongoing unexplained chest pain with the "spell," think of unstable angina pectoris, MI, PE
   b. A very ill or toxic appearance, or there is any suggestion of an impending emergency e.g. abnormal vital signs
   c. Any significant respiratory difficulty, think of PE, anaphylaxis, pulmonary edema (noncardiac or cardiac)
   d. Any unexplained confusion associated with fever, think of thyroid storm, infective endocarditis, metastatic thrombophlebitis
   e. Headache and transient loss of monocular vision (amaurosis fugax) in a patient

Chapter 16 Spells

>50 y/o, think of TA
2. Admit at once to the ED or hospital if there is:
   a. Onset of spells in a patient >60 y/o and there is any sign of organic disease e.g. TIA, stroke, seizure
   b. Hypoglycemia in a diabetic patient on a long-acting β-cell stimulator e.g. glyburide (even though blood sugar is now 100 mg/dL with intravenous glucose), think of recurrence of hypoglycemia
3. Admit to the hospital or have a specialist consult as soon as appropriate if there is:
   a. Spell with loss of bladder control or loss of consciousness, think of seizure
   b. A spell in a nondiabetic patient with low serum glucose, think of insulinoma, exogenous insulin
   c. Associated motor (twitching of thumb) or positive sensory symptoms (tingling paresthesias of hand), think of simple partial seizure
   d. Witnessed unusual automatic behaviors (automatisms) during a spell that the patient doesn't remember, think of complex partial seizure
   e. Associated feeling of about to "pass out," but only upon standing up from sitting or supine, think of orthostatic hypotension, POTS
   f. New onset of spells in a patient >50 y/o, think of brain tumor, TIA, complex partial seizure
   g. An association of the spell with exercise (including sexual intercourse), and discomfort or tingling located anywhere between the umbilicus and ears, think of angina pectoris
   h. Unexplained cause of orthostatic hypotension, think of Addison's disease, pheochromocytoma, cardiac pump failure
   i. Associated palpitations and lightheadedness, think of cardiac arrhythmia causing presyncope
   j. Severe headache associated with sweating at rest, think of pheochromocytoma
   k. Cutaneous flushing, wheezing, watery diarrhea, think of carcinoid syndrome
   l. Cutaneous flushing and hypotension, think of mastocytosis

C. **Make a quick diagnosis if it's obvious.** Is it an easily diagnosed condition or a medication side effect causing the spells? In most patients you will be highly confident of a common cause of the symptom by now. If not, one or more of the following tests may exclude an organic disease and increase your confidence in your working diagnosis: ESR, TSH, glucose

---

Recognize any easily diagnosed cause of the spells:
1. Hyperthyroidism, hypoglycemia, migraine headache
2. Flushing related temporally to intake of alcohol, meals or beverages
3. Drug withdrawal (alcohol, corticosteroids, anabolic steroids, benzodiazepines, clonidine)
4. Medication side effects– temporal association

---

1. Hyperthyroidism may present with resting pulse > 90 bpm, sweating without flushing, and weight loss without decreased food intake. Markedly suppressed TSH level confirms the diagnosis
2. Cutaneous flushing ("dry flush") may be caused by:
   a. Alcohol intake
      (1) Beer drinking after exposure to occupational chemicals e.g. industrial solvents
      (2) Fermented beverages e.g. sherry or port containing tyramine or histamine
      (3) Simultaneous medications e.g. disulfiram, chlorpropamide, metronidazole, cephalosporins
      (4) Provokes flushing of carcinoid or mastocytosis or

perimenopause.
  b. Food additives–nitrites in cured meats; sulfites; monosodium glutamate in Chinese food
  c. Meals–hot beverages; foods (cheeses, chocolate, lemon, hot spices, chili peppers); high carbohydrate meal resulting in a dumping syndrome 30-60 minutes after eating; spoiled fish or cheese containing histamine
3. Drugs almost always cause a "dry flush"
  a. Substance abuse and withdrawal states– anabolic-androgenic steroid abuse, ethanol, corticosteroids (JAMA 261, 1731, 1989), benzodiazepines, clonidine, β-blockers
  b. Medications causing anxiety
    (1) Amphetamines and related drugs (phentermine, phenylpropranolamine, methylphenidate)
    (2) Bronchodilators e.g. β-agonists
    (3) CNS stimulants e.g. caffeine excess ("caffeinism") in normals; caffeine or theophylline may aggravate symptoms of GAD or panic disorder
    (4) Illegal drugs e.g. LSD, MDMA or ecstasy, phencyclidine (PCP), cannabis, cocaine
    (5) Antidepressants–TCAs (protriptyline), SSRIs (especially fluoxetine), venlafaxine
    (6) Benzodiazepines
    (7) Buspirone–anxiolytic after 2-3 weeks, but acutely it may cause marked dysphoria (anxiety, restlessness) and at high doses can cause panic attack
    (8) Anti-infective drugs
      (a) Intramuscular procaine penicillin (Hoigne's syndrome) may cause extreme apprehension and fear of death within one minute of injection, but it is not anaphylaxis
      (b) Interferons
      (c) Mefloquine or chloroquine
  c. Medications causing flushing–vasodilators, CCBs, niacin (nicotinic acid), bromocriptine, tamoxifen, cyclosporin, rifampin, amyl or butyl nitrite (recreational drugs)

D. **Identify your patient's worries and wants.** Spells occur very commonly (e.g. up to 30% of adults have had at least one panic attack), and very few people with symptoms of spells consult about it. During your interview and exam try to intuit or discover why your patient is here today, and not previously, for this problem. Don't necessarily ask directly, but try to get some ideas from your patient's responses to questions about her perception of the spells themselves. You can't completely help your patient unless you know what she really worries about and wants from you. That's why she is here to see you–to satisfy her worries and wants! Here are only some of the possible worries and wants of your patient with spells. You must discover her specific, unique ones

---

During your exam, discover your patient's worries (stroke, brain tumor, seizure) and wants ("an MRI," treatment), so that you can respond to her specific needs as soon as possible.

---

1. Common worries:
  a. That the cause of the spells is a dangerous etiology e.g. stroke, heart attack, epilepsy, brain tumor

b. That the etiology is some rare disease, e.g. WNV encephalitis, MS
   c. What other fears or anxieties might be troubling your patient? For example, she may have had spells at other times, and only with this one does she come for help. What has changed? Perhaps a friend or relative, who had similar spells, recently has been diagnosed with a brain tumor. There are many other possibilities–think of them
2. Your patient wants:
   a. You to perform a thorough physical exam focused on possible causes of the spells and she wants appropriate tests and imaging studies
   b. A plausible explanation of the cause of the spells
   c. Confident reassurance from you that it is not a dangerous or rare etiology. Tell her, "The good news, it's not multiple sclerosis" (or whatever you believe her real worry is)
   d. To know the prognosis, short term (effects on job, home life, marriage; how soon she will be back to normal) and long term (if recurrences are possible; how to prevent recurrences; if it will cause any disability)
   e. Treatment to stop the spells now and to prevent recurrences.
   f. A specialist referral if she believes you are not confident of the diagnosis

E. Know the symptoms that differentiate the 3 common causes of spells.
1. The commonest cause of spells is panic attack

> The common causes of spells:
> 1. Panic attack–onset <40 y/o man or woman; anticipatory anxiety; rapid onset of sympathetic hyperarousal symptoms
> 2. Perimenopause–woman 35-50 y/o; abrupt onset hot flash, then facial flushing, sweating and tachycardia occur; if there are cyclic menses, flushing may occur before or during the period
> 3. Spells associated with an underlying chronic psychological disorder (GAD, MD, somatization)

   a. Characteristics of a panic attack
      (1) Onset of attacks in a man or woman <35-40 y/o
      (2) There are 3 important criteria to look for in your patient:
         (a) Rapid onset (<10 minutes to peak symptoms) of subjective feelings of intense anxiety or apprehension about what might or could happen (anticipatory anxiety), or even overwhelming fright or terror
         (b) Somatic symptoms reflecting sympathetic hyperactivity *viz* palpitations, tachycardia, sweating, trembling, SOB (but not dyspnea), chest pain or discomfort, dizziness, chills or hot flushes, paresthesias, feeling of choking or globus, abdominal discomfort, nausea, a smothering sensation. Often associated with these autonomic physical symptoms are the cognitive symptoms of fear of dying, feelings of unreality or feelings of being detached from oneself, and especially being totally out of control or going "crazy"
         (c) Behaviorally, there is an overwhelming urge to flee or escape the situation in any way possible
      (3) Panic attacks often occur situationally or in the context of a trigger e.g. standing in line, crowded environment, riding in a car over bridges or in tunnels. Nocturnal panic attacks are very common and awaken the patient with a "nightmare"

(4) Panic disorder
  (a) The patient not only has panic attacks, but additionally there is almost constant fear of having the next panic attack; necessary for the diagnosis of panic disorder there must be cognitive symptoms (e.g. fear of dying, loss of control) with the panic attacks. Also the panic attacks always are sudden and unexpected i.e. they are not situational. Panic disorder may be associated with aversions or phobias, especially agoraphobia; and there should be at least 4 of the 13 somatic symptoms listed at 1.a.(2)(b) above to diagnose panic disorder
  (b) "Limited symptom attacks" is the diagnosis if other criteria for panic disorder are met, but <4 of the somatic symptoms listed above are present
  (c) "Nonfearful panic disorder" (NFPD) may be very common in the office patient
    (i) Severe anxiety or discomfort as in a panic attack
    (ii) In contrast, the distress is focused primarily on only one of the hyperarousal symptoms, especially chest pain or SOB e.g. in COPD; the other physical symptoms are not emphasized and very importantly, the cognitive symptoms of dying, going crazy or losing control are absent
    (iii) In one study about 40% of patients with chest pain and negative angiography had evidence of panic attacks
(5) Other chronic psychiatric disorders commonly have associated panic attacks
  (a) GAD–75% have panic attacks; the anxiety is diffuse and not related to a fear of panic attacks or specific stimuli
  (b) MD and somatization disorder–>80% of patients with these disorders have associated panic attacks
  (c) Situational "triggers" of panic attacks
    (i) Social phobia–panic attack is provoked by fear of a social situation that might cause humiliation or embarrassment
    (ii) Specific phobia–panic attack is provoked by fear of a specific item or event
    (iii) Posttraumatic stress disorder–panic attack is provoked by similar circumstances to a previous real threat e.g. rape, shooting
    (iv) Obsessive-compulsive disorder–panic attack only in relation in some way to her obsession or compulsion
  (d) Dissociative episodes–spacey feelings like a panic attack but differs in having complete memory loss
b. What suggests it might not be a panic attack
  (1) Anytime there is an associated symptom or sign suggesting a dangerous cause (see above, Section B)
  (2) If there is not a rapid onset (<10 minutes to peak symptoms), if the somatic symptoms are not intense or if symptoms are not those of sympathetic arousal
2. Common look-alikes causing spells and how each differs from a panic attack
  a. Perimenopause (or "menopause transition")
    (1) Onset in a woman >35-40 y/o
    (2) Symptoms are abrupt onset of hot flashes in the face and upper body, followed by vasodilitation (cutaneous flush), sweating

("wet flush") and reflex tachycardia
    (3) During the same time frame, menses are becoming farther apart (longer cycles), there is decreased menstrual flow, and there are no diagnostic serum hormone changes, i.e. it is a clinical diagnosis
  b. Chronic psychological disorders–onset of each of these psychological disorders begins in a man or woman <35-40 y/o; panic attacks are very common (>50% of patients) in these disorders
    (1) GAD
      (a) The patient worries about things that might happen in the future, and they are rather minor things from an observer's view. Commonly she worries into the night so she has trouble falling asleep. She has always been the "worry wart" in the family. Importantly, the worrying is uncontrollable, and it has pervaded her thoughts most of the day for a number of months. In addition there is anxious apprehension–her total body is in a constant state of tension, ready to confront the imagined danger
      (b) GAD is not associated with symptoms of autonomic hyperarousal; instead, the symptoms reflect intense anxiety, and 3/6 of the following symptoms diagnose GAD by DSMIV criteria: restless or feeling "on edge," irritable, muscle tension, easily fatigued, insomnia in the early night, and difficulty concentrating or her mind just goes blank. About 70% of patients with a primary diagnosis of GAD, also meet criteria for other disorders especially mood disorders, MD, panic disorder with agoraphobia, phobias, alcoholism
      (c) Acute anxiety reaction occurs when the "anxious apprehension" happens episodically; there may be mild symptoms of autonomic arousal relative to baseline conditions, but less than a panic attack
    (2) MD
      (a) Key to diagnosis is that the patient almost always exhibits some significant degree of anhedonia, so search carefully for unexplained, diminished experience of any one of her usual pleasurable activities, that is, decreased "appetite" for sex, good foods, music, sports, work. Symptoms of MD may overlap with GAD. For example, patients with MD worry a lot just like those with GAD, but it is about past events, i.e. guilt over their past actions. Also, she has much more difficulty concentrating than does a patient with GAD, she has early awakening insomnia, and she does not have symptoms of muscle tension
      (b) Spells may be inferred by a family member witnessing psychomotor agitation or retardation or an anxiety reaction which is common in MD
    (3) Somatization disorder
      (a) Insidious onset of somatization occurs in <30 y/o adults and pain in multiple organs dominates the clinical picture–head, abdomen, back, joints, chest, rectum; and pain during intercourse, urinating, menstruating. Also non-pain symptoms occurring in the GI tract and in sexual functioning may be

important components
- (b) These patients may also have pseudoneurological symptoms that may suggest a spell e.g. new onset incoordination or imbalance, localized weakness or paralysis, dysphagia or globus, aphonia, hallucinations, loss of sensations, isolated diplopia

F. Use this summary for efficient diagnosis of a common cause. With the above information from Sections A-E in mind, here is the rapid approach to diagnosis of the cause of spells

1. You already have determined:
   a. In Section A, by H&P, that it is a spell consisting of episodes of an unusual complex of symptoms. The symptoms are perplexing, because they don't suggest disease of any one organ, and she is essentially well in between spells.
   b. In Section B, that there is no evidence in the H&P of any one dangerous cause of the spells.
   c. In Section C, that there is neither an easily diagnosed condition, nor a drug withdrawal or medication side effect that is likely responsible for the spells.
2. From the focused H&P almost always you should quickly be confident of a working diagnosis. Confident final diagnosis is made only in followup the next weeks, months or years when the response to treatment or nontreatment is appropriate to your working diagnosis.
   a. If each attack has a rapid onset (<10 minutes to peak severity) of unexpected intense symptoms suggesting autonomic hyperarousal and the spells began when she was <35-40 y/o, it likely is a panic attack.
   b. If the spells are in a woman >35-40 y/o and they start with a sudden hot flash followed by cutaneous flushing and tachycardia, it likely is due to perimenopause.
   c. If there are chronic symptoms characteristic of GAD or MD or somatization, and occasional episodes of spells, but not intense autonomic hyperarousal symptoms, the symptoms likely are due to the underlying psychological disorder. Panic attacks also occur commonly in each of these disorders.
3. Answer your patient's worries and wants that you determined early on during the exam (Section D). Have you done everything you can to help her?
4. You now have a working diagnosis, but only with followup, sometimes for months or years, can you be confident it is correct. In return visits you are always testing by H&P that your working diagnosis is correct.

G. Abandon your working diagnosis and look for an uncommon cause only if:

1. Any one dangerous symptom or sign (see above, Section B) occurs in followup of weeks, months, or years. Quickly obtain a consult or send your patient to the hospital as appropriate
2. Your patient's response to therapy is not as you expect or if the natural history of your working diagnosis does not occur

Don't spend time and money looking for one of the following etiologies until you are sure your patient doesn't have one of the above 3 common causes of spells.

Chapter 16 Spells

Nevertheless, it may be she has an uncommon or rare cause of the spells. These are important to identify, because each has different treatment or prophylaxis
a. Causes of spells having hyperadrenergic symptoms:
   (1) Pheochromocytoma–many similarities to a panic attack i.e. sympathetic hyperarousal symptoms but no anticipatory anxiety or phobic anxiety or agoraphobia; pallor (not flushing) i.e. marked sweating without flushing occurs with pheochromocytoma; order 24 hour urine metanephrines and catecholamines

> If your patient's symptoms do not respond as expected to your management, he may have an uncommon or rare cause listed in Section G.2 that you can diagnose and treat. Or you may want to refer your patient to a specialist.

   (2) Autonomic (diencephalic) epilepsy–paroxysmal HTN, tachycardia, flushing, history of seizures
   (3) Essential HTN–labile or "hyperdynamic circulation" in a young adult
   (4) Orthostatic hypotension–dizziness (presyncope) related to change of position, sweating, blurred vision, pallor
   (5) POTS–not orthostatic hypotension but tachycardia (>120/bpm absolute rate, and pulse increased on standing >30/bpm), lightheadedness, SOB
   (6) AIP–tachycardia, sweating, hyper- or hypotension, anxiety, abdominal pain, nausea, vomiting
   (7) OSA–may be confused with nocturnal panic attacks, both of which are very common
b. Causes of cutaneous flushing--almost always these have a "dry flush" (must exclude a malignant carcinoid tumor)
   (1) Carcinoid syndrome--upper body flushing, wheezing, large volume diarrhea; order a 24 hr urine 5-HIAA and serum serotonin
   (2) Mastocytosis–flushing and facial warmth, large volume diarrhea, hypotension, urticaria; order a plasma tryptase
   (3) MTC–diarrhea, thyroid nodule, cervical nodes; increased plasma calcitonin
   (4) Pancreatic tumors (VIPoma)–large volume diarrhea, hypokalemia, high plasma vasoactive intestinal peptide
   (5) Male hypogonadism (pseudocarcinoid syndrome)–sublibido, small soft testes
   (6) Renal cell carcinoma–hematuria, flank pain, high ESR
   (7) Migraine variants–history of associated migraine headaches
   (8) Idiopathic flushing (Arch Int Med 148, 2614, 1988)–palpitations, hypotension, syncope
c. Wilson's disease--dyskinesia, tics, elevated liver enzymes

H. Use the glossary for precise thinking and accurate diagnosis.

1. **Agitated** (Latin *agitare* meaning "to hurry.") Now it means an exceedingly restless patient with mental distress of anxiety or fear.
2. **Agoraphobia** (Greek *agora* meaning "marketplace or field" and *phobein,* "to be frightened by.") It is fear either of traveling alone away from the safety of home (familiar controlled place) or of being in crowded places.
3. **Angst** (German word for anxiety.)
4. **Anxiety** (Latin *anxietas* meaning "trouble, worry.") Anxiety implies worry or apprehension about future unpleasant experiences that may or may not be likely to occur; in contrast, fear is an alarm reaction to a recognized and real danger.
5. **Automatisms** (Greek *automotismos* meaning "self-action.") Now they are nonreflex acts that occur without conscious initiation of the act.
6. **Autonomic (nervous system)** (Greek *auto* meaning "self" and *normos*, "law.") It suggests "a law unto itself," because it was thought not to be under control of higher centers of the brain. Interestingly, the word *autonomy* in moral values theory means "self" and "law" or "control," meaning the person is under the control of herself.
7. **Cataplexy** (Greek word meaning "abrupt weakness, hypotonia.")
8. **Depression** (Latin *de* meaning "down" and *premere*, "to press.") The depression overwhelms her.

9. **Diaphoresis** (Greek word meaning "profuse sweating" or perspiration.) Same usage today.
10. **Dysphoria** (Greek word meaning "excessive pain, anguish, agitation.") Now it means any changed behavior ranging from malaise to restlessness.
11. **Emotion** (Latin *emovere* meaning "to disturb.") It is any state of mental excitement. All emotions (surprise, happy, sad, melancholy, anger, fear) have 3 characteristics: subjective feelings, physiological responses, and resulting changes in behavior of the person feeling the emotion.
12. **Flush** (Middle English *fluschen* meaning "to fly up.") Blood flow spreads suddenly into the face and upper body i.e. a transient episodic redness, either with or without sweating.
13. **Narcolepsy** (Greek *narke* meaning "numbness, torpor" and *lepsis*, "a seizure.") It refers to a sudden compulsion to sleep.
14. **Panic.** In Greek mythology, Pan was the god of all nature. Pan had a habit of sleeping near roads, and roused from sleep, he let out a blood-curdling cry that would cause such overwhelming terror or fright in the person, that many died from it.
15. **Spell** (Greek *apiele* meaning "a boast.") Medically a spell refers to abrupt or rapid onset of a complex of symptoms, and they are not readily explainable by disease of a single organ.
16. **Phobia** (Greek *phobos* meaning "fear.") It is a morbid fear of something perceived by the patient as being very dangerous to herself. In itself the object is not dangerous e.g. noctiphobia, fear of darkness.
17. **Ruminative** worry (Latin *rumen* meaning "the gullet" and *ruminare*, "to think, to meditate.") In present medical usage it refers to constant, excessive dwelling on certain ideas.
18. **Somatic** (Greek *soma* meaning "a body, dead or living.") Soma is opposed to *psyche*, the soul. Anything somatic pertains to the body, such as somatic symptoms (pain, dyspnea, palpitations, dizziness); in contrast, cognitive symptoms (from Latin *cognoscere*, "to know") arise via the mind e.g. fear of dying or losing control or going crazy, *vis a vis* panic disorder.
19. **Stereotypic** (Greek *stereos* meaning "solid" and *typos*, "type.") It is a distinctive pattern ("solid type") of symptoms that recur in an individual patient.
20. **Stress** (Old French *estrece* meaning "straitness or oppression.") It contrasts with the word strain, from Latin *stringere*, "to draw tight." Stress refers to a potentially injurious action, whereas strain is the resulting injury. For example, twisting one's arm is a stress, which may or may not lead to a strain of the arm muscles. This concept now has been applied to mental "stress," which can lead to other problems.
21. **Sympathetic** nervous system (Greek *sym* or *syn*, both meaning "together with, invested or endowed with, or in connection with" and *pathos*, "feeling or suffering.") As one part of the autonomic nervous system, and because it served the viscera, the idea of the "sympathies" of the viscera were thereby aroused. (Parasympathetic adds the Greek *para* meaning "beside"). *Pathos* or *pati* is the root word for patient also. The patient is one who suffers; in distinction, the word "client," used by car dealers and lawyers, is from Latin meaning "one who is dependent upon or protected by" another more powerful person.
22. **Temperament** (Latin *temperamentum* meaning "mixture," the peculiar physical character and mental cast of a person.) Formerly all of medicine was divided into the temperaments--the disease was either bilious or choleric; or lymphatic or phlegmatic; or melancholic; or sanguineous; or nervous.
23. **Volition** (Latin *velle* meaning "to will.") It is the conscious willing of an action.

CHAPTER 17 SUBLIBIDO
Questions on Sublibido

A. In your 50 y/o man having "a problem with sex," the most important information is
  1. In the history :
  2. From the physical exam:

B. Your 60 y/o patient says "I have erectile dysfunction and I'd like to try Viagra."
  1. Is there anything wrong with just giving him some samples of Viagra?

  2. You can quickly approach the cause of his problem by :

C. Your 47 y/o normal weight patient (BMI=24) has "erectile dysfunction" and you discover gynecomastia on exam. You know that this is not typical of erectile dysfunction; the gynecomastia suggests:

D. Your 40 y/o patient says he has "erectile problems." You determine by history that it definitely is sublibido, and you find soft testes measuring 2.5 cm length.
  1. At this point, you consider:
  2. A total serum testosterone level is 135 (normal >240) and he has a normal serum FSH level. Now you consider:
  3. You now must order the following tests:

Answers on Sublibido

A. Be certain of the symptom and its distinguishing characteristics
   1. Normal sexual function in men consists of 3 necessary sequential factors–1) normal libido (the need or drive to have sex) requires intact hormonal and psychological functioning; 2) next, adequate erection requires intact neurological and vascular function; and 3) normal orgasm and ejaculation requires intact neurological functioning. So you must, if necessary, spend some focused effort to ascertain that the original "sex problem" was either decreased libido or unchanged libido but difficulty maintaining an erection sufficient for intercourse
   2. Palpate his testes for quantity and quality. Normal testes are firm and >3 cm in length. Soft or small testes suggest a hormonal cause for the sublibido. An abnormal testicular mass suggests a possible estrogen-secreting tumor or cancer
B. All male sexual problems are not treatable by Viagra or similar medications
   1. Viagra and other 5'phosphodiesterase inhibitors act only to treat erectile dysfunction, that is, except for a placebo effect, Viagra will not enhance libido. Also, erectile dysfunction could be due to a brain tumor, which grows more while he is "trying Viagra"
   2. Physiologically, think of an erection as a "psychohormonal-neurovascular reflex." Remembering this provides you an immediate differential diagnosis. If he has sublibido think of psychological causes or hormonal causes; if he has erectile dysfunction only, think of neurological or vascular diseases
C. Another reason not to just treat with Viagra
   Significant gynecomastia along with erectile dysfunction suggests a possibly unusual cause of the sexual problem, e.g. estrogen-secreting tumor in the testes
D. Another dangerous cause of male sexual dysfunction
   1. His history of sublibido suggests either a psychological cause or hormonal cause. His small, soft testes increase the likelihood it is due to a hormonal cause, rather than psychological
   2. The low serum testosterone confirms the hypogonadism. If it were primary hypogonadism, that is, disease of the testes causing low production of testosterone, the FSH should be significantly higher than the normal range, so the FSH is "inappropriately normal." You must assume he has a secondary cause of the hypogonadism i.e. hypothalamic or pituitary dysfunction
   3. You must be certain there is no identifiable tumor, so order an MRI of the pituitary. Because up to 50% of functioning adenomas of the pituitary may not be visible on MRI, always get a morning serum prolactin (small prolactinoma) and a 24 hour urine free cortisol (Cushing's disease)

Chapter 17 Sublibido   213

Sublibido (decreased or absent libido)

Differential diagnosis: the 4 common causes of sublibido
1. Endocrine (hypogonadism, hyperprolactinemia, thyroid disease) serum testosterone is low or prolactin is high or TSH is abnormal
2. Psychological–GAD, MD, somatization disorder
3. Chronic disease (may be undiagnosed) or general bad health
4. Nonmedical problems–bad relationship, financial problems, work stresses, wife's illness

A. **Be certain of the symptom and its distinguishing characteristics.** Your patient's problem or chief complaint is "I'm having a problem with sex." Often, however, it is not the patient volunteering this. Either his wife raises the problem or you discover it by asking all men >40 y/o–"Almost all men your age have some problem with sex; is there anything you want to talk about?" Often he does have a problem, and he is glad you asked
1. Recognize that, in the patient's mind, "a problem with sex" is the same as "erectile dysfunction." Normal male sexual function is a 3 part sequence, however, and each prior step is necessary for the next step to occur, that is, any one of the 3 functions can go wrong causing "a sexual problem"
   a. First, there must be a need or a drive to have sex i.e. libido, which requires intact psychological and hormonal functions
   b. Second, ability to achieve and maintain an erect penis, which requires intact neurological and vascular functions
   c. Finally, orgasm and ejaculation, which require intact neurological function
   A "sexual problem," therefore, may be a problem at one or more of these levels, thus there may be dysfunction with:
   a. Libido–absence or decreased drive to have sex, i.e. sublibido; or
   b. Erection–insufficient hardness of the penis to actually begin and complete intercourse satisfactorily, i.e. erectile dysfunction; or
   c. Orgasm and ejaculation–premature, retrograde, or no ejaculation.
   An erection is a psychohormonal-neurovascular reflex event and that fact can help you with approach to diagnosis; sublibido suggests a psychological or hormonal etiology, whereas erectile dysfunction suggests either neurological or vascular disease is causative
2. First, be sure it is not an ejaculation problem or infertility about which he is complaining. That leaves a potential problem either of sublibido or erectile dysfunction, or both. "Mr. Smith, most people today think that having a problem with sex is the same as erectile dysfunction or insufficient hardness of your erection to have sex. But for many men the problem is the step before getting the erection, that is, the man just has little or no drive to have sex any more. Tell me specifically about your problem"
3. If the problem is lack of sufficient erection (erectile dysfunction), and there is also decreased desire, ask him–"Compared to before

your problem with sex began, how do you think your need or drive for sex was? In other words, can you remember which came first–the decreased need to have sex, or the ability of the penis to get hard?" "How often does the problem occur–every time, or occasionally?" Did the difficulty come on gradually and is it progressively worsening or did the problem begin recently, that is, rapid onset? Did the problem start with obvious causes–death of his wife, significant medical or surgical event, new medication, problems financially, insecurity at work or at home?

Be certain:
1. That your patient has sublibido, i.e. decreased or absent desire or drive to have sex
2. Whether it is new onset or episodic or chronic, persistent sublibido
3. Whether onset was gradual (days-weeks) or insidious
4. If associated erectile dysfunction either preceded or followed the sublibido

---

4. Physical examination
   a. Search carefully for evidence of chronic pain, or chronic known or occult diseases of heart, lung, liver, or kidneys that may suppress normal libido
   b. Palpate the testes; normal is >3cm in length and <u>firm</u> consistency and no masses; palpate for gynecomastia in the peri- and subareolar areas
   c. Auscultate for bruits and also palpate: femoral and lower extremity arteries, carotid and renal arteries
   d. When doing the prostate exam, test for a normal bulbocavernosus reflex indicating intact S_{2-4}

By now you should be confident that your patient has sublibido, whether it is new onset or episodic or chronic, persistent sublibido, and whether onset was rapid or insidious. In almost all instances you now have the information you need for diagnosis of the obvious causes (Section C) and the common causes (Section E). In the rare instance that your patient appears different clinically from the usual office patient with sublibido, be certain (Section B) that he does not have a symptom or sign of a dangerous disease

B. **Be confident it's not a dangerous disease.**
1. Send immediately to the ED by ambulance if there is:
   a. Back pain and bowel or urinary dysfunction (incontinence) with gradual (days-weeks) onset of the sex problem, think of cauda equina syndrome
   b. Abrupt onset of headache, change in vision, stupor or ophthalmoplegia, think of pituitary apoplexy
2. Admit to the hospital or have a specialist consult as soon as appropriate to the clinical situation if there is:
   a. Erectile dysfunction as well as low back or leg pain with rapid walking, think of Leriche syndrome (PVD of the lower aorta and common iliac arteries)
   b. Progressively worsening headache or one that awakens him at night, think of pituitary tumor
   c. Bizarre symptoms like "flashbacks", automatisms, sensory illusions, think of complex partial seizures (temporal lobe epilepsy)

Chapter 17 Sublibido 215

    d. Pain with erection, or bent penis when erect, Peyronie's disease
    e. Bilateral neurological signs or symptoms e.g. lower limb weakness and paresthesias, think of spinal cord tumor, transverse myelitis
    f. Bladder symptoms in a middle aged man, think of multiple system atrophy, transverse myelitis, spinal cord compression (tumor, arteriovenous malformation)

Be certain in the first minutes of your exam that there is no evidence of any <u>one</u> dangerous symptom or sign associated with the sublibido:
1. Occult systemic disease
2. Progressively worsening headache
3. Gynecomastia
4. Focal or worsening neurological symptom or sign

Any suggestion of a dangerous disease, send the patient to the ED.

---

    g. Testicular mass and erectile dysfunction, think of Leydig cell tumor
    h. Unexplained weight loss due to anorexia, think of malignancy, PMR, anorexia nervosa, Addison's disease
    i. Loss of erection only with pelvic thrusting, think of pelvic steal syndrome
    j. Gynecomastia, think of estrogen excess (feminizing adrenal carcinoma, testicular tumor, obesity, drugs)

C. **Make a quick diagnosis if it's obvious.** Is it an easily diagnosed cause or a medication that is responsible for his sexual problem? In most patients you will be <u>highly</u> confident of a common cause of the symptom by now. If not, one or more of the following tests may exclude an organic disease and increase your confidence in your working diagnosis: creatinine, albumin, UA, TSH, electrolytes, glucose (2 hr postprandial)

Recognize any easily diagnosed sexual problem:
1. Erectile dysfunction with normal libido
2. Longstanding erectile dysfunction with subsequent sublibido, i.e. problem getting an erection preceded the sublibido
3. Psychogenic erectile dysfunction i.e. intact libido
4. Medication side effect or substance abuse

---

1. Either erectile dysfunction with intact libido or long standing erectile dysfunction with subsequent loss of libido due to frustration, depression, performance anxiety. If your patient has erectile dysfunction, either without sublibido, or with sublibido which only occurred after the erectile dysfunction, then he needs therapy with an inhibitor of type 5 phosphodiesterase, e.g. sildenafil. See Section G.3 for caveats regarding this therapy with Viagra
    a. Vascular causes of erectile dysfunction e.g. systemic HTN, DM, atherosclerosis (CAD, stroke, PVD), past or current cigarette smoker of <u>any</u> amount; caveat–erectile dysfunction may precede the symptoms of T2DM, CAD, PVD, so be alert to diagnose these occult entities in your patient with new erectile dysfunction

b. Neurological etiologies e.g. Parkinson's disease, Alzheimer's disease, spinal cord injuries, MS (late stage), peripheral or autonomic neuropathies (DM, alcohol)
2. Psychogenic erectile dysfunction often has its onset in a healthy man <40-50 y/o on no medications. There is intact libido, often rapid onset or episodic erectile dysfunction, and no sexual problem masturbating or having sex with another partner
3. Medications–Any <u>new</u> medication, even if it is not mentioned in the PDR as causing either sublibido or erectile dysfunction, may do so in your individual patient
   a. Medications causing only sublibido–niacin, amiodarone, phenothiazines, thioridazine, mesoridazine, fluphenazine, alprazolam
   b. Medications causing both sublibido and erectile dysfunction
      (1) Cardiovascular–spironolactone, methyldopa, reserpine, propranolol, metoprolol, chlorthalidone (but <u>not</u> acebutolol, amlodopine, doxazosin, see Hypertension 29, 8, 1997)
      (2) Psychiatric–TCAs, SSRIs, antipsychotics, benzodiazepines, lithium
      (3) Miscellaneous–cimetidine, phenytoin, gemfibrozil, H2 blockers, metoclopramide, narcotics, stimulants (e.g. cocaine, amphetamines), anabolic-androgenic steroids, finasteride, GnRH analogues e.g. goserelin, leuprolide
   c. Medications causing only erectile dysfunction
      (1) Cardiovascular–thiazides, clonidine, guanethidine, hydralazine, verapamil, α-blockers
      (2) Psychiatric–risperidone, butyrophenones, phenothiazines
      (3) Miscellaneous–NSAIDs, disulfiram, marijuana, statins, fibrates, carbamazepine, barbiturates, primidone, methotrexate

D. **Identify your patient's worries and wants.** Sexual problems, especially sublibido and erectile dysfunction, occur in more than 50% of men >40 y/o, and only a few consult about it. During your interview and exam try to intuit or discover why your patient is here today, and not previously, for this problem. Don't necessarily ask directly, but try to get some ideas from your patient's responses to questions about his perception of the problem itself. You can't completely help your patient unless you know what he really worries about and wants from you. That's why he is here to see you--to satisfy his worries and wants! Here are only some of the possible worries and wants of your patient with a sexual problem. You must discover his specific, unique ones

> During your exam, discover your patient's worries (e.g. tumor, neurological disease, "losing my manhood") and wants ("Viagra"), so that you can respond to his specific needs as soon as possible.

1. Common worries:
   a. That the cause of his sexual problem is a dangerous etiology e.g. HIV, brain tumor, cancer, CAD
   b. That the etiology is some rare disease e.g MS, Shy-Drager syndrome
   c. What other fears or anxieties might be troubling your patient? For example, he may have had a sex problem for many years, and only now does he come for help. What has changed? Perhaps a friend or relative, who had a similar problem, recently has been diagnosed with a pituitary tumor. There are many other possibilities–think of them
2. Your patient wants:

Chapter 17 Sublibido 217

    a. You to perform a thorough physical exam focused on possible causes of the sex problem and he wants appropriate tests and imaging studies
    b. A plausible explanation of the cause of his problem
    c. Confident reassurance from you that it is not a dangerous or rare etiology. Tell him--"The good news, it's not a brain tumor" (or whatever you believe his real worry is)
    d. To know the prognosis, short term (effects on job, home life, marriage; how soon he will be back to normal) and long term (if recurrences are possible; how to prevent recurrences; if it will cause any disability)
    e. Treatment to cure his problem of erectile dysfunction now and to prevent recurrences, *viz* sildenafil (Viagra), or to treat his sublibido with testosterone
    f. A specialist referral if he believes you are not confident of the diagnosis and treatment

E. Know the symptoms that differentiate the 4 common causes of sublibido.

1. Although not the commonest etiology, an endocrine cause of sublibido is most important to identify first because there is specific effective treatment

---

Common causes of most sublibido:
1. Endocrine (hypogonadism, hyperprolactinemia, thyroid disease) serum testosterone is low or prolactin is high or TSH is abnormal
2. Psychological–GAD, MD, somatization disorder
3. Chronic disease (may be undiagnosed) or general bad health
4. Nonmedical problems–bad relationship, financial problems, work stresses, wife's illness

---

    a. Characteristics of an endocrine etiology
      (1) Your patient's testes may be <3 cm in length or soft in consistency, or he may have signs or symptoms of thyroid disease
      (2) Either early morning, fasted serum testosterone is decreased, <u>or</u> serum prolactin is increased above normal <u>or</u> serum TSH is abnormally low or high
    b. What suggests it might not be an endocrine cause of the sublibido
      (1) Anytime there is an associated symptom or sign suggesting a dangerous cause (see above, Section B)
      (2) If the early morning total testosterone concentration is normal and the prolactin is not increased above normal range, and the TSH level is normal. (Recent data suggest a normal FTI (fT4) and a TSH level >2.0 may indicate subclinical hypothyroidism; replacement L-thyroxine might reverse the associated sublibido)
2. Common look-alikes causing or associated with sublibido:
    a. Psychological etiologies
      (1) MD almost always has associated anhedonia, including markedly decreased or absent libido; the depression preceded the sublibido
      (2) GAD–he is the "worry wart" of the family, and there may be some new overwhelming worry or stress in his life, and he "worries all day" that the "catastrophe" may occur
      (3) Other psychiatric entities e.g. somatization
    b. Any chronic disease or general bad health–recent onset sublibido may be an early sign of occult disease e.g. T2DM, atherosclerosis,

malignancy
- (1) Chronic pain e.g. arthritis, IBS
- (2) Chronic disease e.g. cardiac, pulmonary, liver, kidney, HIV
c. Nonmedical problem– commonest causes of sublibido, but they almost never are volunteered–you have to intuit or ask about them; often you will need to spend some length of time talking with the couple, together and separately, to get some idea of the source of the sublibido. Some common underlying problems are:
- (1) Psychosocial stressors–financial difficulties, work stress, wife's illness, his illness
- (2) Lack of attraction for his sexual partner e.g. weight gain of his wife, ageing
- (3) Bad relationship–they just dislike each other, wife's lack of interest in sex, infidelity by either partner

F. Use this summary for efficient diagnosis of a common cause.
With the information from Sections A-E in mind, here is the rapid approach to diagnosis of sublibido.
1. You have already determined:
   a. In Section A, by H&P, that absent or diminished libido is present.
   b. In Section B, that there is no evidence in the H&P of any one dangerous cause of the sexual problem.
   c. In Section C, that it is neither erectile dysfunction only nor a drug or medication that is likely responsible for the sexual problem.
2. From the focused H&P almost always you should quickly be confident of a working diagnosis. Confident final diagnosis is made only in followup the next months or years when the response to treatment or nontreatment is appropriate to your working diagnosis.
   a. If there is any suggestion of an endocrine etiology by H&P, order morning fasted blood levels of total testosterone, prolactin, free thyroxine, TSH; laboratory evidence suggesting an endocrine cause for the sublibido is any one of the following:
   - (1) Hypogonadism–if total testosterone is low, you may get a SHBG level to exclude low SHBG artifactually lowering the testosterone. If your patient is <40-50 y/o, the serum LH values should be increased, but hypogonadal patients >50 y/o commonly do not have increased LH (which suggests a hypothalamic etiology). The lower the testosterone, or if the early morning prolactin is elevated significantly, or there are other symptoms or signs of hypopituitarism, then an MRI should be done to exclude a pituitary tumor.
   - (2) Hyperprolactinemia–elevated serum prolactin in a fasted patient, early morning.
   - (3) Hyperthyroidism–fT4 (or FTI) that is elevated with an appropriately low TSH.
   - (4) Hypothyroidism–decreased fT4 (or FTI) and appropriately increased TSH of primary hypothyroidism. Subclinical hypothyroidism (normal fT4 and TSH >2.0) may indicate a trial of replacement L-thyroxine. Caution: secondary or central hypothyroidism also has a low fT4 but it may have either low TSH or an inappropriately normal or even slightly elevated level of TSH (biologically inactive TSH).
   Treatment for sublibido due to endocrine causes is not Viagra, but

normalization of hormone levels.
  b. If the endocrine studies are normal and there is evidence of MD or GAD present, treat appropriately (see Section G.3.f).
  c. If there is known or possibly occult disease responsible for the sublibido, diagnose and treat optimally. Especially important in patients with chronic disease is alleviation of pain.
  d. Explore thoroughly for any psychosocial problems (bad relationship with his wife, work stresses) causing the sublibido, and counsel appropriately.
3. Answer your patient's worries and wants that you determined early on during the exam (Section D). Have you done everything you can to help him? All the Viagra in the world will not help a patient in an unhappy relationship, nor will it increase libido except by placebo effect.
4. You now have a working diagnosis, but only with followup can you be confident it is correct. In followup visits you are always testing by H&P that your working diagnosis is correct.

G. Abandon your working diagnosis and look for an uncommon cause only if:
1. Any one dangerous symptom or sign (see above, Section B) occurs in followup of weeks or months. Quickly obtain a consult or send your patient to the hospital as appropriate

If your patient's symptoms do not respond as expected to your management, he may have an uncommon or rare cause listed in Section G.2 that you can diagnose and treat. Or you may want to refer your patient to a specialist.

2. Your patient's response to therapy is not as you expect or if the natural history of your working diagnosis does not occur.
   Don't spend time and money looking for one of the following etiologies until you are sure your patient doesn't have one of the 4 common causes of sexual problems above. Nevertheless, it may be that he has an unusual cause. These are important to recognize, because each has different treatment or prophylaxis
   a. Rare endocrine diseases--Cushing's syndrome, acromegaly, Addison's disease, hypopituitarism, Langerhan's cell histiocytosis, hypothalamic or pituitary sarcoidosis, adrenal or testis feminizing tumor, testicular Leydig cell tumors, adrenal cortical tumor, choriocarcinoma
   b. Other diseases–
      (1) Medical diseases e.g. hemochromatosis, celiac disease, scleroderma, pernicious anemia, OSA, amyloidosis, zinc deficiency, thalassemia, sickle cell anemia
      (2) Psychiatric diseases e.g. schizophrenia, anorexia nervosa.
      (3) Neurological diseases e.g. Alzheimer's disease, parkinsonism, spinal cord tumor, temporal lobe disease, myotonic muscular dystrophy, adrenoleukodystrophy, Parkinson's-plus syndromes e.g. Shy-Drager syndrome, multiple system atrophy
      (4) Vascular diseases–e.g. HTN, aortoiliac atherosclerosis, Leriche syndrome, arteritis
3. Caveats in using Viagra (Urology 60 (Suppl B), 28, 2002):
   a. There must be no cigarette smoking or alcohol intake in the few hours before using Viagra. Never prescribe Viagra in a patient taking nitrates, and not without cardiology consult if he has markedly depressed systolic function
   b. The partner must be involved in all aspects of diagnosis and therapy, and should understand the increasing reliance on reflexogenic erection as the man gets older. That is, there must be much greater penile sexual stimulation (oral or manual)

before intercourse
- c. The Viagra is taken 30-60 minutes before anticipated sex activity. Faster onset of action occurs with an empty stomach, and a prior heavy fat, gourmet meal may adversely affect the action of Viagra. The effect of Viagra may persist 3-5 hours, so inadequate effect of Viagra at 1 hour, possibly may be followed by good effect 1-2 hours later
- d. Start initially with 50 mg Viagra, then titrate up to 100 mg if there is an inadequate response, or down to 25 mg if an adequate response
- e. Explain that a positive response to Viagra may occur with the first 1 or 2 doses, but it may take up to 7 or 8 trials on different days for adequate response. First attempts may be emotionally charged, and high anxiety for both partners, especially if erectile dysfunction has been long term
- f. Regarding MD and erectile dysfunction, recognize the following:
  - (1) Erectile dysfunction may have caused "secondary" depression. Treat first with Viagra, because SSRI therapy may lead to much more severe erectile dysfunction
  - (2) MD may be primary and erectile dysfunction is just one of its symptoms. Initial therapy is for depression, but SSRI may cause worsening of erectile dysfunction even while relieving the other depressive symptoms. Patients will stop the effective SSRI therapy unless your careful followup detects the worsening erectile dysfunction and you treat it with Viagra

H. Use the glossary for precise thinking and accurate diagnosis.

1. **Acromegaly** (Greek *akron* meaning "extremity" and *megas,* "large.") Excess growth hormone after epiphyseal closure causes enlarged cranium, hands, feet, jaw (loose teeth)
2. **Andropause** (Greek *andro* meaning "man" an *pause*, "cessation.") An unfortunate term recently coined to be the counterpart of menopause ("cessation of menses.") The term signifies decreased serum testosterone with ageing, not decreased maleness.
3. **Anorexia nervosa** (Greek *an* meaning "lack of" and *orexis*, "appetite.") *Nervosa* implies a neurological etiology, which is controversial.
4. **Choriocarcinoma** (Greek *chorion* meaning "membrane" and *carkinos,* "crab, cancer.") Now it refers to malignant epithelial cells of the placental trophoblastic cells.
5. **Erectile dysfunction**– Inability to achieve and maintain an erection sufficient for sex; of itself it says nothing about libido.
6. **Hemochromatosis** (Greek *haima* meaning "blood" and *chroma,* "color or complexion.") Originally the bronze color of skin and other organs was thought due to discoloration by iron from blood. Now we know the accumulated iron is from exogenous sources.
7. **Impotence**–Formerly used as a medical term for all male sexual problems, even infertility. More recently it referred to both lack of desire (sublibido) and inability to get an erection (erectile dysfunction); it no longer is a useful term with our current understanding of normal function.
8. **Leukodystrophy (adrenal)** (Greek *leukos* meaning "white" and *dys*, "abnormal" and *trephein,* "to nourish.") It is disease thought to be due to faulty nutrition causing demyelination of central hemispheres
9. **Paraphilia** (Greek *para* meaning "resembling or abnormal" and *philein*, "to love.") It is an abnormal craving for or attraction to the object denoted by the word stem; the word suffix, "-philia" is used in similar fashion, but opposite in meaning, to the word suffix "-phobia," e.g. pedophilia.
10. **Sarcoidosis** (Greek *sarkos* meaning "flesh" and *osis*, "abnormal increase.") A disease characterized by nonmalignant granulomas or noncasecting tubercles in various tissues
11. **Sublibido** (Latin *sub* meaning "under" or abnormally low, and *libido,* "desire, lust, rut.") It means decreased or absent libido.

Chapter 18 Tremor

Questions on Tremor

A. In a patient complaining of "my hand shakes," the most important information you want to find
  1. In the history :
  2. From the physical exam:
B. List the kinds of tremor:
  1.
  2.
     a.
     b.
C. In the office, the 2 common causes of chronic tremor and their major distinguishing characteristics are:
  1.
     a.
     b.
     c.
     d.
  2.
     a.
     b.
     c.
     d.

Answers on Tremor
A. Be certain of the symptom and its distinguishing characteristics
   1. "How does the tremor affect your daily life?" A patients with essential (idiopathic) tremor (ET) complains of difficulty with tasks requiring hand movements, especially drinking from a cup or glass. He commonly spills liquids to such a degree as to avoid social situations or even eating at restaurants. The patient with idiopathic Parkinson's disease (IPD) has no problem drinking from a cup, it just may take a long time i.e. he doesn't spill liquids
   2. While he is sitting, have him hold his hands outstretched straight in front of him, extended at the elbows, palms down. A patient with essential tremor will have bilateral tremor of his fingers, and no resting tremor. The patient with early IPD complaining of tremor will have minimal tremor (as does everybody) with this maneuver, but also he will have a tremor of his fingers at rest i.e. with the arms and hands supported against gravity. IPD has a unilateral tremor the first few years, but he may only consult after he began having it in both hands
B. The kinds of tremor are simple, but usual nomenclature can be confusing
   1. Rest tremor–occurs in the fingers while hands and arms are supported against gravity
   2. Non-resting tremor, that is, tremor with some movement. Movement tremors are called action or kinetic, meaning the same thing i.e. tremors brought on or exaggerated by some movement. There are 2 kinds of action (non-resting) tremor
      a. Postural tremor–arms and hands held outstretched, unsupported against gravity
      b. Intention tremor–hand moves to touch a target, e.g. finger-to-nose, heel-to-shin
   Watch for dysmetria i.e. the finger misses the target (nose)
C. Common causes of tremor
   Both essential tremor and the rest tremor of IPD disease have insidious onset and chronic, daily tremor; they differ:
   1. Essential (idiopathic) tremor (ET)
      a. Onset of tremor in a patient <40-50 y/o
      b. Postural tremor
      c. At onset, bilateral upper extremities are affected, but commonly asymmetrical severity
      d. Tremor is an isolated symptom
   2. Parkinson's disease (IPD)
      a. Onset of tremor in a patient >40-50 y/o
      b. Rest tremor, early on
      c. Unilateral rest tremor at onset (and it remains unilateral for 2-5 years)
      d. Other symptoms may dominate the clinical picture i.e. bradykinesia, rigidity, gait difficulty

Chapter 18 Tremor

Tremor

> **Differential diagnosis: the 2 common causes of chronic tremor**
> 1. Essential tremor (ET)–postural (non-resting) tremor; it starts bilaterally in the hands; no other symptoms
> 2. IPD–rest tremor; starts unilaterally in the hands; typical associated symptoms e.g. bradykinesia, rigidity, gait difficulty

A. **Be certain of the symptom and its distinguishing characteristics.** Your patient's problem or chief complaint is "My hands shake"
1. First, be certain the problem is tremor, and whether it is either a new or episodic or chronic, daily tremor. Have him demonstrate the tremor, because it almost always will be present. "Show me what you mean by shakiness"
    a. By definition a tremor is a movement of some body part, and it is rhythmical <u>and</u> involuntary <u>and</u> oscillatory. If the involuntary movement is not rhythmical i.e. it is irregular, then it is not a tremor. It may be a dystonia, myoclonus, tic, athetosis, clonus, asterixis, but it is not a tremor
    b. Very important is the body part he chooses to show you the tremor, and the specific way he activates the tremor. The body part almost always is the arms and hands and the shaking occurs either:
       (1) The limb is at rest and supported against gravity (forearms resting in his lap or on a table edge) and his fingers shake i.e. a rest tremor; or
       (2) When there is no support against gravity, for example, arms and hands outstretched in front of him, i.e., a postural tremor. Tremor occurring during any voluntary movement is called a kinetic or action (non-resting) tremor, so a postural tremor is a form of action tremor.
       (3) Another specific type of action (non-resting) tremor is an intention tremor, which is manifest when you test for target-directed movements, e.g. finger to nose maneuver. Postural tremor commonly has an equally severe or lesser amplitude tremor when you test for an intention tremor. The amplitude of an intention tremor may significantly increase at the termination of the movement, that is, as the finger approaches the nose. A dominant intention tremor that worsens (increases in amplitude) as the finger approaches the target, suggests cerebellar disease, and dysmetria (i.e. he misses the target) confirms cerebellar disease

    At this point you have determined your patient has a tremor, and you have identified the type of tremor as either resting or non-resting tremor (postural or intention tremor with dysmetria)
2. Ask him "When did you first notice the shaking?" If he can tell you fairly specifically, then it likely had a recent onset. "Is it possible the tremor was there before, and you just had not noticed it?" A

negative answer confirms a likely recent onset of the tremor. Recent tremors of abrupt onset include all potentially dangerous etiologies (see Section B), as well as the benign psychogenic tremor, whereas the common etiologies of tremor have insidious onset and chronic course. Age at the start of the tremor is very important, but almost always it is in retrospect and may not be accurate. Still try to determine when the tremor began

> Be certain:
> 1. That your patient has a tremor, i.e. movement that is rhythmical, involuntary and oscillatory
> 2. Whether it is new onset tremor or chronic daily tremor
> 3. Whether the onset was abrupt or insidious
> 4. If the dominant tremor is either rest tremor or non-resting tremor (postural tremor or intention tremor with dysmetria)
> 5. Of his age when it started and if it was unilateral or bilateral at onset

3. Physical exam–always do a thorough neurological exam, but primarily:
   a. Test for rest tremor. Have him sit relaxed, arms resting in his lap, eyes closed and counting down from 100 slowly to bring on the rest tremor. If the legs are tested for rest tremor, they must be completely supported against gravity
   b. Test for postural tremor, patient standing or sitting, arms and hands outstretched horizontally forward, palms down, with fingers comfortably spread. Balancing a piece of paper on each hand, alternately, magnifies the tremor for better observation and estimation of amplitude and frequency. If large amplitude it is called a "coarse" tremor, and if small amplitude, it is a "fine" tremor
   c. Remove the paper and test for intention tremor by finger to nose maneuver, again alternately. An isolated postural tremor commonly has an intention tremor of about the same amplitude and frequency as the postural tremor, and there is no dysmetria. An intention tremor suggests a cerebellar lesion if:
      (1) A postural tremor significantly worsens on kinetic target-directed testing, e.g. finger-nose maneuver; or
      (2) There is no postural tremor, but only a significant intention tremor; or
      (3) Anytime dysmetria occurs, i.e. his finger misses the nose or target
   d. Test for bradykinesia by watching for slowed onset and slowed gait while he walks in the hall (look for reduced arm swing and difficulty pivoting) and slowed finger to thumb opposition movements

By now you should be confident it is a tremor, whether it is new onset or chronic tremor, if it was abrupt or insidious onset, and if it is a rest tremor or non-resting tremor (postural tremor or intention

Chapter 18 Tremor

tremor with dysmetria). In almost all instances you now have the information you need for diagnosis of the obvious causes (Section C) and the common causes (Section E). In the rare instance that your patient appears different clinically from the usual office patient with tremor, be certain (Section B) that he does not have a symptom or sign of a dangerous disease

B. **Be confident it's not a dangerous disease.**
1. Send immediately to the ED by ambulance if there is:
   a. Fever or <u>any</u> mental status change in a patient with possible hyperthyroidism (goiter, stare, weight loss, rapid arrhythmia), think of thyroid storm

---

Be certain in the first minutes of your exam that there is no evidence of any <u>one</u> dangerous symptom or sign associated with the tremor:
1. Acutely ill patient
2. Fever >104°F
3. Rapid onset of weakness
4. Altered sensorium
5. Rapid onset of severe, symptomatic tremor

Any suggestion of a dangerous disease, send the patient to the ED.

---

   b. Fever >104°, rigidity and resting tremor in a patient treated with antipsychotic drugs, think neuroleptic malignant syndrome (e.g. haloperidol, thiothixene)
   c. Rapid onset weakness, areflexia, and tremor (postural and intention), think of GBS
   d. Rapid onset of tremor with hypothermia, think of hypoglycemia (treated diabetic, insulinoma, alcoholic hypoglycemia)
   e. Chronic alcoholic patient with altered sensorium and signs and symptoms of sympathetic hyperactivity including rapid onset tremor, think of delirium tremens
2. Admit at once to the ED or hospital if there is:
   a. Recent or rapid onset of postural and intention tremor, think of poisoning by mercury, carbon monoxide, arsenic, lead, manganese, DDT, dioxins, lindane, toluene
   b. Rapid onset of rest tremor (also other parkinsonism signs), think of recreational drugs (like MPTP), household organophosphates
   c. Rapid onset of postural tremor in a susceptible patient, think of drug withdrawal, especially ethanol or sedative-hypnotics
3. Admit to the hospital or have a specialist consult as soon as appropriate if there is:
   a. Rapid onset of rest tremor and bradykinesia in a patient on neuroleptic agents (phenothiazines or butyrophenones), think of drug-induced parkinsonism
   b. Rapid onset of intention tremor, think of intoxications (phenytoin, barbiturates, lithium, ethanol), cerebellar disease
   c. Rapid onset of intention tremor and dysmetria, think of cerebellar vascular lesion
   d. Hypertensive patient with "spells" and postural tremor, think of pheochromocytoma, panic attack, GAD
   e. Rapid onset of a coarse intention tremor of an arm and leg on one side, think of Holmes' tremor syndrome (stroke, tumor, vascular malformation of the contralateral midbrain or thalamus)
   f. Peripheral neuropathy and a postural tremor that may be paroxysmal, think of porphyria, psychogenic tremor

C. **Make a quick diagnosis if it's obvious.** Is it an easily diagnosed condition or a medication that is responsible for the tremor? In most patients you will be <u>highly</u> confident of a common cause of the symptom by now. If not, one or more of the following tests may exclude an organic disease and increase your confidence in your working diagnosis: TSH, glucose
1. Physiologic tremor occurs in almost everybody. The patient may

notice it with outstretched hands, but it causes no particular problem. You may be asked about it by certain patients. You should wonder why he is concerned about it, what his worry is
2. Enhanced physiologic tremor is common to a spectrum of conditions ranging from anxiety and fatigue, to hyperthyroidism, or endogenous and exogenous intoxications. It is a <u>postural</u> tremor, and it is a small amplitude, high frequency tremor of the hands and arms. Different from ET or IPD, the tremor is recent onset and treatment of the disorder e.g. anxiety or hyperthyroidism, "cures" the tremor

---

Recognize any easily diagnosed <u>new</u> tremor:
1. Enhanced physiologic tremor e.g. hyperthyroidism, anxiety disorder
2. Medication side effect

---

3. Drugs or toxins causing new or worsening postural tremor
   a. Sympathomimetics e.g. epinephrine, isuprel, β2-agonists (bronchodilators), theophylline, dopamine, caffeine
   b. Centrally acting agents e.g. neuroleptics, metoclopramide, TCAs, lithium, cocaine, ethanol, amphetamines, salbutamol
   c. Steroids e.g. prednisone, tamoxifen, medroxyprogesterone
   d. Miscellaneous e.g. valproate, amiodarone, procainamide, mexiletine, calcitonin, thyroxine, hypoglycemic agents, chemotherapeutic agents
   e. Drug withdrawal states–CNS-acting drugs e.g. alcohol, cocaine, illicit drugs

D. **Identify your patient's worries and wants.** Physiological tremor occurs in almost everybody, and essential tremor has a prevalence of 6% (20-fold more common than Parkinson's disease). During your interview and exam try to intuit or discover why your patient is here today, and not previously, about his tremor. Most tremors will have been present for months or years. Don't necessarily ask directly, but try to get some ideas from your patient's responses to questions about the tremor itself. You can't completely help your patient unless you know what he really worries about and wants from you. That's why he is here to see you–to satisfy his worries and wants! Here are only some of the possible worries and wants of your patient with tremor. You must discover his specific, unique ones

---

During your exam, discover your patient's worries (stroke, infection, Parkinson's disease) and wants (reassurance, treatment to stop the tremor) so that you can respond to his specific needs as soon as possible.

---

1. Common worries are:
   a. That the cause of the tremor is a dangerous etiology e.g. brain tumor, stroke, or a frightening disease *viz* Parkinson's disease
   b. That the etiology is some rare disease e.g. WNV, toxic chemicals, carbon monoxide, MS
   c. What other fears or anxieties might be troubling your patient? For example, he has had a tremor for years, and only now does he come for help. What has changed? Perhaps a friend or relative, who had similar chronic tremors, recently

Chapter 18 Tremor

has been diagnosed with a brain tumor. There are many other possibilities–think of them
2. Your patient wants:
   a. You to perform a thorough physical exam focused on possible causes of the tremor and he wants appropriate tests and imaging studies
   b. A plausible explanation of the cause of the tremor
   c. Confident reassurance from you that it is not a dangerous or rare etiology. Tell him--"The good news, it's not Parkinson's disease" (or whatever you believe his real worry is)
   d. To know the prognosis, short term (effects on job, home life, marriage; how soon he will be back to normal) and long term (if recurrences are possible; how to prevent recurrences; if it will cause any disability)
   e. Treatment to stop the tremor now and to prevent recurrences (e.g. propranolol or primidone for essential tremor)
   f. A specialist referral (neurologist) if he thinks you are not confident of the diagnosis

E. Know the symptoms that differentiate the 2 common causes of tremor.
1. The commonest etiology is essential tremor (ET)

> The 2 common causes of <u>chronic</u>, daily tremors:
> 1. ET–postural tremor; it starts bilaterally in the hands; no other symptoms
> 2. IPD–rest tremor; starts unilaterally in the hands; typical associated symptoms e.g. bradykinesia, rigidity, gait difficulty

   a. Characteristics of ET
      (1) It is not a new tremor, that is, it is a chronic daily tremor
      (2) It almost always begins in a patient <u><40-50 y/o</u>, although commonly he does not consult about it until years after its onset
      (3) It is a <u>bilateral</u> (but it may be asymmetrical in severity) postural tremor of hands and forearms (often with an intention tremor of similar or lesser amplitude and frequency)
      (4) The tremor occurs in <u>isolation,</u> i.e. there are no other significant symptoms or signs
      (5) After a number of years from onset, there may be an associated voice or head tremor (no-no direction)
   b. What suggests it might not be ET
      (1) Anytime there is an associated symptom or sign suggesting a dangerous cause (see above, Section B)
      (2) If the tremor <u>begins</u> only on one side, or if there is more than one kind of tremor, the dominant tremor either occurs at rest or on movement toward a target, i.e. an intention tremor
      (3) If there is another neurologic symptom e.g. rigidity, bradykinesia, associated gait disturbance, or any <u>one</u> focal neurological sign
2. Common look-alike causing tremor and how it differs from ET
   a. Idiopathic Parkinson's disease (IPD)
      (1) It also is a chronic, daily tremor like ET, but its onset is later, most being in patients <u>>40-50 y/o</u> (5% present <40 y/o)
      (2) A "pill rolling" rest tremor is characteristic of IPD, but no rest tremor may occur in some IPD patients. Nevertheless, an <u>asymmetrical</u> rest tremor can be detected in at least 80% on

proper physical exam at presentation
- (3) The chief complaint in 60% of IPD patients, however, is postural tremor, similar to ET. IPD differs from ET:
  - (a) It begins in one hand and arm (or leg), and only becomes bilateral in 2-5 years, at which time it often affects the ipsilateral leg
  - (b) When the arms are extended to elicit postural tremor, frequently there is a latency period (3-5 seconds) before the tremor begins
  - (c) There also may be tremor of legs, eyelids, jaw, chin (but <u>not</u> head) with IPD
- (4) The four cardinal signs of IPD are rest tremor, bradykinesia, rigidity, disturbed gait and posture (late symptom)
  - (a) Rigidity is called "lead pipe" because it is constant during the full ROM passive testing. If there is a significant postural tremor present (that occurs along with rest tremor), the rigidity will take on a cogwheel character, like a ratcheting
  - (b) Bradykinesia or slowness in starting and performing voluntary movements, such as walking, occurs only 50% of the time on presentation
- (5) Prevalence of IPD is 2% of people >65 y/o. The difficulty in diagnosis of IPD is apparent when you realize that extrapyramidal signs are common in the "normal" elderly; 15% of those 65-74 y/o and more than 50% of all people >85 y/o have mild extrapyramidal features present e.g. hypomimia and reduced arm swing during walking. Confident diagnosis of IPD requires the presence of at least 2 of the 3 cardinal signs–bradykinesia, rigidity, rest tremor

F. Use this summary for efficient diagnosis of a common cause.
With the above information from Sections A-E in mind, here is the rapid approach to diagnosis of the cause of tremor.
1. You already have determined:
   a. In Section A, by H&P, that it is tremor and not another movement disorder.
   b. In Section B, that there is no evidence in the H&P of any <u>one</u> dangerous cause of the tremor.
   c. In Section C, that it is neither an easily diagnosed cause nor a medication that likely is responsible for the tremor.
2. From the focused H&P almost always you should quickly be confident of a working diagnosis. Confident final diagnosis is made only in followup the next months or years when the natural history of the tremor or its response to treatment or nontreatment is appropriate to your working diagnosis.
   a. If your patient has onset of the tremor <40-50 y/o and he has a chronic bilateral, isolated (no other neurological symptoms) postural tremor, it is likely ET.
   b. If your patient is >40-50 y/o and there is a unilateral rest tremor, or bilateral if it started 2-5 years ago, and there is another neurological sign (e.g. bradykinesia, rigidity), it likely is IPD.
   c. Sometimes a confident diagnosis cannot be made in a patient with recent onset tremor without other neurological symptoms. Either diagnose it as "indeterminate tremor syndrome" or refer your

Chapter 18 Tremor 229

patient to a neurologist, who probably will give the same diagnosis.
3. Answer your patient's worries and wants that you determined early on during the exam (Section D). Have you done everything you can to help him?
4. You now have a working diagnosis, but only with followup can you be highly confident it is correct. In return visits you are always testing by H&P that your working diagnosis is correct.

G. Abandon your working diagnosis and look for an uncommon cause only if :

1. Any one dangerous symptom or sign (see above, Section B) occurs in followup of weeks, months, and years. Quickly obtain a neurology consult or send your patient to the hospital as appropriate

> If your patient's symptoms do not respond as expected to your management, he may have an uncommon or rare cause listed in Section G.2 that you can diagnose and treat. Or you may want to refer your patient to a specialist.

2. Your patient's response to therapy is not as you expect or if the natural history of your working diagnosis does not occur. ET has excellent response either to propranolol or primidone, and almost all IPD patients (confirmed by postmortem diagnosis) respond to levodopa; if there is no response, question the diagnosis of IPD

   Don't spend time and money looking for one of the following etiologies until you are sure your patient doesn't have one of the 2 common causes above. Nevertheless, it may be he has an uncommon or rare cause of the tremor. These are important to recognize, because each has different treatment or prophylaxis
   a. About 25% of patients who had definite diagnosis of IPD postmortem, while living had fewer than 2 of 3 cardinal signs (rest tremor, rigidity, bradykinesia) needed for clinical diagnosis of IPD. Also, about 25% of patients who do have 2 of 3 cardinal signs are misdiagnosed as IPD, and have one of the following atypical parkinsonism syndromes
      (1) Characteristics of these syndromes, differing from IPD, are the following:
         (a) Multisystem atrophy (MSA)--early orthostatic hypotension, early dysarthria, frequent ataxia and early falls
         (b) Progressive supranuclear palsy (PSP)--tremor is uncommon, rigidity is symmetrical, early dysarthria, early falls, limited vertical gaze, especially downward
         (c) Corticobasal degeneration—early apraxia (hand can become useless or "phantom"), early dysarthria, early falls
      (2) Characteristics suggesting you should question the diagnosis of IPD in your patient:
         (a) Onset <40 y/o or, at onset, bilateral signs or symmetrical signs
         (b) Poor initial response to adequate dose of levodopa
         (c) Other CNS symptoms--early autonomic failure; pyramidal tract or eye signs
         (d) Rapidly progressive disease
         (e) Family history of another movement disorder
   b. Wilson disease–think of it with onset of a prominent tremor in anybody <50 y/o; it may be rest, postural or intention tremor, or all three; "wing-beating" tremor (tremor of shoulder joint when arms abducted, elbows flexed, then up-down tremor of the forearms) is classical. Think of Wilson disease every time you think of psychogenic tremor, because each has a bizarre presentation. Look for abnormal LFTs, choreoathetosis, open-mouth grimace. Obtain blood for serum copper and ceruloplasmin levels
   c. Task specific tremors may occur during writing ("primary writing tremor"); others occur in typists or musicians; etiology is controversial

d. Dystonic tremor syndromes–it is a postural tremor that is clinically indistinguishable from enhanced physiologic tremor or ET; tremor may occur only in the dystonic body part or in a body part not affected by dystonia e.g. in spasmodic torticollis
   e. Primary orthostatic tremor--subjective feeling of unsteadiness only during stance, not during gait; visible or palpable rippling of leg muscles during stance
   f. Isolated voice tremor–tremulous vocalization only, no other tremor of the body parts
   g. Holmes' tremor--may have rest, intention and postural tremors; they are less rhythmic than usual tremors; midbrain or thalamic lesion; it may follow a stroke
   h. Palatal tremor syndrome–rhythmic movements of the soft palate may follow a brain stem or cerebellar stroke
   i. Tremor with peripheral neuropathy–all postural tremor
      (1) Chronic demyelinating neuropathies
      (2) Gammopathies (IgM, IgG)
      (3) Polyneuropathies e.g. DM, uremia, porphyria (paroxysmal tremor), chemicals (mercury, lead, arsenic, alcohol, lindane, dioxins)
      (4) Malabsorption neuropathy–associated diarrhea, weight loss
   j. Metabolic–all postural or intention tremor
      (1) Low glucose, Mg, Ca, Na
      (2) Chronic hepatocerebral degeneration–occurs in patients with repeated episodes of hepatic coma; resembles Wilson disease, i.e. it may include all three tremors, plus choreoathetosis, ataxia, dysarthria
      (3) Hepatic encephalopathy, CRF, B12 deficiency, eosinophilic-myalgia syndrome, HIV, Klinefelter's syndrome
   k. Infections–all rest, postural, or intention tremor
      (1) MS--intention tremor with dysmetria and titubation (head and trunk tremor seen while standing) occurs late in the disease; tremor usually is no aid in diagnosis
      (2) Neurosyphilis, neuroborreliosis (Lyme disease)
   l. RSD–rest or postural tremor; extremity pain and edema usually precede the tremor
   m. Non-tremors
      (1) Rhythmic myoclonus–intermittent, brief muscle jerks that resemble tremor, especially Holmes' tremor and its variants
      (2) Cortical tremor--closely resembles a high frequency postural tremor
      (3) Asterixis–negative myoclonus with sudden lapses of innervation; if focal, it suggests contralateral hemisphere lesion; if bilateral, metabolic dysfunction or intoxication
   n. Psychogenic tremor
      (1) It may be a "bizarre" presentation e.g. generalized body shaking, which makes the diagnosis easy, because he can't maintain it long--it wears him out. Alternatively, and more commonly, the tremor complained of and elicited on exam is in an extremity, and it may be either rest, postural or intention tremor, or all three together. But there often is some discrepancy in how the tremor occurs on your exam, e.g. varying severity
      (2) Almost always the tremor has an abrupt or rapid onset, and also a sudden remission; or it may be intermittently present. A clue to diagnosis is complaint of tremor, but it is "not there now"
      (3) On exam, distraction or voluntary movement of the contralateral hand produces significant variation in tremor frequency. Two important signs of psychogenic tremor were reported recently (Mov Disord 13 294 1998):
         (a) Coactivation sign of psychogenic tremor–tremor occurs only in the presence of increased muscle tone, and disappears when a body part is totally relaxed
         (b) Absence of finger tremors on exam, when the complaint is upper limb postural tremor
         (c) Tremor may increase with attention and decrease with distraction (just the opposite of organic tremor)

H. Use the glossary for precise thinking and accurate diagnosis.

1. **Akinetic** (Greek *a* meaning "negative" and *kinesis,* "motion." It refers to absence or poverty of movements or reduced movement initiation.
2. **Apraxia** (Greek word meaning "a not acting.") A sign of cortical dysfunction referring to an inability to perform some action, e.g. to use a pencil properly, when paresis or paralysis is not present.
3. **Ataxia** (Greek *a* meaning "without" and *taxis,* "order or arrangement.") It is lack of smooth, ordered movements or incoordination, and it refers especially to gait.
4. **Athetosis** (Greek word *athetos* meaning "lacking a fixed position.") It refers to

Chapter 18 Tremor 231

involuntary writhing movements, especially of the hands and arms.
5. **Bradykinesia** (Greek *brady* meaning "slow" and *kinesis,* "movement.") It refers to slow or sluggish physical and mental responses.
6. **Chorea** (Greek word meaning "dancing.") It now indicates involuntary convulsive-like twitchings and jerky movements.
7. **Cogwheel** (rigidity) It is rhythmic brief on-and-off resistance during passive movement about a joint, and it is a ratcheting like a cogwheel.
8. **Dyskinesia** (Greek *dys* meaning "difficult or disordered" and *kinesis,* "movement.") It refers to any abnormal voluntary movements, for example, movements are fragmented or incomplete.
9. **Dysmetria** (Greek *dys* meaning "difficult or disordered" and *metron,* "measure.") It is difficulty in measuring distance in a muscular act, that is, under- or over-shooting in a reaching movement e.g in the finger to nose maneuver the finger misses the nose.
10. **Dystonia** (Greek *dys* meaning "disordered" and *tonos,* "tonicity.") It is disordered tonicity of muscle *viz* sustained muscle contractions causing twisting and repetitive movement or abnormal postures.
11. **Essential** (tremor) (Latin *essentia* meaning "quality or being.") The necessary or inherent part of a thing. As a descriptive adjective "essential" was first used originally as "essential hypertension," because the high BP in the elderly was thought necessary or essential to force blood through hardened, nonelastic arteries. "Essential" now has been mindlessly transferred from essential hypertension and applied to mean "any unknown cause."
12. **Hypomimia**—Facial immobility, due to combined rigidity and bradykinesia.
13. **Hypophonia** (Greek *hypo* meaning "under" or below normal and *phone,* "voice.") It is defective speech in that it is soft or whispered.
14. **Idiopathic** (Greek *idios* meaning "one's own" and *pathos,* "disease.") Originally it referred to a disease peculiar to that individual or originating within that person. Now it is used to denote any disease of unknown causation.
15. **Kinetic** (tremor) (Greek *kinein* meaning "to move.") It refers to anything pertaining to motion, e.g. tremor occurring during some motion or movement, either postural or intention tremors.
16. **Myoclonus** (Greek *myos* meaning "muscle" and *klonos,* "turmoil.") It indicates involuntary contractions of a muscle or group of muscles, e.g. he can't release a handshake.
17. **Palsy** (French word *paralysie* means "paralysis.") Palsy is the Anglicized contraction of *paralysie.*
18. **Tardive** (French word for "tardy or late.") It refers to a disease in which the characteristic lesion appears only late in the course of the disease.
19. **Titubation** (Latin *titubatio* meaning "a staggering" or stumbling gait.) It is shaking of the head or trunk, as seen in cerebellar disease or essential tremor, but not in PD.
20. **Tremor--** (Latin word meaning "shaking, trembling.") Now it is used as a noun rather than adjective.

Chapter 19 Vertigo

Questions on Vertigo

A. In a patient complaining of dizziness to determine vertigo is present, the most important information to get is a
  1. History of:
  2. Physical exam finding:
B. Before you can be confident it is vertigo, however, you must be sure it is not one of the other 2 major types of "dizziness." They are:
  1.
     a. History:
     b. Physical exam:
  2.
     a. History:
     b. Physical exam:
C. The commonest cause of vertigo seen in the office and its distinguishing characteristics are:
  1.
     a.
     b.
     c.
D. The 2 other common causes of vertigo seen in the office and their distinguishing characteristics are:
  1.
     a.
     b.
     c.
  2.
     a.
     b.
     c.
E. Your 55 y/o patient just moved to Amarillo from Tucumcari, NM. She is well but on her ROS she notes "a little dizziness that is getting worse." On exam you find decreased hearing in her left ear and a Weber test that lateralizes to her right ear. She believes the "meclizine is no longer working" and wants "a higher dose." Your management now is:

Chapter 19 Vertigo   233

Answers on Vertigo
A. Be certain of the symptom in a patient with "dizziness"
   1. Vertigo is a spinning or rotational sensation. It is not a feeling of about to pass out (presyncope) and not a problem of imbalance when standing still or walking (disequilibrium). Whether it is the patient or her surroundings that seem to be spinning is of no use in diagnosis, so don't waste time asking
   2. The Dix-Hallpike maneuver may provoke the identical dizziness (vertigo) of which she is complaining. If not, spinning the patient on a swiveling stool will reproduce vertigo
B. The other 2 common kinds of dizziness and their distinguishing characteristics
   1. Presyncope
      a. She feels as if she is going to pass out or lose consciousness
      b. No exam or test provokes the presyncopal feeling, but orthostatic hypotension is a common cause of presyncope
   2. Disequilibrium
      a. The "dizziness" occurs only on standing or walking. It is not truly a dizzy feeling in her head (as it is with presyncope or vertigo), but it is a feeling of her being about to fall or of imbalance
      b. Romberg test may be positive
C. The commonest cause of vertigo
   1. Benign paroxysmal positional vertigo (BPPV)
      a. It is episodic (i.e. paroxysmal)
      b. It lasts <1 minute, and most episodes last <20-30 sec
      c. Vertigo is an isolated symptom
D. The other 2 common causes of vertigo seen in office patients
   1. Vestibular neuronitis (labyrinthitis)
      a. It is new onset vertigo
      b. It is very severe vertigo for 1-2 days, then it lessens over the next days to weeks
      c. Often there is nausea and prominent vomiting but no associated ear findings of hearing loss, ear fullness or tinnitus during the vertigo
   2. Meniere's disease
      a. It is episodic vertigo
      b. Each episode lasts a few hours
      c. During each attack there may be ipsilateral decreased hearing, ear fullness, tinnitus
E. Recognize possibly dangerous signs and symptoms of vertigo
   The combination of progressively worsening "dizziness," unilateral left ear hearing loss, and a Weber test that lateralizes to her good right ear (suggesting sensorineural loss of the affected left ear), is acoustic neuroma until proven otherwise. If you are confident of your exam, an MRI should be done. If you are uncertain about the hearing loss, a test for auditory acuity could be done first. Increasing the dose of meclizine and followup in 6-12 months would be very bad judgment by the clinician and dangerous for the patient

Vertigo

Differential diagnosis: the 3 common causes of vertigo
1. BPPV–<u>episodic</u>; lasts < 1 minute; no other symptoms
2. Vestibular neuronitis–<u>new</u> onset; lasts <u>days</u>-weeks; prominent associated vomiting early
3. Meniere's–<u>episodic</u>; lasts a few <u>hours</u>; ipsilateral ear symptoms during the attack, e.g. tinnitus, ear fullness, decreased hearing

A. **Be certain of the symptom and its distinguishing characteristics.** Your patient's problem or chief complaint is "I'm dizzy all the time." Most dizziness is not vertigo, an illusion of spinning or rotation or rising or tilting. Vertigo indicates a lesion located between the vestibular apparatus and the brainstem or cerebellum. <u>Central lesions</u> (brainstem, cerebellum) are dangerous and have <u>associated neurological symptoms or signs</u>; peripheral lesions present either with vertigo alone (isolated), or with associated symptoms of cochlear disease (hearing loss or tinnitus or ear fullness). Ask, "Tell me about the very first time you got the dizziness" and also "Tell me exactly what a typical attack at present is like." Don't let her use the word "dizzy" or "vertigo" in her description. "Do you feel anything else before or while you are dizzy?" Look for autonomic symptoms (nausea, vomiting, sweating, pallor) or cochlear symptoms (tinnitus, temporary loss of hearing, ear fullness) that may occur with vertigo but rarely with other types of dizziness
1. Listen carefully to determine it is vertigo, a spinning or rotating sensation. Be sure it is not one of the other 3 types of dizziness:
   a. Disequilibrium–imbalance while standing or turning or walking
   b. Presyncope–feeling about to pass out e.g. faint or orthostatic hypotension or cardiac arrhythmia
   c. Lightheadedness–giddy or swimming sensation in the head, often occurring in a young healthy person
2. "Does anything happen just before you get dizzy, for example, do you associate anything with its onset?" Head movement may induce vertigo, or the vertigo may occur spontaneously, that is, without a precipitating cause. But head movement <u>always</u> makes vertigo worse; if head movement does not affect intensity, it's not vertigo. Extremely importantly, "Precisely how long does the vertigo last, <u>not</u> the associated nausea or unsteadiness, but just the spinning?"
3. Physical examination–in every patient with complaint of "dizziness" quickly do the following tests to provoke the patient's symptom of dizziness and to get more confidence it is vertigo
   a. Dix-Hallpike maneuver should provoke vertigo in BPPV; an abnormal Romberg test suggests disequilibrium; observe gait and pivoting for multiple sensory deficits in the elderly
   b. Blood pressure and pulse, supine (taken after she is supine at least 10 minutes) and standing (taken immediately and every 30-45 sec

Chapter 19 Vertigo 235

for 5-10 min as necessary); on standing, ask "How does that make you feel?"; orthostatic hypotension (decreased mean arterial pressure and appropriate symptoms) indicates it is presyncope, not vertigo; postural dizziness (dizziness lasting seconds immediately on standing) is very common and suggests a hypersensitivity to somatic sensations e.g. lightheadedness, anxiety

---

Be certain:
1. The symptom is vertigo and not presyncope or disequilibrium
2. Whether it is either new onset vertigo or episodic vertigo or chronic, daily vertigo
3. If it is episodic vertigo, whether an episode lasts either <1 min or 2-30 min or hours-days
4. If there are any concomitant symptoms e.g. unilateral tinnitus, ear fullness, hearing loss

---

    c. If you still are uncertain whether it is vertigo, spin her 10-15 times while she sits on a revolving stool. Ask her: "How does that make you feel?" If she has vertigo, she will volunteer "That's it"
    d. Otologic and neurological exam, especially cerebellum and cranial nerve exam; look into both ears by otoscope; whisper or rub your fingers together near her ear to test grossly for decreased hearing; always do both Rinne and Weber tests, especially to screen for decreased hearing and otosclerosis; look for papilledema; while looking in one eye with overhead lights on, have your nurse cover the other eye, to detect nystagmus with fixation removed. During the Dix-Hallpike maneuver, with her head extended and down, nystagmus and vertigo both last <20 sec and each disappears on repeat testing 3-4 times, so by the 5th time, there is no provoked nystagmus or vertigo if it is a peripheral cause of vertigo
    e. Signs of abnormal nystagmus
        (1) Anytime nystagmus is vertical i.e. up-beating or down-beating, when her gaze is up or down
        (2) Gaze-evoked nystagmus i.e. the direction of rapid beating changes with change in gaze direction
        (3) Visual fixation does not lessen or stop the nystagmus (nurse covers the eye, see above)

By now you should be confident it is vertigo, if it is either new, episodic or chronic daily vertigo, and whether it lasts <1 minute, 2-30 minutes or hours-days. In almost all instances you now have the information you need for diagnosis of the obvious causes (Section C) and the common causes (Section E). In the rare instance that your patient appears different clinically from the usual office patient with vertigo, be certain (Section B) that she does not have a symptom or sign of a dangerous disease.

B. **Be confident it's not a dangerous disease.**
1. Send immediately to the ED by ambulance if there is:
    a. Abrupt onset vertigo that lasts minutes or hours and unilateral deafness or tinnitus, think of labyrinthine (internal auditory) artery occlusion or hemorrhage
    b. Abrupt onset vertigo that lasts hours but without deafness or brainstem signs,

       think of anterior vestibular artery ischemia (or infarction)
- c. Inability to stand or walk alone, even with your insistence that she try, think of cerebellar infarct
- d. Vomiting, brain stem signs, but no loss of hearing, think of posterior inferior cerebellar artery syndrome (Wallenberg's)
- e. Vomiting, unilateral hearing loss, ipsilateral facial weakness and ipsilateral ataxia, think of anterior inferior cerebellar artery (AICA) occlusion
- f. Same as (e) but also headache, nuchal rigidity, inability to stand or walk, think of cerebellar hemorrhage (fatal unless decompressed quickly by surgery)
- g. Vomiting (without hearing loss), truncal ataxia, dysmetria of extremities, think of cerebellar infarction

---

Be certain in the first minutes of your exam that there is no evidence of any <u>one</u> dangerous symptom or sign associated with the vertigo:

1. Abrupt onset vertigo either with new, severe headache or vomiting
2. Any brain stem symptoms (6 Ds) e.g. diplopia or blurred vision, dysphagia, dysarthria, dysesthesias, dysmetria, disequilibrium (ataxia)
3. Any one focal neurologic sign
4. Syncope
5. Weakness (not just fatigue)
6. Vertical nystagmus or nonfatigable nystagmus
7. Vertigo is so severe she cannot walk or stand alone

Any suggestion of a dangerous disease, send the patient to the ED.

---

2. Admit at once to the ED or hospital if there is:
   - a. Abrupt onset of vertigo in a patient with risk factors for stroke (DM, smoking, HTN, known atherosclerotic disease), think ischemia or infarction in the vertebrobasilar artery system
   - b. Abrupt onset of vertigo (lasting minutes) with one or more brain stem signs and symptoms (diplopia, dysarthria, dysphagia, dysmetria, dysesthesia, drop attacks, visual loss or visual hallucinations), think of vertebrobasilar TIA
   - c. Vertigo associated with progressive involvement of the brain stem nuclei (6D's), think of brain stem tumor, e.g. glioma
   - d. Positional vertigo associated with abnormal positional nystagmus (vertical nystagmus, prolonged >20 sec, nonfatigable), progressively worsening headache, gait imbalance, think of tumor, MS, strokes
   - e. Recent or chronic otitis media and new onset vertigo, think of bacterial labyrinthitis
   - f. Any dizziness associated with syncope (loss of consciousness), think of drop attacks, absence seizure, complex partial seizure
3. Admit to the hospital or have a specialist consult as soon as appropriate if there is:
   - a. Abrupt onset of isolated vertigo lasting 2-30 minutes in a patient >50 y/o, think of TIA
   - b. Abrupt onset of vertigo lasting 2-30 minutes in a patient <50 y/o think of migraine headache, partial seizure, perilymphatic fistula
   - c. Vertigo, or more frequently disequilibrium, associated with progressively worsening unilateral hearing loss and tinnitus, think of acoustic neurinoma
   - d. Vertigo and hearing loss following head trauma, even days later, think of labyrinthine concussion
   - e. Cough, straining, barotrauma or head trauma associated with a "popping" sound in one ear along with sudden hearing loss, vertigo, tinnitus, think of perilymphatic fistula
   - f. Bilateral sensorineural hearing loss, oscillopsia and disequilibrium (but <u>not</u> vertigo), positive Romberg test, think of ototoxicity e.g. aminoglycoside drug

Chapter 19 Vertigo

 g. Mild vertigo (or disequilibrium) with facial weakness or numbness and ipsilateral extremity dysmetria, think of acoustic neurinoma
 h. Deep burning ear pain followed by vertigo, decreased hearing, facial weakness, and vesicles in the external auditory canal, think of *H. zoster* (Ramsay Hunt syndrome)
 i. Conductive hearing loss, think of cholesteatoma, otosclerosis, serous otitis

C. **Make a quick diagnosis if it's obvious.** Is it an easily diagnosed cause or a medication causing the dizziness? In most patients you will be <u>highly</u> confident of a common cause of the symptom by now. If not, one or more of the following tests may exclude an organic disease and increase your confidence in your working diagnosis: CBC, FTA-ABS

Recognize any easily diagnosed cause of dizziness:
1. Postural dizziness (isolated symptom)
2. Postural tachycardia syndrome (POTS)
3. Post head trauma, post ear surgery, external ear foreign body or cerumen, otitis media; before (aura) or during migraine headache
4. Medications

---

1. Postural dizziness is an isolated symptom and very common. It immediately follows change in position e.g. standing from supine or sitting, bending over, squatting, and it lasts seconds. BP is unchanged on standing i.e. there is no orthostatic hypotension when the dizziness is occurring and pulse rate increase is <20 bpm
2. Postural tachycardia syndrome (POTS) also has <u>no</u> orthostatic hypotension, but the pulse rate increases >30 bpm or the absolute pulse rate is >120 bpm (see chapter on Fatigue)
3. Spot diagnoses are external ear blockage by cerumen or foreign body; underlying acute or chronic otitis media; also post ear surgery or post head trauma, including "whiplash" injury; cholesteatoma suggested by an abnormality of the tympanic membrane; associated with migraine headache
4. Medications–the following classes of drugs have been associated with "vertigo" of central origin–alcohol, anticonvulsants, hypnotics, tranquilizers, analgesics. Also, more than 90% of the drugs in the PDR have dizziness listed as a side effect, so any recently begun medication may potentiate your patient's sense of dizziness from any etiology. Stopping or decreasing the dose of the new medication may alleviate her vertiginous symptoms

D. **Identify your patient's worries and wants.** Dizziness occurs in almost everybody at some time in life, and yet few consult about it. During your interview and exam try to intuit or discover why your patient is here today, and not previously, for the dizziness. Don't necessarily ask directly, but try to get some ideas from your patient's responses to questions about her perception of the dizziness itself. You can't completely help your patient unless you know what she really worries about and wants from you. That's why she is here to see you–to satisfy her worries and wants! Here are only some of the possible worries and wants of your patient with dizziness. You must discover her specific, unique ones
1. Common worries are:
 a. That the cause of the dizziness is a dangerous cause e.g. brain tumor, stroke, HTN
 b. That the etiology is some rare disease e.g. WNV encephalitis, MS
 c. What other fears or anxieties might be troubling your patient? For example, she may have had vertigo at other times, and only now does she come for help. What

has changed? Perhaps a friend or relative, who had similar dizziness, recently has been diagnosed with a brain tumor. There are many other possibilities–think of them

2. Your patient wants:
   a. You to perform a thorough physical exam focused on possible causes of the vertigo and she wants appropriate tests and imaging studies
   b. A plausible explanation of the cause of the vertigo
   c. Confident reassurance from you that it is not a dangerous or rare etiology. Tell her–"The good news, it's not MS" (or whatever you believe her real worry is)

> During your exam, discover your patient's worries (stroke, brain tumor) and wants (reassurance, symptom relief), so that you can respond to her specific needs as soon as possible.

   d. To know the prognosis, short term (effects on job, home life, marriage; how soon she will be back to normal) and long term (if recurrences are possible; how to prevent recurrences; if it will cause any disability)
   e. Treatment to stop the vertigo now and to prevent recurrences (e.g. low salt diet for Meniere's syndrome; propranolol for migraines)
   f. A specialist referral (neurologist, ENT) if she believes you are not confident of the diagnosis

E. Know the symptoms that differentiate the 3 common causes of vertigo.
   1. The commonest cause is benign paroxysmal positional vertigo (BPPV)

> Common causes of most complaints of <u>new or episodic</u> vertigo:
> 1. BPPV–<u>episodic</u>; lasts < 1 minute; no other symptoms
> 2. Vestibular neuronitis–<u>new</u> onset; lasts <u>days</u>-weeks; prominent associated vomiting early
> 3. Meniere's–<u>episodic</u>; lasts a few <u>hours</u>; ipsilateral ear symptoms during the attack, e.g. tinnitus, ear fullness, decreased hearing

   a. Characteristics of BPPV
      (1) It is recent onset vertigo, and it is <u>episodic</u>, that is 1-2 times daily
      (2) The vertigo is <u>positional</u>, that is, it recurs specifically with head movement; the vertigo usually lasts seconds, and almost never >1-2 minutes; sensations of motion sickness (nausea, unsteady feelings), however, may continue for hours, but the vertigo itself does not; an occasional patient may say she had the dizziness for several days when she means she felt she <u>might</u> get dizzy or unsteady if she were to move in certain ways–but that is not vertigo; you must be certain that the vertigo (spinning) itself lasts not >1-2 minutes, though nausea or unsteadiness may last longer
      (3) Vertigo is the only auditory-related symptom of BPPV, except occasionally mild nausea
      (4) Effective treatment is by "particle-repositioning" (Epley) maneuver, and good response to treatment is strong confirmatory evidence of a correct diagnosis of BPPV

Chapter 19 Vertigo   239

    b. What suggests it might not be BPPV
      (1) Anytime there is an associated symptom or sign suggesting a dangerous cause (see above, Section B)
      (2) If you cannot identify head movement as precipitating each episode of vertigo, that is, in BPPV the vertigo does not occur spontaneously
      (3) If the duration of vertigo (not the nausea or "dizzy or unsteady feeling") lasts longer than 1-2 minutes (in the elderly, think of TIA if the vertigo lasts >2-30 minutes)
      (4) If there is any one associated cochlear symptom during the vertigo–either unilateral decreased hearing or tinnitus or ear fullness
  2. Common look-alikes causing vertigo, and how each differs from BPPV
    a. Vestibular neuronitis (or labyrinthitis)
      (1) It is new vertigo; there is no identifiable precipitating event, that is, it is spontaneous, and it is constant, severe vertigo; she wants to lie still, but with urging and help, she can stand and walk alone
      (2) The vertigo reaches peak severity over 1-2 hours, often with associated vomiting, and like BPPV, there is no concomitant auditory symptom i.e. no tinnitus, loss of hearing or ear fullness
      (3) Vertigo may be severe for 1-2 days, and then there is gradual lessening in intensity over days to weeks
      (4) It is the only cause of vertigo that is not episodic, but some patients with vestibular neuronitis later have episodes of BPPV that may occur episodically for years
      (5) Signs suggesting a cerebellar cause
        (a) If she cannot stand alone with her eyes open, or
        (b) If the nystagmus is either vertical or it does not markedly decrease or disappear with visual fixation, or
        (c) If there is bidirection gaze-evoked nystagmus (rapid phase changes as gaze changes to the right or left)
    b. Meniere's disease
      (1) Except for the first attack, this is not new vertigo but it recurs as discrete episodes that may be separated by months or years
      (2) The attacks always are spontaneous in onset, meaning there is no identifiable event that predictably precedes the attack; vertigo lasts a only few hours, but a sense of dizziness or unsteadiness may last days
      (3) Different from both BPPV and vestibular neuronitis, there are auditory-associated symptoms before or during the vertigo: unilateral decreased hearing or ear fullness or tinnitus. Permanent hearing loss detectable between attacks may only occur after repeated attacks and many months or even years after the initial episode of vertigo
      (4) Screen every patient diagnosed as Meniere's disease for syphilis and autoimmune inner ear disease (FTA-ABS, sed rate, anticochlear antibodies); episodic, spontaneous attacks of vertigo without other evidence suggesting Meniere's, think of migrainous vertigo and treat as for migraine

F. Use this summary for efficient diagnosis of a common

cause. With the above information from Sections A-E in mind, here is the rapid approach to diagnosis of vertigo.
1. You already have determined:
   a. In Section A, by H&P, that it is vertigo, and not presyncope or disequilibrium.
   b. In Section B, that there is no evidence in the H&P of any <u>one</u> dangerous cause of the vertigo.
   c. In Section C, that there is neither an easily diagnosed cause nor a medication that is likely responsible for the vertigo.
2. From the focused H&P almost always you should quickly be confident of a working diagnosis. Confident final diagnosis is made only in followup the next few days or weeks when the response to treatment or nontreatment is appropriate to your working diagnosis.
   a. If the vertigo is precipitated <u>only</u> by change in head position, and it occurs in isolation (i.e. no concomitant vomiting or cochlear symptoms of tinnitus, earfulness, or hearing loss) and the vertigo lasts <1 minute, then the patient likely has BPPV.
   b. If there are <u>episodes</u> of vertigo, separated by weeks or months, the vertigo is constant for a <u>few hours</u> and there is hearing loss or tinnitus or ear fullness before or during the vertigo, then the patient likely has Meniere's disease.
   c. If there is gradual onset (hours to peak severity) of almost constant severe vertigo without cochlear symptoms, and the vertigo begins to lessen in intensity at least by 24-48 hours, the likely diagnosis is vestibular neuronitis. (Caution if there is abrupt onset and peak severity vertigo in seconds-minutes <u>or</u> the patient absolutely cannot stand or walk <u>or</u> there are abnormal neurological symptoms <u>or</u> abnormal nystagmus).
3. Answer your patient's worries and wants that you determined early on during the exam (Section D). Have you done everything you can to help her?
4. You now have a working diagnosis, but only with followup, sometimes long term, can you be highly confident it is correct. In return visits you are always testing by H&P that your working diagnosis is correct.

G. Abandon your working diagnosis and look for an uncommon cause only if:

1. Any <u>one</u> dangerous symptom or sign (see above, Section B) occurs in followup of days, weeks, or months. Quickly obtain a neurology or ENT consult or send your patient to the hospital as appropriate

> If your patient's symptoms do not respond as expected to your management, he may have an uncommon or rare cause listed in Section G.2 that you can diagnose and treat. Or you may want to refer your patient to a specialist.

2. Your patient's response to therapy is not as you expect or if the natural history of your working diagnosis does not occur. Patients with each of these 3 common causes of vertigo above should be "well" or back to normal when there is not an ongoing vertiginous episode
<u>Don't</u> spend time and money looking for one of the following etiologies until you are

Chapter 19 Vertigo 241

sure your patient doesn't have one of the 3 common causes of vertigo above. Nevertheless, it may be she has an uncommon or rare cause of the vertigo. These are important to recognize, because each has different treatment or prophylaxis

a. Migraine–vertigo occurs in about one-fourth of patients with migraine. Basilar migraine may have vertigo associated with posterior fossa symptoms of dysarthria, diplopia and ataxia. Although it can occur at any age, basilar migraine is more commonly seen in adolescent women during menstruation. A patient with "Meniere's disease" not responding to treatment, and who also has any photophobia or phonophobia during a vertiginous episode deserves a trial of migraine prevention therapy. Previous diagnoses of "benign recurrent vertigo of adulthood" and "vestibular Meniere's disease" probably are due to migraine.
  If your patient has episodic vertigo of no known cause, think of migraine (migraine sine cephalgia, migraine equivalent). Trial of prophylactic antimigraine therapy e.g. Diamox 250 mg bid or propranolol 80-160 mg/d
b. Horizontal canal variant of BPPV--rare compared to the common posterior canal variant discussed above. The vertigo also is caused by position change in and out of bed, but it may occur with head turning while walking or standing or even sitting and leaning back
c. Otosclerosis–vertigo, hearing loss and tinnitus may occur. Rinne test is negative (bone conduction is greater than air conduction) and Weber test lateralizes to the ear with hearing loss, indicating conductive hearing loss. Conductive hearing loss without past history of ear trauma or otitis media suggests otosclerosis, which occurs clinically in up to 2% of the population, mostly elderly
d. Autoimmune inner ear disease–indistinguishable clinically from Meniere's disease. Very different from Meniere's is the natural history, that is, autoimmune disease quickly becomes bilateral and symptoms rapidly progress in weeks to months without treatment; any patient diagnosed with Meniere's disease must have blood drawn for sed rate (vasculitis) and anticochlear antibodies
e. Syphilitic labyrinthitis–cannot be distinguished clinically from Meniere's disease. Any patient with symptoms suggestive of Meniere's disease must have an FTA-ABS test
f. Bilateral idiopathic vestibulopathy–complains of oscillopsia (jiggling of objects while she walks, runs or drives a car) and disequilibrium, worse in the dark. She may have had Meniere's disease, autoimmune ear disease, otosyphilis or bilateral acoustic neuroma in the past, who they now have bilateral loss of vestibular function. Ototoxicity (aminoglycosides, cisplatinum, furosemide) also may be the cause, but a history of vertigo almost always is lacking in cases of ototoxicity, because the vestibular damage is bilateral
g. Serous labyrinthitis–a complication of acute or chronic middle ear infections; occasionally vertigo and subtle hearing loss
h. Perilymphatic fistula–vertigo, hearing loss, tinnitus may be caused by head trauma, barotrauma, loud noise, cough, sneeze, after ear surgery; diagnosis is by history of trauma and treatment is symptomatic
i. Recurrent vestibulopathy–recurrent episodes of spontaneous vertigo (similar to Meniere's disease), but unlike Meniere's there are no auditory or neurological symptoms or signs
j. Familial vestibulopathy–of two kinds, but both respond to acetazolamide; first type has episodes of vertigo lasting minutes, and after several years they develop oscillopsia and disequilibrium; the second type has migraine and essential tremor with vertigo lasting up to a few hours, and disequilibrium does not occur
k. Psychological etiologies either may be responsible for the "vertigo" or they may potentiate vertigo. Being totally confident the dizziness is vertigo in some of these patients may be difficult, as the history may be inconsistent. So always look for one of these disorders also, because treatment of the psychological disorder may cure or alleviate the vertigo
    (1) GAD--"worry wart" of the family; worries about things that conceivably could happen, but they are extremely unlikely to occur; she worries about a specific problem most of the day for weeks or months, and often she can't get to sleep at night for worrying about that problem
    (2) MD–search for any anhedonia-- "What do you do for enjoyment (hobbies, symphony, sports)?" Is she doing them now with the same frequency as in the past? Why not? She "worries" also about actions, but about past actions i.e. guilt, different from GAD. Depressed mood is common
    (3) Panic attack–sudden onset of fear and symptoms of sympathetic arousal (tachycardia, palpitations, diaphoresis) with peak in <10 minutes, and she focuses on how to escape or flee the particular situation or environment
    (4) Somatization syndrome–pain in multiple systems, "Do you have any pains? Tell

me about them"
l. Leukoaraiosis–ischemic white matter disease in patients with DM or HTN; symptoms suggest parkinsonism, but she is unresponsive to levodopa
m. Superior canal dehiscence (Am J Otology 21, 9, 2000)--resembles BPPV in that there are brief episodes of dizziness with change in head position; it is not vertigo, but unsteadiness (disequilibrium) and it is chronic, often for years; refer to ENT
n. Vestibular paroxysmia (Lancet 343, 798, 1994)–frequent brief attacks of vertigo, unilateral hyperacusis or tinnitus; treatment with carbamazepine
o. Cogan's syndrome–interstitial keratitis (like tertiary syphilis), and vertigo, hearing loss, like Meniere's disease
p. Phobic postural vertigo (Neurology 46, 1515, 1996)–disturbed balance while standing or walking and momentary vertigo; occurs in specific places or situations and there is associated severe anxiety.

H. Use the glossary for precise thinking and accurate diagnosis.

1. **Aphasia** (Greek *a* meaning "negative" and *phasis*, "speech.") It refers to an inability of the patient to comprehend the other person's speech or writing, or to express herself in speech or writing. It is due to injury or disease of brain centers of comprehension or speech, usually a left brain lesion of or near Broca's area.
2. **Apoplexy** (Greek word *apoplexia* meaning a "seizure" due to being "struck down.") The ancients believed that one seized by sudden disability was being "struck down" by the gods.
3. **Ataxia** (Greek *a* meaning "negative" and *taxis*, "order.") It is failure of muscular coordination causing inaccurate, clumsy movements.
4. **Cholesteatoma** (Greek *chole* meaning "bile" and *steatos*, "fat" and *oma*, "tumor.") It is a middle ear fatty tumor containing cholesterol debris.
5. **Cholesterol** (Greek *chole* meaning "bile" and *stereos*, "solid.") It is the main constituent of common gallstones; only much later was cholesterol a chemical name.
6. **Cochlea** (Latin word meaning "snail"and it is from the Greek word *kochlias* meaning "a small spiral shell.")
7. **Diaphoresis** (Greek word for "profuse sweating.") We still use it this way.
8. **Diplopia** (Greek *diplo* meaning "double or twice" and *opsis*, "sight or vision.") It refers to seeing two images of a single object.
9. **Disequilibrium** (Latin *dis* meaning "deprived of" and *aequus*, "equal" and *libra*, "balance.") It refers to imbalance standing or walking. Note the distinction of Latin *dis*, meaning "deprived of" as opposed to Greek *dys*, "difficult or abnormal."
10. **Dizzy** (Anglo-Saxon *dysig* meaning "foolish." Originally it connoted strange behavior under divine influence.
11. **Dysarthria** (Greek *dys* meaning "difficult or disturbed" and *arthroun*, "to utter distinctly" and *ia* "state or condition.") It is poor articulation of words due to neuromuscular disease, usually CNS or peripheral nerve disease.
12. **Dysdiadochokinesia** (Greek *dys* meaning "difficult or abnormal" and *diadochos*, "succeeding" and *kinesis*, "motion.") It refers to difficulty performing alternating opposite motor movements e.g. alternating pronation and supination of outstretched arms. It is loss of the ability to stop one movement and immediately follow it by its opposite movement.
13. **Dysesthesias** (Greek *dys* meaning "abnormal" and *aisthesis*, "perception.") It refers to an unpleasant abnormal sensation produced by normal stimuli e.g. numbness, paresthesia
14. **Dysmetria** (Greek *dys* meaning "abnormal" and *metron*, "measure.") It is an inaccurate measuring of distance in a muscular action, that is, <u>missing the target</u> in touching finger to nose or heel to shin. Dysmetria suggests cerebellar disease.
15. **Fistula**, perilymphatic (Latin word for "pipe or tube.") It is a drainage tract by which an abnormal communication has occurred; specifically it is a hole in the round window between the inner and middle ear.
16. **Giddy** (Old English *gydig* meaning "mad" or "god-possessed.")
17. **Leukoaraiosis** (Greek *leukos* meaning "white.") Now it refers to ischemic white matter diseases.
18. **Matutinal** vertigo (Latin *matutinalis* meaning "in the morning.") It is vertigo on first arising from sleep.
19. **Nystagmus** (Greek *nystakes* meaning "nodding or drowsy.") In ancient times, it referred to an involuntary drooping of the eyes as a sign of sleepiness. Now it is involuntary, repetitive to and fro movements of the eyes, often due to neurological disease.
20. **Ophthalmoplegia** (Greek *ophthalmos* meaning "the eye" and *plege*, "stroke.") It is

paralysis of one or more eye muscles
21. **Orthostatic** (Greek *orthos* meaning "straight or erect" and *statikos,* "causing to stand.") Postural implies onset of a symptom with any change in position, so an orthostatic change is one kind of postural change, i.e. symptoms on standing from supine or sitting position.
22. **Oscillopsia** (Greek *oscillare* meaning "to swing" and *opsis*, "vision.") Now it means that while she walks or runs, viewed objects jerk up and down uncontrollably.
23. **Otolith** (Greek *otos* meaning "the ear" and *lithos*, "stone.") It refers to calcareous inner ear stone-like masses, responsible for BPPV.
24. **Otosclerosis** (Greek *otos* meaning "the ear" and *skleros*, "hard or tough.") It refers to abnormal new bone formation immobilizing the stapes and decreasing hearing acuity.
25. **Paroxysm** (Greek *paroxysmos* meaning "abrupt recurrence or intensification of some symptoms.")
26. **Prodrome** (Greek *pro* meaning "in front of" and *dromos*, "a running.") It refers to minor or nonspecific symptoms preceding the dominant symptoms characteristic of that disease. A syndrome (*syn* meaning "together") may include prodromal symptoms or it just may be the dominant symptoms alone.
27. **Tabes dorsalis** (tertiary syphilis) (Latin word *tabes* means "decay or wasting.") Originally tabes meant any wasting disease. Discovery that syphilis destroyed the posterior columns of the spinal cord and caused ataxia led to the present terminology.
28. **Tinnitus** (Latin word meaning "a ringing or tinkling sound" in the ears.) Now it is any sound repetitively "heard" without an external inciting sound.
29. **Titubation** (Latin *titubatio* meaning "a staggering.") It is a stumbling gait with shaking of the head and trunk, or just a rhythmic rocking of the trunk and head, back and forth or side to side, usually due to cerebellar disease.
30. **Vertigo** (Latin *vertere* meaning "to turn" and *igo,* "a condition.") It refers to an illusion of movement or spinning. Whether the spinning is of self or of surrounding objects is not useful for diagnosis.
31. **Vestibule** (Latin word meaning "entrance.") In anatomy, vestibule is a cavity at the entrance of a canal or vessel, and the ear vestibule is the cavity in the middle of the bony labyrinth.

Chapter 20 Weakness

Questions on Weakness

A. Your patient likely has weakness (suggesting organic disease), compared to either fatigue (suggesting a syndrome of nonorganic illness) or malaise (possibly organic disease) if you find
   1. By history
      a. Weakness:
      b. Malaise:
      c. Fatigue:
   2. By physical exam
      a. Weakness:
      b. Malaise:
      c. Fatigue:
   3. By which organs are diseased in each
      a. Weakness:
      b. Malaise:
      c. Fatigue:
B. The commonest cause of "weakness" in office patients and its distinguishing characteristics are:
   1.
      a.
      b.
C. The other 2 common causes of weakness and their distinguishing characteristics:
   1.
      a.
      b.
   2.
      a.
      b.
D. Weakness indicates disease either of neurological or muscular systems. Once you are certain it is weakness, a quick approach to diagnosis of etiology is
   1. Muscular vs neurological:
   2. Neurological subgroups:
E. If your patient complains of weakness and you find an UMN sign present, the following signs help to localize the lesion
   1. Quadriparesis (arms and legs):
   2. Paraparesis (legs only):

Chapter 20 Weakness

Answers on Weakness
A. Be certain the symptom is weakness
 1. By history:
    a. Weakness: He complains of inability to do some specific action that he previously could do quite easily e.g. comb his hair, lift things overhead, walk upstairs, stand from sitting. Often he can tell you when the weakness started
    b. Malaise: He complains of "I just feel sick (or ill)" or "I'm not myself, something is wrong." There are no tasks he can't do, and he is not just tired all the time. He often is able to date accurately the onset of his complaint or "sick" feeling
    c. Fatigue: No specific task he can't do, he simply is too tired to do anything; he goes to sleep tired and awakens tired; he is tired just thinking about doing something. He can't remember when his "weakness" began
 2. By physical exam:
    a. Weakness: You can demonstrate weakness of certain specific muscles or muscle groups by testing strength
    b. Malaise: There may be no objective findings on exam
    c. Fatigue: No objective findings on exam, except possibly bilateral tender points of fibromyalgia
 3. Organs diseased in each
    a. Weakness: Neurological or muscular system
    b. Malaise: Systemic disease may be occult, and no specific organic disease demonstrable
    c. Fatigue: None
B. The commonest cause of complaint of "weakness" in office patients and its distinguishing characteristics
 1. Deconditioning syndrome
    a. Onset in a patient <60 y/o
    b. Some combination of smoking tobacco, obesity, increasing age, extreme sedentary lifestyle
C. The other 2 common causes
 1. MD
    a. Onset in a patient <60 y/o
    b. Presence of anhedonia and depressed mood
 2. Sarcopenia
    a. Onset in a patient >60 y/o
    b. Aggravating factors may be sedentary lifestyle, obesity, smoking, MD, but none is necessary for sarcopenia to occur
D. Approach to diagnosis of weakness
 1. Muscular vs neurological: Muscle disease (myopathy) affects predominantly proximal muscles, and neuropathy predominantly affects distal muscle groups
 2. Neurological subgroups: Immediately look for symptoms and signs of an UMN lesion (spasticity, hyperreflexia, Babinski sign) indicating a lesion proximal to the anterior horn cell i.e. brain or spinal cord. LMN signs indicate disease of the anterior horn cell and distally; symptoms and signs are flaccidity, hypo- or areflexia, atrophy of muscles, fasciculations
E. Pattern of weakness can suggest the site of a lesion in the spinal cord
 1. Quadriparesis (arms and legs): Spinal cord lesion, at or above the cervical level

2. Paraparesis (legs only): Spinal cord lesion, at or below upper thoracic level

UMN signs are present in both quadriparesis and paraparesis. Be certain there is no suggestion that the lesion might be cortical e.g. presence of drowsiness, confusion, seizure, which dictates brain MRI rather than spinal MRI

Weakness

DDx: the 3 common causes of chronic, generalized weakness
1. Deconditioning syndrome–<60 y/o patient; obesity, smoker, sedentary
2. MD–patient <60 y/o; anhedonia and depressed mood
3. Sarcopenia–patient >60 y/o

A. Be certain of the symptom and its distinguishing characteristics. Your patient's problem or chief complaint is "I'm so weak I can't do anything."

First, be certain your patient's problem is weakness, that is, loss of strength in one or more arms or legs and not malaise or fatigue or SOB or dizziness. If he has weakness, there are specific movements or actions that he cannot do as well as he could in the recent past. Fatigue, in contrast, is present even before starting exercise or muscle contractions. Such a patient is "tired all the time" (he goes to sleep tired and awakens tired) and he is "weak all over." It is not a lack of muscle power, but rather a lack of energy, so that is not weakness. Weakness also may occur episodically after only a few repeated contractions e.g. MG, compared to the recent past when he could perform many more contractions without difficulty. Your patient with malaise volunteers "I'm just not well" or "I feel sick." Commonly such a patient has an occult disease, so look carefully for it

1. To determine if weakness is present, in your H&P you are looking for one of the following:
    a. Proximal weakness
       (1) Upper limbs–brushing or washing his hair, lifting objects overhead
       (2) Lower limbs–rising from a stool or toilet, climbing stairs
    b. Distal weakness
       (1) Upper limbs–difficulty with finger movements e.g. buttons, keys, coins, door knobs
       (2) Lower limbs–foot drop, tripping over the carpet
    c. Generalized weakness–similar weakness but in more than one region
2. Ask your patient–"Tell me what the problem is, and don't use the word, weak." "Tell me exactly what you want to do, that you cannot do," and "Why specifically can you not do it?"; "When is the first time you noticed this problem?" and if the weakness is episodic, "Have you found anything that brings on the weakness?" "What are you doing in the hours and minutes before the weakness begins?"
3. Ask him–"What are things you really enjoy doing? What do you do for fun?" and "How often have you been doing them lately?" Look for any evidence of anhedonia to explain totally or partially his "weakness." "If you had no weakness, would you be completely well?" You want to identify any other symptoms associated with his "weakness"

4. Physical examination–assuming from these answers that you conclude it might be weakness, by focused exam demonstrate that weakness (loss of strength) is present now; a neurological principle is that signs of weakness usually precede the symptom of weakness, therefore bilateral or generalized weakness may be present even as the patient complains of a focal weakness, e.g. unilateral leg weakness. If it is focal weakness, next determine where the lesion (nerve or muscle) is and what the cause is. Caution– if there is significant pain in the extremity, antalgic weakness (he may seem to be weak only because of the pain) may be present, so you will not get a valid test of strength

---

Be certain:
1. That the symptom is weakness and not fatigue or malaise
2. Whether it is new weakness, episodic weakness, or chronic, persistent, daily weakness
3. Of the age at onset, and whether it was rapid or insidious
4. If there are any associated symptoms of anhedonia or depressed mood

---

  a. Which extremities and which muscles are involved, and is the weakness symmetrical? Quickly test for strength each of the following movements (note how easy it is to remember–for all joints test for flexion and extension; for shoulders, fingers, hips, test also for abduction and adduction):
  (1) Shoulder abduction (C_5); elbow flexion (C_5) and extension (C_6, $_7$); wrist flexion and extension (C_6); and finger extension (C_7), flexion (C_8) and abduction (T_1)
  (2) Hip flexion ($L_{1, 2}$), adduction (L_3) and abduction (L_5); knee extension ($L_{3, 4}$) and flexion (L_5, S_1); ankle extension (L_4) and flexion (S_1); toe extension (L_5) and flexion (S_1)
  (3) If it is episodic weakness, have him exercise the involved area without resting e.g. hold the arms abducted at 90° or keep the eyes looking upward or laterally (blinking allowed) for 2-3 minutes
  b. Once you are certain there is weakness:
  (1) Are there signs of an UMN lesion *viz* hyperreflexia, hypertonia or spasticity (clonus), Babinski sign, slowing of rapid alternating movements, or unilateral absence of cutaneous abdominal or cremasteric reflexes?
  (2) Are there signs of a LMN lesion *viz* flaccidity, areflexia, fasciculations, and early atrophy of distal muscles?
  (3) Are there signs of a primary myopathy, which differs from a LMN lesion *viz* minimal atrophy, fasciculations absent, proximal muscles most prominently diseased and normal DTRs in early disease?

Quick Interpretation of Weakness

	Involved limbs	Causes if UMN signs are present	Causes if LMN signs are present
Monoparesis	Any one limb	Discrete CNS lesion	Radiculopathy, plexopathy, mononeuropathy
Hemiparesis	One side of body	Contralateral CNS lesion	-----
Quadriparesis	Arms <u>and</u> legs	Spinal cord, at or above the cervical level	Distal weakness–polyneuropathy; Proximal weakness–myopathy
Paraparesis	Legs	Spinal cord, thoracic or upper lumbar levels	Polyneuropathy or myopathy; GBS; cauda equina syndrome

By now you should be confident it is weakness, whether it is either new, episodic or chronic daily weakness, if its onset was rapid or insidious, whether it is a myopathy or neuropathy, and if there are important associated symptoms. In almost all instances you now have the information you need for diagnosis of the obvious causes (Section C) and the common causes (Section E). In the rare instance that your patient appears different clinically from the usual office patient with weakness, be certain (Section B) that he does not have a symptom or sign of a dangerous disease

B. Be confident it's not a dangerous disease.
1. Send immediately to the ED by ambulance if there is:
   a. Evidence of a catastrophic illness presenting with weakness e.g. tachypnea, syncope, hypotension, diaphoresis, pallor, dyspnea, pain, think of MI, sepsis, hypovolemia, Addisonian crisis
   b. Symptoms of dyspnea or tachypnea with generalized weakness, think of GBS, MG crisis, polymyositis, ALS, amyloid myopathy
   c. Any evidence of progression of weakness i.e. descending weakness (think of botulism) or ascending weakness, think of GBS, tick paralysis
   d. New cranial nerve symptoms of hoarseness or nasal voice, difficulty swallowing fluids, drooling, along with descending weakness, think of botulism, MG crisis, MS
   e. Progressive, symmetrical weakness and markedly decreased (or absent) DTR's, think of GBS, tick paralysis
   f. Any rapid onset weakness, think of GBS, botulism, MG, Addisonian crisis, organophosphate poisoning
   g. Rapid onset of flaccid paresis, think of stroke, trauma, CNS tumor, GBS, MG, WNV encephalitis, poliomyelitis, Japanese encephalitis
   h. New onset of generalized weakness and change in consciousness or mentation, think of brain lesion

i. Progressively worsening lower extremity weakness and autonomic symptoms (fever, hyper- or hypotension, tachy- or bradycardia), think of emergency GBS
j. Abrupt onset of generalized flaccid paralysis, think of poisoning with a neuromuscular blocker
2. Admit at once to the ED or hospital if there is:
    a. Evidence of an UMN lesion (hyperreflexia or positive Babinski or increased muscle tone in the affected limbs), think of transverse myelitis
    b. Evidence of a LMN lesion in the affected limbs (hyporeflexia or absent DTR's, decreased or flaccid muscle tone, negative Babinski), think of GBS

Be certain in the first minutes of your exam that there is no evidence of any <u>one</u> dangerous symptom or sign associated with the weakness:
1. Progressively worsening weakness
2. Abrupt onset
3. Dyspnea i.e. respiratory distress
4. Changes in mentation, confusion
5. Autonomic symptom e.g. hypotension
6. Rapid onset generalized flaccid paralysis
7. Abrupt onset of fluctuating weakness
8. Sensory level
9. Impaired bowel, bladder or sexual function

Any suggestion of a dangerous disease, send the patient to the ED.

---

c. Evidence of neuromuscular or muscle lesions (negative Babinski, DTR's not increased or absent, muscle tone decreased or flaccid), think of electrolyte imbalance, MG, periodic paralysis, Lambert-Eaton, botulism, tick paralysis
d. Significant dysphagia, think of MG, tetanus, polymyositis, ALS
e. Increased muscle tone (or spasms) centrally (masseter muscles, neck, chest), think of tetanus
f. Blurred vision or diplopia with weakness, think of botulism, MG, MS
g. Abrupt onset of temporary focal, unilateral weakness that lasts 2-30 minutes, think of TIA (elderly) or migraine (young person)
h. Gradual evolution over minutes to hours of bilateral symptoms including weakness, depressed level of consciousness or seizures, think of cerebral vein thrombosis
i. Marked lower extremity weakness with either a sensory level (impaired sensation below a specific spinal level on the trunk) or normal strength in the upper extremities, think of a spinal cord lesion
j. Lower extremity weakness with neck or back pain and impaired bowel, bladder or sexual function, think of spinal cord lesion
k. Focal back pain and tenderness with unexplained fever, think of spinal or epidural abscess
l. New onset weakness of the face or neck with ophthalmoplegia, think of Fisher variant of GBS, brain stem stroke, botulism, MG
m. New onset of weakness with a rapidly progressive mixed sensory and motor neuropathy, think of neurotoxins e.g. heavy metals, chemicals, plant or animal toxins
n. Weakness, weight loss, orthostatic hypotension, think of Addison's disease, PMR, apathetic hyperthyroidism
3. Admit to the hospital or obtain a neurology consult as soon as appropriate if there is:
    a. New onset of weakness associated with <u>any</u> significant muscle trauma, think of rhabdomyolysis (always get creatine kinase levels in any patient with trauma causing bruising)
    b. New onset hemiparesis, think of polycythemia, thrombocytosis, TA, stroke
    c. Evidence of weakness and cachexia, think of malignancy, chronic infection, inflammatory disease, malnutrition, PMR
    d. Weakness only following exercise, think of MG, glycogen storage disease (McArdle's syndrome), paroxysmal myoglobinuria, PVD (claudication) of the

Chapter 20 Weakness 251

legs, spinal stenosis
   e. Gradual evolution over 5-10 minutes of unilateral weakness beginning in the hand and spreading to the arm, then face, think of migraine without headache (migraine sine cephalgia)
   f. Focal weakness after an unwitnessed possible seizure, think of Todd's paralysis
   g. Weakness of all four limbs with complete sparing of the face, think of an upper cervical cord lesion
   h. Fluctuating or episodic weakness, think of MG (bulbar muscles e.g. diplopia) or Lambert-Eaton myasthenic syndrome (proximal muscles of legs and shoulders, rarely bulbar paralysis)

C. **Make a quick diagnosis if it's obvious.** Is it an easily diagnosed chronic disease or a medication causing the weakness? In most patients you will be <u>highly</u> confident of a common cause of the symptom by now. If not, one or more of the following tests may exclude an organic disease and increase your confidence in your working diagnosis: CBC, ESR, UA, CPK, LFTs, TSH, glucose, electrolytes, creatinine, Ca, P, 25-hydroxyVitD, albumin, CXR

Recognize any easily diagnosed cause of the weakness:
1. Chronic systemic disease e.g. heart, lung, kidney, infection, arthritis, DM
2. Medications–onset of weakness is temporally related to starting the medication

---

1. Systemic diseases–
   a. Any chronic disease especially cardiac, pulmonary, renal, liver, anemia
   b. Infections, acute or chronic–HIV, TB, UTI
   c. Rheumatologic diseases–RA, PMR, SLE
   d. Endocrine diseases–especially hyper- or hypothyroidism; Cushings syndrome, hypoadrenalism, diabetic neuropathy
   e. Metabolic alterations–DM (uncontrolled); hypo- or hyperkalemia; hypercalcemia; osteomalacia (low serum Ca, P, or 25-hydroxyVitD)
2. Medications causing:
   a. Myopathies: glucocorticoids, diuretics, laxatives, amiodarone, β-blockers, penicillamine, cyclosporine, statins, excess L-thyroxine, colchicine, vincristine, rifampin, zidovudine, labetolol; chronic ethanol
   b. Neuropathies: antibiotics (INH, ethambutol, metronidazole, dapsone, chloramphenicol); antineoplastics (vinca alkaloids, doxorubicin, cisplatin, thalidomide); miscellaneous (gold, antiretrovirals, amiodarone, phenytoin, pyridoxine, procainamide, colchicine, tacrolimus, nitric oxide)
   c. Neuromuscular junction disorder: neuromuscular blockers, organophosphate, carbamates

D. **Identify your patient's worries and wants.** "Weakness" occurs in more than 40% of the general population, and only a few consult about it. During your interview and exam try to intuit or discover why your patient is here today, and not previously, for this problem. Don't necessarily ask directly, but try to get some ideas from your patient's responses to questions about his perception of the weakness itself. You can't completely help your patient unless you know what he really worries about and wants from you. That's why he is here to see you–to satisfy his worries and wants! Here are only some of the possible worries and wants of your patient with weakness. You must discover his specific, unique ones

> During your exam, discover your patient's worries (cancer, heart disease, stroke) and wants (treatment, reassurance), so that you can respond to his specific needs as soon as possible.

1. Common worries are:
   a. That the cause of the weakness is a dangerous etiology e.g. malignancy, anemia, stroke
   b. That the etiology is some rare disease e.g. WNV, inhalation anthrax, ALS
   c. What other fears or anxieties might be troubling your patient? For example, he may have had weakness at other times, and only now does he come for help. What has changed? Perhaps a friend or relative, who had similar episodes of weakness, recently has been diagnosed with CHF? There are many other possibilities–think of them
2. Your patient wants:
   a. You to perform a thorough physical exam focused on possible causes of the weakness and he wants appropriate tests and imaging studies
   b. A plausible explanation of the cause of the weakness
   c. Confident reassurance from you that it is not a dangerous or rare etiology. Tell him--"The good news, it's not cancer" (or whatever you believe his real worry is)
   d. To know the prognosis, short term (effects on job, home life, marriage; how soon he will be back to normal) and long term (if recurrences are possible; how to prevent recurrences; if it will cause any disability)
   e. Treatment to stop the weakness now and to prevent recurrences
   f. A specialist referral if he believes you are not confident of the diagnosis

E. Know the symptoms that differentiate the 3 common causes of weakness.

1. The commonest cause is deconditioning syndrome

> Common causes of most <u>chronic, generalized</u> weakness in office patients:
> 1. Deconditioning syndrome–<60 y/o patient; obesity, smoker, sedentary
> 2. MD–patient <60 y/o; anhedonia and depressed mood
> 3. Sarcopenia–patient >60 y/o

   a. Characteristics of deconditioning syndrome
      (1) Typically, onset of weakness is in a <40-50 y/o sedentary, very obese patient ("couch potato"). Weakness is aggravated by alcohol and cigarette use and other symptoms, e.g. SOB, aches and pains, lightheadedness, add to his feeling of weakness
      (2) The weakness is a form of disuse atrophy of muscles, i.e. a deconditioning syndrome. As these patients approach middle age, they no longer can compensate as they did when younger, and weakness becomes apparent in everyday activities
      (3) Quick history, "Tell me about a typical day's activities"; both work day and weekend is often enough to identify these patients. A 2 week diary of daily life activities is helpful, both in diagnosis and suggestions for therapy
      (4) Bedrest causes loss of muscle mass and protein catabolism of 8 gm/day, and absolute bedrest or immobilization may result in 5% loss of strength daily; sedentary lifestyle can result in 5%

loss of muscle strength yearly
   b. What suggests it might not be generalized weakness due to deconditioning:
      (1) Anytime there is an associated symptom or sign suggesting a dangerous cause (see above, Section B)
      (2) Anytime there is any suggestion the weakness is localized, for example, to one or more extremities
      (3) Anytime the patient can tell you exactly when the "weakness" began, especially if it is recent ("It started 3 weeks ago on Tuesday afternoon")
      (4) Anytime there is associated with the weakness any malaise ("For the past 3-4 weeks, I just feel ill all the time")
      (5) If the weakness fluctuates or is diurnal
2. Common look-alikes causing weakness and how each differs from deconditioning syndrome
   a. MD
      (1) Onset in a patient <60 y/o; caution–he may not be motivated to make a full effort in strength testing
      (2) Look for evidence of anhedonia, that is, lack of appetite for any one of his usual pleasurable activities–food, sex, work, hobbies, music, sports; or depressed mood
      (3) MD may occur concomitantly and worsen either deconditioning syndrome or sarcopenia
   b. Sarcopenia
      (1) Onset of weakness in a patient >60 y/o
      (2) It is age-related decreased skeletal muscle mass; loss of muscle mass usually begins at age 30 y/o (on average a 70 y/o man has lost 25 lb of muscle), there is 1-2% per year loss of strength. In men >60 y/o prevalence of sarcopenia may be 25%
      (3) The association between sarcopenia and age-related hypogonadism ("andropause") is currently controversial. Any suggestion of concurrent sublibido or erectile dysfunction indicates need for fasting blood levels of total testosterone (T) and prolactin. If (T) is low, get serum LH, FSH and SHBG, the latter to determine if low (T) is due to low SHBG (e.g. obesity). Consider pituitary MRI if low LH, FSH, bioactive T or high prolactin

F. **Use this summary for efficient diagnosis of a common cause.** With the above information from Sections A-E in mind, here is the rapid approach to diagnosis of the cause of weakness.
   1. You already have determined:
      a. In Section A, by H&P, that your patient has weakness, and that it is either localized in one or more extremities, or it is generalized weakness.
      b. In Section B, that there is no evidence in the H&P of any one dangerous cause of the weakness.
      c. In Section C, that there is neither an easily diagnosed systemic disease nor a medication that is likely responsible for the weakness.
   2. From the focused H&P almost always you should quickly be confident of a working diagnosis. Almost all patients with weakness that is localized or of new onset either will be admitted to the hospital or referred as quickly as appropriate to a neurologist.

Common causes in the office have generalized weakness of insidious onset. Confident final diagnosis of these common causes is made only in followup the next weeks or months when the response to treatment or nontreatment is appropriate to your working diagnosis.
- a. If your <60 y/o patient has some combination of an extreme sedentary lifestyle, cigarette smoker, and obesity, diagnose deconditioning syndrome and treat by helping him reverse his aberrant lifestyle e.g. exercise program, low calorie diet.
- b. If your patient <60 y/o has new onset of symptoms of anhedonia or depressed mood, diagnose and treat MD.
- c. If your patient is >60 y/o with a normal exam for his age, diagnose and treat sarcopenia by exercise strength training (Med Sci Sports Exer 31, 12, 1999) and exogenous testosterone only if he is hypogonadal (sublibido and low active testosterone).

3. Answer your patient's worries and wants that you determined early on during the exam (Section D). Have you done everything you can to help him?
4. You now have a working diagnosis, but only with followup can you be confident it is correct. In return visits you are always testing by H&P that your working diagnosis is correct.

G. Abandon your working diagnosis and look for an uncommon cause only if:

1. Any one dangerous symptom or sign (see above, Section B) occurs in followup of weeks, months, or years. Quickly obtain a neurology consult or send your patient to the hospital as appropriate

If your patient's symptoms do not respond as expected to your management, he may have an uncommon or rare cause listed in Section G.2 that you can diagnose and treat. Or you may want to refer your patient to a specialist.

2. Your patient's response to therapy is not as you expect or if the natural history of your working diagnosis does not occur. Deconditioning syndrome does not worsen symptomatically, and in fact, an appropriate strengthening exercise program (write exercise and diet prescriptions) can "cure" the weakness.

Don't spend time and money looking for one of the following etiologies until you are sure your patient doesn't have one of the 3 common causes of generalized weakness above. Nevertheless, it may be he has an uncommon or a rare cause of the weakness. These are important to recognize, because each has different treatment or prophylaxis.

Causes of new onset generalized weakness without localizing signs are the following:
- a. Motor neuron
  - (1) ALS–UMN and LMN deficits; diplopia, dysphagia, weakness and wasting of limb/muscles
  - (2) Postpolio syndrome–new onset weakness, fasciculations and further atrophy of muscles initially involved 20-40 years earlier
- b. Spinal root
  - (1) Lyme disease–history of tick bite and rash
  - (2) Compressive (entrapment) e.g. cervical myelopathy, spinal stenosis
  - (3) GBS–ascending symmetric weakness and loss of DTRs in legs
- c. Neuropathies–think of them if there is distal > proximal constant, progressive weakness, any sensory loss, any pain, any atrophy or fasciculations, decreased or absent DTRs:

Chapter 20 Weakness 255

- (1) Diphtheric polyneuropathy–may resemble GBS; follows by 6-8 weeks the acute illness, so chronic cough may still be present or worsening
- (2) Porphyric neuropathy–recurrent attacks of colicky abdominal pain and vomiting, sometimes with confusion and delirium; arms weaker than legs
- (3) Lead neuropathy--arms predominantly affected
- (4) Nutritional deficiencies (B12, alcohol, pellagra)
- (5) Toxic neuropathy
- (6) Chronic inflammatory demyelinating polyradiculopathy (CIDP) may begin like GBS, but then has a protracted relapsing course; look for MM, dysproteinemias
- (7) Subacute combined degeneration (B12 deficiency)–myelopathy (paresthesias of hands and feet, loss vibration sense, positive Romberg sign) and often peripheral neuropathy with loss of DTRs

  d. Neuromuscular junction disorders–think of them if variable or fluctuating weakness:
  - (1) MG–fluctuating diplopia or dysphagia; power decreases with sustained contractions
  - (2) Lambert-Eaton syndrome–proximal limb muscle weakness; power increases with sustained contractions
  - (3) Toxins e.g. botulism, organophosphate

  e. Myopathies–think of them if proximal >distal, constant, progressive weakness; creatine kinase elevation; none of the above listed symptoms or signs of neuropathy i.e. no muscle wasting or loss of DTRs
  - (1) Polymyositis (dermatomyositis)–muscle pain and tenderness, high CPK (rash)
  - (2) Inclusion body myositis–patient >50 y/o; weakness and atrophy distal muscles
  - (3) Myositis (inflammatory myopathy) associated with sarcoidosis, PMR, eosinophilia-myalgia syndrome, IBD, HIV, toxoplasmosis
  - (4) Trichinosis–weakness with muscle pain, fever, high ESR, marked eosinophilia
  - (5) Metabolic disorders–electrolyte disorders (K, Mg, Ca, P)
  - (6) Toxins (alcohol, drugs)
  - (7) Muscular dystrophies with onset adolescent or adult
    - (a) Fascioscapulohumeral–face, shoulders, distal legs; arms weaker than legs
    - (b) Myotonic–face, neck, distal muscles; characteristic myotonia
  - (8) Myopathy secondary to osteomalacia of any cause e.g. phenytoin interfering with vitamin D metabolism, celiac sprue (low urine Ca)
  - (9) Amyloid myopathy (Ann Neurol 43, 719, 1998)–think of amyloidosis if no known cause of weakness; fluorescent Congo red stain for muscle biopsy diagnosis
  - (10) Malignancy-associated myopathy

H. **Use the glossary for precise thinking and accurate diagnosis.**
1. **Antalgic** weakness (Greek *anti* meaning "against" and *algos*, "pain.") It is apparent weakness (not weakness) due to decreased muscle contraction because of the pain caused by the muscle contraction.
2. **Apoplexy** (Greek *apoplexia* meaning "seizure" and it referred to being struck down by the gods.) Now some use it only for hemorrhagic stroke, others use it also for occlusive stroke. There is sloppy usage of "apoplectic" by some neurologists to mean simply "abrupt onset of symptoms."
3. **Bulbar** (Greek *bolbos* meaning "rounded mass.") It refers to medulla oblongata and its lesions of bulbar palsy causing weakness and atrophy or fasciculations of the tongue, pharynx or palate; dysphagia, dysarthria, regurgitation of food and difficulty protruding the tongue.
4. **Clonus** (Greek *klonos* meaning "violent motion.") Ancients used the term for epileptic convulsions. Now it is the rapid alternating jerking (rigidity and relaxing) e.g. at the ankle joint.
5. **Dysphonia** (Greek *dys* meaning "difficult, impaired" and *phone*, "voice.") It is disturbed voice production secondary to vocal cord pathology or vagal nerve damage, as opposed to aphasia (language dysfunction) and dysarthria (articulation problem).
6. **Fasciculation** (Latin *fascis* meaning "bundle.") It refers to a small moving raised area on skin representing local involuntary muscle contractions. It is the root word of "Fascism" as well.
7. **Flaccid** (Latin *flaccidus* meaning "weak or lax.")
8. **Gegenhalten** (German word meaning going and stopping, "involuntary resistance to passive movement.") It is a sign of extrapyramidal disease.
9. **Jake palsy**–acute peripheral neuritis causing weakness.

10. **Malaise** (French word meaning a "vague feeling of bodily discomfort.") Your patient with malaise volunteers "I feel ill," and new onset of malaise suggests organic disease, as opposed to fatigue, which is usually due to a nonorganic illness.
11. **Myasthenia** (gravis) (Greek *myos* meaning "muscle" and *astheneia*, "weakness.") It means literally muscular weakness.
12. **Myotonia** (Greek *myos* meaning "muscle" and *tonos*, "tension.") It is decreased ability of a muscle group to relax after contraction, with tonic spasm, e.g. he shakes hands and he can't release his grip.
13. **Palsy** (anglicized contraction of the French word *paralysie* meaning "paralysis.").
14. **Paralysis** (Greek *paralytikos* meaning "one's side was lax," derived from *para* meaning "one side" and *lysis*, "loosening or disruption.")
15. **Paraplegia** (Greek word *para* meaning "along the side of" and *plege*, "a stroke.") Originally paraplegia meant "stroke on one side," which we now call hemiplegia. Now paraplegia is used to represent paralysis of both lower limbs due to a spinal cord lesion.
16. **Paresis** (Greek word meaning "slackening" or loss of strength.) Formerly the term referred specifically to syphilitic weakness, now it means any partial loss of motor function, short of paralysis.
17. **Rhabdomyolysis** (Greek *rhabdotos* meaning "striped" and *mys*, "muscle" and *lysis*, "dissolution.") It is breakdown of striated voluntary muscle resulting in myoglobinuria. Note that leiomy- refers to smooth or involuntary muscle (Greek *leios*, "smooth").
18. **Sarcopenia** (Greek *sarkos* meaning "flesh" and *penia*, "poverty, need.") It refers to gradual decreased skeletal muscle mass and strength that occurs in the elderly.
19. **Spondolysis** (Greek *spondylos* meaning "vertebra" and *osis*, "a disease process," which often connotes an abnormal increase.) Spondylosis refers to osteoarthritis of vertebral joints.

Chapter 20 Weakness   257

INDEX

Abdominal pain ... 12-14, 17-31, 39, 49-51, 54, 55, 57, 58, 70, 71, 73-76, 78-80, 82, 83, 111, 115, 133, 154, 158, 166, 191, 192, 209, 255

Anxiety (see GAD also)
.... 6, 16, 43, 102, 103, 106, 152, 158, 186, 200, 201, 204-207, 209, 215, 220, 226, 235, 242

Chest pain 15, 33-47, 60, 62, 86, 88, 100, 132, 150, 152, 154, 157, 177, 178, 180-182, 184, 185, 189, 192, 202, 205, 206

Constipation 18-21, 27-30, 32, 48-58, 70, 71, 79

Cough 13, 18, 20, 23, 38-40, 59-69, 105, 108, 110, 111, 115, 132, 134, 144, 146, 155, 162, 181, 184, 185, 189, 192-197, 236, 241, 255

Depression (see MD also)
.... 2, 5, 7, 49, 86, 92, 102, 103, 105, 106, 209, 215, 217, 220

Diarrhea 3, 13, 18-21, 24, 27-31, 49, 50, 52-56, 58, 70-84, 94, 101, 108, 110, 111, 115, 116, 133, 157, 173, 192, 203, 209, 230

Dizziness .. 3, 9, 14, 30, 75, 79, 110, 112, 149-159, 191, 199, 201, 205, 210, 232-239, 241, 242, 247

Dyspnea . 6, 16, 18, 22, 33-35, 38-40, 43, 46, 60-63, 65, 67-69, 75, 86, 88-90, 95, 124, 134, 142, 154, 165, 166, 176-186, 191, 196, 205, 210, 249, 250

Edema ... 18, 60, 61, 63, 82, 85-95, 165, 168, 173, 177, 178, 180, 181, 184, 202, 230

Erectile dysfunction 94, 111, 141, 211-218, 220, 253

Fatigue 2, 6, 82, 89, 94, 96-106, 128, 134, 152, 158, 197, 226, 236, 237, 244, 245, 247, 248, 256

Fibromyalgia . 2, 79, 96, 97, 99, 102-105, 109, 112, 114, 121, 122, 124, 125, 127, 128, 131, 139, 245

GAD 6, 97, 103-105, 108, 114, 137, 144, 159, 179, 185, 201, 204, 205, 207, 208, 219, 225, 241

Headache . 2, 3, 5, 12, 19, 20, 24, 27, 30, 38, 40, 67, 71, 73-76, 78, 79, 88, 89, 92, 100, 103, 104, 107-119, 154, 158, 162, 166, 168, 181, 189, 194-196, 199, 201-203, 214, 215, 236, 237, 251

Joint pain 3, 120-135

LBP 7, 31, 79, 82, 89, 128, 130, 132, 136-148

Low back pain (see LBP also) 7, 13, 136, 137, 139, 143

MD ... iv, 7, 13, 49, 53, 76, 97, 100, 103-105, 108, 114, 118, 137, 144, 158, 159, 179, 201, 205-208, 213, 217, 219, 220, 245, 253, 254, 259

Panic attack . 2, 14, 34-36, 39, 43, 44, 46, 150, 158, 159, 178, 179, 181, 184, 185, 200, 201, 204-209, 225

Pharyngitis 2, 40, 65, 68, 166, 181, 188, 190-192, 195-197

Presyncope 9, 25, 38, 39, 149-160, 203, 209, 233, 235, 240

Rash 13, 24, 25, 30, 31, 39, 40, 45, 46, 63, 68, 74, 79, 82, 83, 86, 89, 92, 100, 110, 111, 124, 125, 128, 132, 133, 146, 161-175, 196, 197, 254, 255

Shortness of breath (see SOB also) 7, 33, 35, 176, 177, 179
SOB 7, 24, 35, 40, 43, 46, 98, 152, 157, 158,
176-187, 201, 205, 206, 209, 247, 252
Sore throat (see ST also) 7, 39, 46, 115, 116, 188-198
Spells 52, 111, 199-210, 225
ST . . . . v, 7, 39, 67, 98, 103, 104, 132, 180, 188-197
Sublibido 111, 211-220, 253, 254
Tremor 53, 57, 147, 160, 221-231, 241
Vertigo 6, 9, 111, 150, 152, 153, 158-160, 232-243
Weakness . 14, 51, 58, 63, 75, 96-99, 104, 105, 124-126, 133, 140,
141, 147, 148, 152, 180, 185, 208, 209, 215, 225, 236, 237,
244-256

Ordering Information

JACKHAL BOOKS
PO Box 357
Vega, TX 79092
Phone/fax 806-267-0240
email werner@ama.ttuhsc.edu

8:00 AM to 5:00 PM CST

WERNER'S OFFICE DIAGNOSIS

Harold V. Werner, MD,

Single Copies $ 24.95 US
  Plus Shipping $5.00

(Texas Residents add 8.25% sales tax)

Courses for credit, continuing education materials, and study guide for this text, are available or can be created to fit your specific needs.

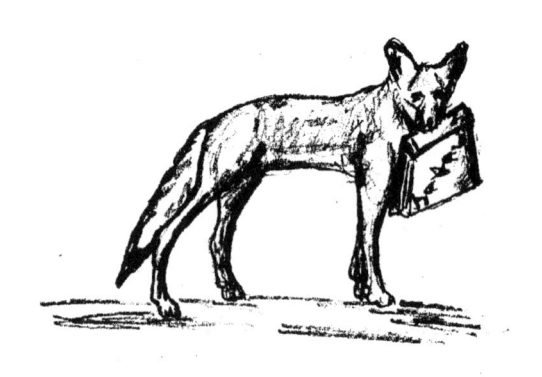